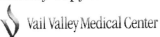

Fitness and Exercise

Exercise

SOURCEBOOK

Second Edition

Health Reference Series

Second Edition

Fitness and Exercise
SOURCEBOOK

Basic Consumer Health Information about the Fundamentals of Fitness and Exercise, Including How to Begin and Maintain a Fitness Program, Fitness as a Lifestyle, the Link between Fitness and Diet, Advice for Specific Groups of People, Exercise as It Relates to Specific Medical Conditions, and Recent Research in Fitness and Exercise

Along with a Glossary of Important Terms and Resources for Additional Help and Information

Edited by
Kristen M. Gledhill

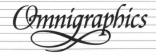

615 Griswold Street • Detroit, MI 48226

Bibliographic Note

Because this page cannot legibly accommodate all the copyright notices, the Bibliographic Note portion of the Preface constitutes an extension of the copyright notice.

Each new volume of the *Health Reference Series* is individually titled and called a "First Edition." Subsequent updates will carry sequential edition numbers. To help avoid confusion and to provide maximum flexibility in our ability to respond to informational needs, the practice of consecutively numbering each volume will be discontinued.

Edited by Kristen M. Gledhill

Health Reference Series

Karen Bellenir, *Series Editor*
Peter D. Dresser, *Managing Editor*
Maria Franklin, *Permissions Assistant*
Joan Margeson, *Research Associate*
Dawn Matthews, *Verification Assistant*
Jenifer Swanson, *Research Associate*
EdIndex, Services for Publishers, *Indexers*

Omnigraphics, Inc.

Matthew P. Barbour, *Vice President, Operations*
Laurie Lanzen Harris, *Vice President, Editorial Director*
Kevin Hayes, *Production Coordinator*
Thomas J. Murphy, *Vice President, Finance and Controller*
Peter E. Ruffner, *Senior Vice President*
Jane J. Steele, *Marketing Coordinator*

Frederick G. Ruffner, Jr., Publisher

© 2001, Omnigraphics, Inc.

Library of Congress Cataloging-in-Publication Data

Fitness and Exercise Sourcebook / edited by Kristen M. Gledhill.-- 2nd ed.
    p. cm. -- (Health reference series)
    "Basic consumer health information about the fundamentals of fitness and exercise, including how to begin and maintain a fitness program, fitness as a lifestyle, the link between fitness and diet, advice for specific groups of people, exercise as it relates to specific medical conditions, and recent research in fitness and exercise; along with a glossary of important terms and resources for additional help and information."
    Includes bibliographical references and index.
    ISBN 0-7808-0334-5 (lib. bdg. : alk. paper)
    1. Physical fitness--Handbooks, manuals, etc. 2. Exercise--Handbooks, manuals, etc. I. Gledhill, Kristen M. II. Health reference series (Unnumbered)
GV436 .F53 2001
613.7--dc21
                          2001021453

∞

Table of Contents

Part III: Fitness for Specific Groups of People

Part IV: Exercise and Specific Medical Conditions

Preface

About this Book

Physical activity tops the list of the Department of Health and Human Services' leading health indicators in its *Healthy People 2010: Understanding and Improving Health*. Regular physical activity, the report states, is associated with lower death rates for adults of any age, even when only moderate levels of physical activity are performed.

As important as it is to the health of adults, however, regular physical activity is important throughout the life cycle, from childhood to old age. In children, the main effects are on attitudes and habit formation. During adolescence, the intensity of physical activity often increases, which results in more physical risks but diminished cardiac risk factors. In adult life, benefits shift to the prevention of work loss and premature death from chronic disease. Finally, in old age, exercise conserves function and improves the quality of life.

Even in the face of overwhelming evidence in favor of regular physical activity, the increased prevalence of obesity and heart disease in the U.S. appears to parallel a decline in physical activity. It is no longer a part of our everyday lives. Technology has reduced job-related physical demands. Labor-saving devices, such as cars, elevators, and remote controls, have removed substantial amounts of physical activity from our lives. Reports from the Centers for Disease Control and Prevention (CDC) suggest participation in vigorous activity by adults, adolescents and children has dropped substantially during the past few decades. Presently, only 22% regularly engage (five times a week for 30 minutes) in sustained physical activity of any intensity during their leisure time.

Distinctions between physical activity, exercise, and physical fitness are useful in understanding health research. According to the CDC, physical activity is "any bodily movement produced by skeletal muscles that results in energy expenditure...." Exercise is "a subset of physical activity that is planned, structured, and repetitive "and is done to improve or maintain physical fitness." Physical fitness is "a set of attributes that are either health- or skill-related, ... including cardiorespiratory endurance, muscular strength and endurance, flexibility, and body composition, balance, agility, power, reaction time, speed, and coordination."

This volume examines physical activity, its effects, benefits, techniques, and risks. On an individual level, there are several things people can do to increase their own personal physical fitness. The second edition of the *Fitness and Exercise Sourcebook* provides people of all ages and abilities with the latest information regarding physical activity and its relationship to healthy living. The material compiled in this volume explores the components of physical fitness, beginning with initiating and maintaining a fitness program. The reader also will find information on the link between fitness and diet and suggestions on how to pair these two factors to maximize overall health. However, because the issues involved with becoming and staying physically fit vary with age and ability, the book also provides relevant information for specific groups of people, including those at risk for or suffering from certain medical conditions. The reader is then introduced to the benefits, risks, requirements, and processes involved with a wide variety of specific sports and activities. Finally, a list of resources for additional help and information directs readers to more information they can use to find their own individual paths to a more physically fit lifestyle. Virtually all of the research included here finds that some exercise is more beneficial than no exercise for overall health, and that more exercise is better than some. The regimen usually prescribed for reaching physical fitness includes 30 minutes of moderate aerobic activity, such as brisk walking, jogging, swimming or even active gardening, on most, if not all, days of the week.

How to Use This Book

This book is divided into parts and chapters. Parts focus on broad areas of interest and chapters on specific topics within those areas.

Part I: *General Fitness and Exercise* gives an overview of the effects and benefits of exercise. It includes the text of Healthy People 2010, the U.S. Department of Health and Human Services' initiative to improve the overall health of Americans. Also included is information on designing a fitness program, avoiding risks associated with exercise, and tips on buying exercise equipment.

Part II: *Fitness and Your Diet* answers the questions most frequently asked about sports nutrition, the role of different nutrients and water in exercise, and how exercise and diet work as components in a weight-loss plan.

Part III: *Fitness for Specific Groups of People* addresses issues surrounding fitness and exercise for children, teenagers, adults, families, older adults, and women.

Part IV: *Exercise and Specific Medical Conditions* considers exercise and its effects on and role in preventing various medical conditions, such as AIDS, arthritis, asthma, cancer, chronic illness, diabetes, fibromyalgia, cardiovascular disorders, hypoglycemia, mental health, obesity, repetitive strain injury, and sarcopenia.

Part V: *Specific Activities* focuses on various exercise activities and how they play a part in overall physical fitness. Included in this part are chapters on everyday fitness, aerobic fitness, walking, water sports, bicycling, skiing, and in-line skating.

Part VI: *Additional Help and Information* provides readers with a glossary of fitness and exercise terms, a comprehensive list of further reading, and resources.

Bibliographic Note

This volume contains documents and excerpts from publications issued by the following U.S. government agencies: the President's Council on Physical Fitness and Sports, National Institute in Aging, National Aeronautic and Space Administration, Federal Trade Commission, Department of Health and Human Services, National Institutes of Health, President's Council on Physical Fitness and Exercise, and Centers for Disease Control and Prevention.

In addition, this volume contains copyrighted documents from the following organizations: Mayo Foundation for Medical Education and Research, Nemours Foundation, National Jewish Medical Research Center, National Multiple Sclerosis Society, National Arthritis and

Musculoskeletal and Skin Diseases Clearinghouse, American Heart Association, Medical Network Inc., National Association of Sport and Physical Education, Shape Up America!, MET-RX Foundation for Health Management, International Fitness Professionals Association, and Weight Control Information Network.

Copyrighted articles from the following publications are also included: *American Fitness, Men's Health, USA Today, Skiing, Current Health 2, Diabetes Forecast, Nutrition Action Health Letter, Tufts University Health and Nutrition Letter, American Family Physician, Science News, The Physician and Sports Medicine*, and *Research Quarterly for Exercise and Sport, Consumer Reports On Health, The Columbia University College of Physicians & Surgeons Complete Home Medical Guide, Saturday Evening Post,* and *About.com.* The documents chosen present basic information regarding physical fitness and exercise for the interested layperson.

Physical fitness is vitally linked to other health-related concerns, such as nutrition and diet, as well as the prevention or management of major chronic medical conditions, including diabetes, cancer and heart disease. The reader is therefore encouraged to consult other related volumes in the *Health Reference Series*, including *Diet and Nutrition Sourcebook, Second Edition, Respiratory Diseases and Disorders Sourcebook, Diabetes Sourcebook, Second Edition, Cardiovascular Diseases and Disorders Sourcebook, Cancer Sourcebook, Third Edition, Physical and Mental Issues in Aging Sourcebook, Healthy Aging Sourcebook, Sports Injuries Sourcebook,* and *Cancer Sourcebook for Women.*

Acknowledgements

The editor wishes to thank the organizations and publications that were especially instrumental in compiling the information in this volume: the Centers for Disease Control and Prevention, the National Institutes of Health, *AIDS Weekly Plus*, Nidus Information Services, the National Arthritis and Musculoskeletal and Skin Diseases Information Clearinghouse, the National Association for Sport and Physical Education, Shape Up America!, MET-RX Foundation for Health Management, Weight Control Information Network, the President's Council on Physical Fitness and Exercise, the Federal Trade Commission, the Department of Health and Human Services, the International Fitness Professionals Association, and the Mayo Foundation for Education and Research. Additionally, the meticulous research efforts of Joan Margeson and Jenifer Swanson and valuable assistance from

Maria Franklin in obtaining reprint permissions for the copyrighted material used in this book are gratefully acknowledged.

Note from the Editor

This book is part of Omnigraphics' *Health Reference Series*. The series provides basic information about a broad range of medical concerns. It is not intended to serve as a tool for diagnosing illness, in prescribing treatments, or as a substitute for the physician/patient relationship. All persons concerned about medical symptoms or the possibility of disease are encouraged to seek professional care from an appropriate health care provider.

Our Advisory Board

The *Health Reference Series* is reviewed by an Advisory Board comprised of librarians from public, academic, and medical libraries. We would like to thank the following board members for providing guidance to the development of this series:

Dr. Lynda Baker, Associate Professor of Library and Information Science, Wayne State University, Detroit, MI

Nancy Bulgarelli, William Beaumont Hospital Library, Royal Oak, MI

Karen Imarasio, Bloomfield Township Public Library, Bloomfield Hills, MI

Karen Morgan, Mardigian Library, University of Michigan-Dearborn, Dearborn, MI

Rosemary Orlando, St. Clair Shores Public Library, St. Clair Shores, MI

Health Reference Series *Update Policy*

The inaugural book in the *Health Reference Series* was the first edition of *Cancer Sourcebook* published in 1990. Since then, the Series has been enthusiastically received by librarians and in the medical community. In order to maintain the standard of providing high-quality health information for the lay person the editorial staff at Omnigraphics felt it was necessary to implement a policy of updating volumes when warranted.

Medical researchers have been making tremendous strides, and it is the purpose of the *Health Reference Series* to stay current with the most recent advances. Each decision to update a volume will be made on an individual basis. Some of the considerations will include how much new information is available and the feedback we receive from people who use the books. If there is a topic you would like to see added to the update list, or an area of medical concern you feel has not been adequately addressed, please write to:

Editor
Health Reference Series
Omnigraphics, Inc.
615 Griswold Street
Detroit, MI 48226

The commitment to providing on-going coverage of important medical developments has also led to some format changes in the *Health Reference Series*. Each new volume on a topic is individually titled and called a "First Edition." Subsequent updates will carry sequential edition numbers. To help avoid confusion and to provide maximum flexibility in our ability to respond to informational needs, the practice of consecutively numbering each volume has been discontinued.

Part One

General Fitness and Exercise

Part One

Chapter 1

Healthy People 2010: Understanding and Improving Health

Editor's Note

Fitness impacts every area of a person's life. It plays a role in the maintenance of health, disease prevention, life expectancy, and the quality of life. But the circumstances of life can also impact a person's ability to achieve fitness. Disease, injury, disbility, hereditary factors, social circumstances, and lifestyle choices can work toward motivating an individual to seek personal fitness, or they can thwart efforts by creating impediments and frustration.

Information about Healthy People 2010, the U.S. Department of Health and Human Services' initiative to improve the overall health of Americans, is presented in this chapter. The initiative's broad scope seeks to help individuals gain the knowledge, motivation, and opportunities they need to make informed decisions about their health. Many of its components are directly related to fitness, and some are related only incidentally. All the components are described here, however, so that the reader can appreciate their widespread implications and the interaction between fitness and other areas of life.

Introduction

Healthy People 2010 outlines a comprehensive, nationwide health promotion and disease prevention agenda. It is designed to serve as

U.S. Department of Health and Human Services. *Healthy People 2010* (Conference Edition, in Two Volumes). Washington, DC: January 2000.

a roadmap for improving the health of all people in the United States during the first decade of the 21st century.

Like the preceding Healthy People 2000 initiative—which was driven by an ambitious, yet achievable, 10-year strategy for improving the nation's health by the end of the 20th century—Healthy People 2010 is committed to a single, overarching purpose: promoting health and preventing illness, disability, and premature death.

The History Behind the Healthy People 2010 Initiative

Healthy People 2010 builds on initiatives pursued over the past two decades. In 1979, *Healthy People: The Surgeon General's Report on Health Promotion and Disease Prevention* provided national goals for reducing premature deaths and preserving independence for older adults. In 1980, another report, *Promoting Health / Preventing Disease: Objectives for the Nation*, outlined 226 targeted health objectives for the Nation to achieve over the next 10 years.

Healthy People 2000: National Health Promotion and Disease Prevention Objectives, released in 1990, identified health improvement goals and objectives to be reached by the year 2000. The Healthy People 2010 initiative continues in this tradition as an instrument to improve health for the first decade of the 21st century.

Healthy People 2010 is about improving health—the health of each individual, the health of communities, and the health of the nation. However, the Healthy People 2010 goals and objectives cannot by themselves improve the health status of the nation. Instead, they should be recognized as part of a larger, systematic approach to health improvement.

This systematic approach to health improvement is composed of four key elements:

- Goals
- Objectives
- Determinants of health
- Health status

Whether this systematic approach is used to improve health on a national level, as in Healthy People 2010, or to organize community action on a particular health issue, such as promoting smoking cessation, the components remain the same. The goals provide a general focus and direction. The goals, in turn, serve as a guide for developing a set of objectives that will actually measure progress within a specified amount of time.

4

The objectives focus on the determinants of health, which encompass the combined effects of individual and community physical and social environments and the policies and interventions used to promote health, prevent disease, and ensure access to quality health care. The ultimate measure of success in any health improvement effort is the health status of the target population. Healthy People 2010 is built on this systematic approach to health improvement.

Healthy People 2010 Goals

Goal 1: Increase Quality and Years of Healthy Life

The first goal of Healthy People 2010 is to help individuals of all ages increase life expectancy and improve their quality of life.

Life Expectancy

Life expectancy is the average number of years people born in a given year are expected to live based on a set of age-specific death rates. At the beginning of the 20th century, life expectancy at birth was 47.3 years. Fortunately, life expectancy has dramatically increased over the past 100 years (see Figure 1.1). Today, the average life expectancy at birth is nearly 77 years.

Life expectancy for persons at every age group has also increased during the past century. Based on today's age-specific death rates, individuals aged 65 years can be expected to live an average of 18 more years, for a total of 83 years. Those aged 75 years can be expected to live an average of 11 more years, for a total of 86 years.

Differences in life expectancy between populations, however, suggest a substantial need and opportunity for improvement. At least 18 countries with populations of 1 million or more have life expectancies greater than the United States for both men and women (see Figure 1.2).

There are substantial differences in life expectancy among different population groups within the United States. For example, women outlive men by an average of 6 years. White women currently have the greatest life expectancy in the United States. The life expectancy for African American women has risen to be higher today than that for white men. People from households with an annual income of at least $25,000 live an average of 3 to 7 years longer, depending on gender and race, than people from households with annual incomes of less than $10,000.

Quality of Life

Quality of life reflects a general sense of happiness and satisfaction with our lives and environment. General quality of life encompasses all aspects of life, including health, recreation, culture, rights, values, beliefs, aspirations, and the conditions that support a life containing these elements. Health-related quality of life reflects a personal sense of physical and mental health and the ability to react to factors in the physical and social environments. Health-related quality of life is inherently more subjective than life expectancy and therefore can be more difficult to measure. Some tools, however, have been developed to measure health-related quality of life.

Global assessments, in which a person rates his or her health as "poor," "fair," "good," "very good," or "excellent," can be reliable indicators of a person's perceived health. In 1996, 90 percent of people in the United States reported their health as good, very good, or excellent.

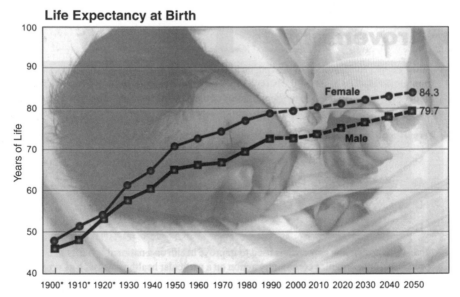

* Death registration area only. The death registration area increased from 10 States and the District of Columbia in 1900 to the coterminous United States in 1933.

Source: U.S. Department of Commerce. Bureau of the Census.

Figure 1.1. *Past and projected female and male life expectancy at birth, United States, 1900-2050.*

Life Expectancy by Country

FEMALE		
Country		Years of Life Expectancy
	Japan	82.9
	France	82.6
	Switzerland	81.9
	Sweden	81.6
	Spain	81.5
	Canada	81.2
	Australia	80.9
	Italy	80.8
	Norway	80.7
	Netherlands	80.4
	Greece	80.3
	Finland	80.3
	Austria	80.1
	Germany	79.8
	Belgium	79.8
	England and Wales	79.6
	Israel	79.3
	Singapore	79.0
	United States	**78.9**

MALE		
Country		Years of Life Expectancy
	Japan	76.4
	Sweden	76.2
	Israel	75.3
	Canada	75.2
	Switzerland	75.1
	Greece	75.1
	Australia	75.0
	Norway	74.9
	Netherlands	74.6
	Italy	74.4
	England and Wales	74.3
	France	74.2
	Spain	74.2
	Austria	73.5
	Singapore	73.4
	Germany	73.3
	New Zealand	73.3
	Northern Ireland	73.1
	Belgium	73.0
	Cuba	73.0
	Costa Rica	73.0
	Finland	72.8
	Denmark	72.8
	Ireland	72.5
	United States	**72.5**

Source: World Health Organization. United Nations. Centers for Disease Control and Prevention. National Center for Health Statistics. National Vital Statistics System. 1990-1995 and unpublished data.

Figure 1.2. *Life expectancy at birth by gender and ranked by selected countries, 1995.*

Healthy days is another measure of health-related quality of life that estimates the number of days of poor physical and mental health in the past 30 days. In 1998, 82 percent of adults reported having no days in the past month where poor physical or mental health impaired their usual activities. The proportions of days that are reported "unhealthy" are the result more often of mentally unhealthy days for younger adults and physically unhealthy days for older adults.

Years of healthy life is a combined measure developed for the Healthy People initiative. The difference between life expectancy and years of healthy life reflects the average amount of time spent in less than optimal health because of chronic or acute limitations. After decreasing in the early 1990s, years of healthy life increased to a level in 1996 that was only slightly above that at the beginning of the decade (64.0 years in 1990 to 64.2 years in 1996). During the same period, life expectancy increased a full year.

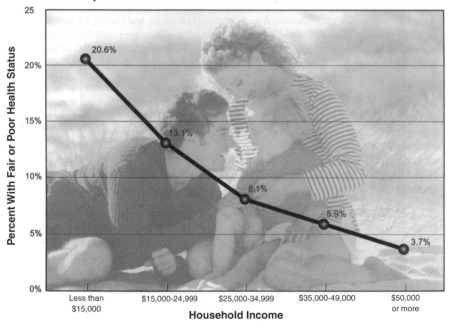

Relationship Between Household Income and Fair or Poor Health Status

Source: Centers for Disease Control and Prevention, National Center for Health Statistics. National Health Interview Survey, 1995.

Figure 1.3. Percentage of persons with fair or poor perceived health status by household income, United States, 1995.

As with life expectancy, various population groups can show dramatic differences in quality of life. For example, people in the lowest income households are five times more likely to report their health as fair or poor than people in the highest income households (see Figure 1.3). A higher percentage of women report their health as fair or poor compared to men. Adults in rural areas are 36 percent more likely to report their health status as fair or poor than are adults in urban areas.

Achieving a Longer and Healthier Life: The Healthy People Perspective

Healthy People 2010 seeks to increase life expectancy and quality of life over the next 10 years by helping individuals gain the knowledge, motivation, and opportunities they need to make informed decisions about their health. At the same time, Healthy People 2010 encourages local and state leaders to develop communitywide and statewide efforts that promote healthy behaviors, create healthy environments, and increase access to high-quality health care. Given the fact that individual and community health are virtually inseparable, it is critical that both the individual and the community do their parts to increase life expectancy and improve quality of life.

Goal 2: Eliminate Health Disparities

The second goal of Healthy People 2010 is to eliminate health disparities among different segments of the population. These include differences that occur by gender, race or ethnicity, education or income, disability, living in rural localities, or sexual orientation. This section highlights ways in which health disparities can occur among various demographic groups in the United States.

Gender

Whereas some differences in health between men and women are the result of biological differences, others are more complicated and require greater attention and scientific exploration. Some health differences are obviously gender specific, such as cervical and prostate cancers.

Overall, men have a life expectancy that is 6 years less than women and have higher death rates for each of the 10 leading causes of death. For example, men are two times more likely than women to die from unintentional injuries and four times more likely than women to die from firearm-related injuries. Although overall death rates for women may currently be lower than for men, women have shown increased death rates over the past decade in areas where men have experienced improvements, such as lung cancer. Women are also at greater risk for Alzheimer's disease than men and twice as likely as men to be affected by major depression.

Race and Ethnicity

Current information about the biologic and genetic characteristics of African Americans, Hispanics, American Indians, Alaska Natives, Asians, Native Hawaiians, and Pacific Islanders does not explain the health disparities experienced by these groups compared with the white, non-Hispanic population in the United States. These disparities are believed to be the result of the complex interaction among genetic variations, environmental factors, and specific health behaviors.

Even though the nation's infant mortality rate is down, the infant death rate among African Americans is still more than double that of whites. Heart disease death rates are more than 40 percent higher for African Americans than for whites. The death rate for all cancers is 30 percent higher for African Americans than for whites; for prostate cancer, it is more than double that for whites. African American women have a higher death rate from breast cancer despite having a mammography screening rate that is higher than that for white women. The death rate from HIV/AIDS for African Americans is more than seven times that for whites; the rate of homicide is six times that for whites.

Hispanics living in the United States are almost twice as likely to die from diabetes than are non-Hispanic whites. Although constituting only 11 percent of the total population in 1996, Hispanics accounted for 20 percent of the new cases of tuberculosis. Hispanics also have higher rates of high blood pressure and obesity than non-Hispanic whites. There are differences among Hispanic populations as well. For example, whereas the rate of low-birth-weight infants is lower for the total Hispanic population compared with whites, Puerto Ricans have a low-birth-weight rate that is 50 percent higher than that for whites.

American Indians and Alaska Natives have an infant death rate almost double that for whites. The rate of diabetes for this population group is more than twice that for whites. The Pima of Arizona have one of the highest rates of diabetes in the world. American Indians and Alaska Natives also have disproportionately high death rates from unintentional injuries and suicide.

Asians and Pacific Islanders, on average, have indicators of being one of the healthiest population groups in the United States. However, there is great diversity within this population group, and health disparities for some specific groups are quite marked. Women of Vietnamese origin, for example, suffer from cervical cancer at nearly five times the rate for white women. New cases of hepatitis and tuberculosis are also higher in Asians and Pacific Islanders living in the United States than in whites.

Income and Education

Inequalities in income and education underlie many health disparities in the United States. Income and education are intrinsically related and often serve as proxy measures for each other (see Figure 1.4). In general, population groups that suffer the worst health status are also those that have the highest poverty rates and least education. Disparities in income and education levels are associated with differences in the occurrence of illness and death, including heart disease, diabetes, obesity, elevated blood lead level, and low birth weight. Higher incomes permit increased access to medical care, enable one to afford better housing and live in safer neighborhoods, and increase the opportunity to engage in health-promoting behaviors.

Income inequality in the United States has increased over the past three decades. There are distinct demographic differences in poverty by race, ethnicity, and household composition (see Figure 1.5) as well as geographical variations in poverty across the United States. Recent health gains for the U.S. population as a whole appear to reflect achievements among the higher socioeconomic groups; lower socioeconomic groups continue to lag behind.

Overall, those with higher incomes tend to fare better than those with lower incomes. For example, among white men aged 65 years, those in the highest income families could expect to live more than 3 years longer than those in the lowest income families. The percentage of people in the lowest income families reporting limitation in activity caused by chronic disease is three times that of people in the highest income families.

The average level of education in the U.S. population has steadily increased over the past several decades—an important achievement given that more years of education usually translate into more years of life. For women, the amount of education achieved is a key determinant of the welfare and survival of their children. Higher levels of education may also increase the likelihood of obtaining or understanding

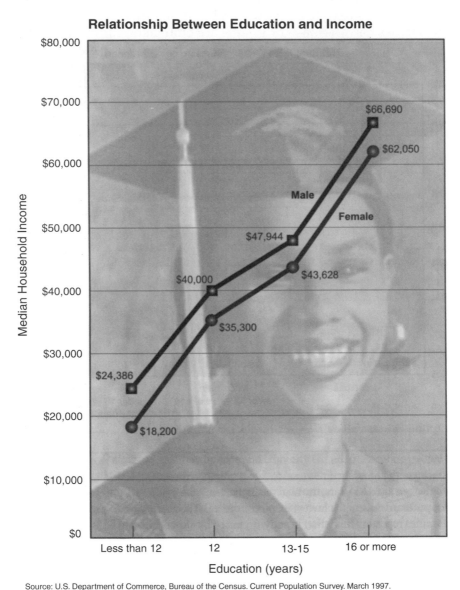

Relationship Between Education and Income

Source: U.S. Department of Commerce, Bureau of the Census. Current Population Survey. March 1997.

Figure 1.4. *Relationship between education and median household income among adults 25 years and older, by gender, United States, 1996.*

health-related information needed to develop health-promoting behaviors and beliefs in prevention.

But again, educational attainment differs by race and ethnicity (Figure 1.6). Among people aged 25 to 64 years in the United States, the overall death rate for those with less than 12 years of education is more than twice that for people with 13 or more years of education. The infant mortality rate is almost double for infants of mothers with less than 12 years of education when compared with those with an education of 13 or more years.

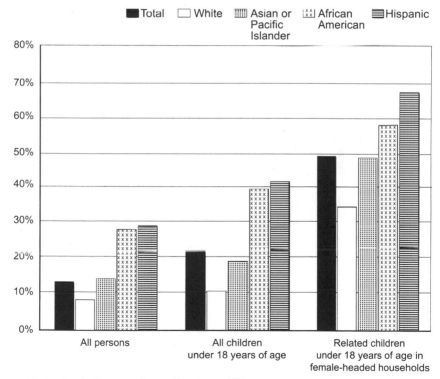

Persons Below the Poverty Level

Source: U.S. Department of Commerce, Bureau of the Census. 1997.

Figure 1.5. *Percentage of persons below the poverty level by race/ethnic group and type of household, United States, 1996.*

13

Disability

People with disabilities are identified as persons having an activity limitation, who use assistance, or who perceive themselves as having a disability. In 1994, 54 million people in the United States, or roughly 21 percent of the population, had some level of disability. Although rates of disability are relatively stable or falling slightly for people aged 45 years and older, rates are on the rise among the

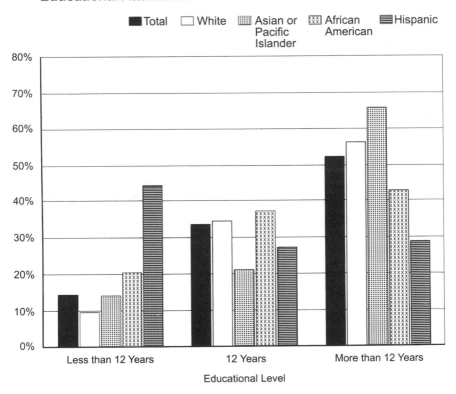

Educational Attainment

Source: U.S. Department of Commerce, Bureau of the Census. Current Population Survey. 1996.

Figure 1.6. *Percentage of adults aged 25 to 64 years by educational level, race and ethnicity, United States, 1996.*

14

younger population. People with disabilities tend to report more anxiety, pain, sleeplessness, and days of depression and fewer days of vitality than do people without activity limitations. People with disabilities also have other disparities, including lower rates of physical activity and higher rates of obesity. Many people with disabilities lack access to health services and medical care.

Rural Localities

Twenty-five percent of Americans live in rural areas, that is, places with fewer than 2,500 residents. Injury-related death rates are 40 percent higher in rural populations than in urban populations. Heart disease, cancer, and diabetes rates exceed those for urban areas. People living in rural areas are less likely to use preventive screening services, exercise regularly, or wear seat belts. In 1996, 20 percent of the rural population was uninsured compared with 16 percent of the urban population. Timely access to emergency services and the availability of specialty care are other issues for this population group.

Sexual Orientation

America's gay and lesbian population comprises a diverse community with disparate health concerns. Major health issues for gay men are HIV/AIDS and other sexually transmitted diseases, substance abuse, depression, and suicide. Gay male adolescents are two to three times more likely than their peers to attempt suicide. Some evidence suggests lesbians have higher rates of smoking, obesity, alcohol abuse, and stress than heterosexual women. The issues surrounding personal, family, and social acceptance of sexual orientation can place a significant burden on mental health and personal safety.

Achieving Equity: The Healthy People Perspective

Although the diversity of the American population may be one of our nation's greatest assets, diversity also presents a range of health improvement challenges that must be addressed by individuals, the community and state in which they live, and the nation as a whole.

Healthy People 2010 recognizes that communities, states, and national organizations will need to take a multidisciplinary approach to achieving health equity that involves improving health, education, housing, labor, justice, transportation, agriculture, and the environment. However, our greatest opportunities for reducing health disparities are in empowering individuals to make informed health care decisions and in promoting communitywide safety, education, and access to health care.

Healthy People 2010 is firmly dedicated to the principle that—regardless of age, gender, race, ethnicity, income, education, geographic location, disability, and sexual orientation—every person in every community across the nation deserves equal access to comprehensive, culturally competent, community-based health care systems that are committed to serving the needs of the individual and promoting community health.

Objectives

The nation's progress in achieving the two goals of Healthy People 2010 will be monitored through 467 objectives in 28 focus areas. Many objectives focus on interventions designed to reduce or eliminate illness, disability, and premature death among individuals and communities. Others focus on broader issues, such as improving access to quality health care, strengthening public health services, and improving the availability and dissemination of health-related information. Each objective has a target for specific improvements to be achieved by the year 2010.

Together, these objectives reflect the depth of scientific knowledge as well as the breadth of diversity in the nation's communities. More importantly, they are designed to help the nation achieve its two overarching goals and realize the vision of healthy people living in healthy communities.

Determinants of Health

The depth of topics covered by the objectives in Healthy People 2010 reflect the array of critical influences that determine the health of individuals and communities.

For example, individual behaviors and environmental factors are responsible for about 70 percent of all premature deaths in the United States. Developing and implementing policies and preventive interventions that effectively address these determinants of health can reduce the burden of illness, enhance quality of life, and increase longevity.

Individual biology and behaviors influence health through their interaction with each other and with the individual's social and physical environments. In addition, policies and interventions can improve health by targeting factors related to individuals and their environments, including access to quality health care (see Figure 1.7).

Biology refers to the individual's genetic makeup (those factors with which he or she is born), family history (which may suggest risk for disease), and the physical and mental health problems acquired during life. Aging, diet, physical activity, smoking, stress, alcohol or illicit drug abuse, injury or violence, or an infectious or toxic agent may result in illness or disability and can produce a "new" biology for the individual.

Behaviors are individual responses or reactions to internal stimuli and external conditions. Behaviors can have a reciprocal relationship to biology; in other words, each can react to the other. For example, smoking (behavior) can alter the cells in the lung and result in shortness of breath, emphysema, or cancer (biology) that may then lead an individual to stop smoking (behavior). Similarly, a family history that includes heart disease (biology) may motivate an individual to develop good eating habits, avoid tobacco, and maintain an active lifestyle (behaviors), which may prevent his or her own development of heart disease (biology).

Personal choices and the social and physical environments surrounding individuals can shape behaviors. The social and physical environments include all factors that affect the life of individuals, positively or negatively, many of which may not be under their immediate or direct control.

The social environment includes interactions with family, friends, coworkers, and others in the community. It also encompasses social institutions, such as law enforcement, the workplace, places of worship, and schools. Housing, public transportation, and the presence or absence of violence in the community are among other components of the social environment. The social environment has a profound effect on individual health, as well as on the health of the larger community, and is unique because of cultural customs; language; and personal, religious, or spiritual beliefs. At the same time, individuals and their behaviors contribute to the quality of the social environment.

The physical environment can be thought of as that which can be seen, touched, heard, smelled, and tasted. However, the physical environment also contains less tangible elements, such as radiation and ozone. The physical environment can harm individual and community health, especially when individuals and communities are exposed to toxic substances; irritants; infectious agents; and physical hazards in homes, schools, and worksites. The physical environment can also promote good health, for example, by providing clean and safe places for people to work, exercise, and play.

Policies and interventions can have a powerful and positive effect on the health of individuals and the community. Examples include

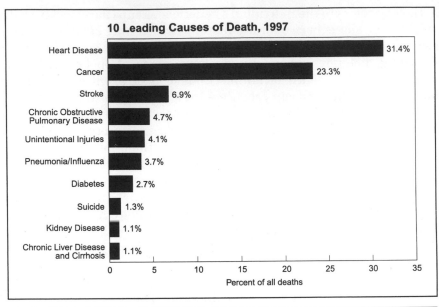

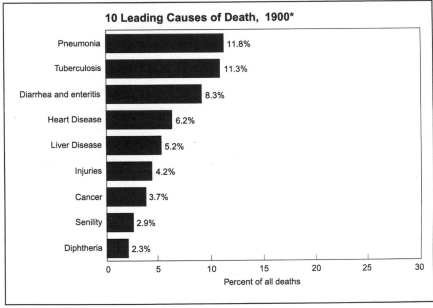

*Not all States are represented.

Source: Centers for Disease Control and Prevention, National Center for Health Statistics, National Vital Statistics System and unpublished data. 1997.

Figure 1.7. *The 10 leading causes of death as a percentage of all deaths in the United States, 1900 and 1997.*

health promotion campaigns to prevent smoking; policies mandating child restraints and seat belt use in automobiles; disease prevention services, such as immunization of children, adolescents, and adults; and clinical services, such as enhancing mental health care. Policies and interventions that promote individual and community health may be implemented by a variety of agencies, such as transportation, education, energy, housing, labor, justice, and other venues, or through places of worship, community-based organizations, civic groups, and businesses.

The health of individuals and communities also depends greatly on access to quality health care. Expanding access to quality health care is important to eliminate health disparities and to increase the quality and years of healthy life for all people living in the United States. Health care in the broadest sense not only includes services received through health care providers but also health information and services received through other venues in the community.

The determinants of health—individual biology and behavior, the physical and social environments, policies and interventions, and access to quality health care—have a profound effect on the health of individuals, communities, and the nation. An evaluation of these determinants is an important part of developing any strategy to improve health.

Our understanding of these determinants and how they relate to one another, coupled with our understanding of how individual and community health determines the health of the nation, is perhaps the most important key to achieving our Healthy People 2010 goals of increasing the quality and years of life and of eliminating the nation's health disparities.

Health Status

To completely understand the health status of a population, it is essential to monitor and evaluate the consequences of the determinants of health.

The health status of the United States is a description of the health of the total population using information that is representative of most people living in this country. For relatively small population groups, however, it may not be possible to draw accurate conclusions about their health using current data collection methods. The goal of eliminating health disparities will necessitate improved collection and use of standardized data to correctly identify disparities among select population groups.

19

Leading Causes of Death by Age Group

Younger than 1 Year	Number of Deaths
Birth defects	6,178
Disorders related to premature birth	3,925
Sudden infant death syndrome	2,991
1-4 Years	
Unintentional Injuries	2,005
Birth defects	589
Cancer	438
5-14 Years	
Unintentional Injuries	3,371
Cancer	1,030
Homicide	457
15-24 Years	
Unintentional Injuries	13,367
Homicide	6,146
Suicide	4,186
25-44 Years	
Unintentional Injuries	27,129
Cancer	21,706
Heart disease	16,513
45-64 Years	
Cancer	131,743
Heart disease	101,235
Unintentional Injuries	17,521
65 Years and Older	
Heart disease	606,913
Cancer	382,913
Stroke	140,366

Source: Centers for Disease Control and Prevention, National Center for Health Statistics. National Vital Statictics Systems. 1999.

Figure 1.8. *The 3 leading causes of death by age group, United States, 1997.*

Health status can be measured by birth and death rates, life expectancy, quality of life, morbidity from specific diseases, risk factors, use of ambulatory care and inpatient care, accessibility of health personnel and facilities, financing of health care, health insurance coverage, and many other factors. The information used to report health status comes from a variety of sources, including birth and death records; hospital discharge data; and health information collected from health care records, personal interviews, physical examinations, and telephone surveys. These measures are monitored on an annual basis in the United States and are reported in a variety of publications, including Health, United States and Healthy People Reviews.

The leading causes of death are frequently used to describe the health status of the nation. The nation has seen a great deal of change over the past 100 years in the leading causes of death (see Figure 1.8). At the beginning of the 1900s, infectious diseases ran rampant in the United States and worldwide and topped the leading causes of death. A century later, with the control of many infectious agents and the increasing age of the population, chronic diseases top the list.

A very different picture emerges when the leading causes of death are viewed for various subgroups. Unintentional injuries, mainly motor vehicle crashes, are the fifth leading cause of death for the total population, but they are the leading cause of death for people aged 1 to 44 years. Similarly, HIV/AIDS is the 14th leading cause of death for the total population but the leading cause of death for African American men aged 25 to 44 years (Figure 1.9).

The leading causes of death in the United States generally result from a mix of behaviors; injury, violence, and other factors in the environment; and the unavailability or inaccessibility of quality health services. Understanding and monitoring behaviors, environmental factors, and community health systems may prove more useful to monitoring the nation's true health, and in driving health improvement activities, than the death rates that reflect the cumulative impact of these factors. This approach has served as the basis for developing the Leading Health Indicators.

Leading Health Indicators

The Leading Health Indicators reflect the major public health concerns in the United States and were chosen based on their ability to motivate action, the availability of data to measure their progress, and their relevance as broad public health issues.

21

The Leading Health Indicators illuminate individual behaviors, physical and social environmental factors, and important health system issues that greatly affect the health of individuals and communities. Underlying each of these indicators is the significant influence of income and education.

The process of selecting the Leading Health Indicators mirrored the collaborative and extensive efforts undertaken to develop Healthy People 2010. The process was led by an interagency work group within the U.S. Department of Health and Human Services. Individuals and organizations provided comments at national and regional meetings or via mail and the Internet. A report by the Institute of Medicine, National Academy of Sciences, provided several scientific models on which to support a set of indicators. Focus groups were used to ensure that the indicators are meaningful and motivating to the public.

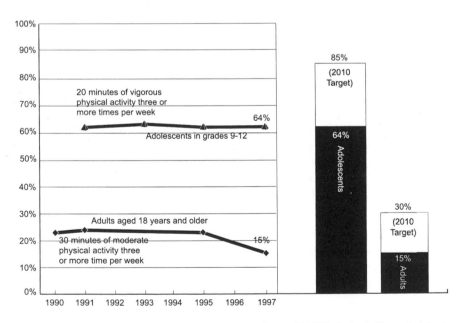

Source: Centers for Disease Control and Prevention. Youth Risk Behavior Survey. 1991-1997. Centers for Disease Control and Prevention, National Center for Health Statistics. National Health Interview Survey. 1990-1997.

Figure 1.9. *Participation in regular physical activity, United States, 1990-1997.*

22

For each of the Leading Health Indicators, specific objectives derived from Healthy People 2010 will be used to track progress. This small set of measures will provide a snapshot of the health of the nation. Tracking and communicating progress on the Leading Health Indicators through national- and state-level report cards will spotlight achievements and challenges in the next decade. The Leading Health Indicators serve as a link to the 467 objectives in Healthy People 2010: Objectives for Improving Health and can become the basic building blocks for community health initiatives.

The Leading Health Indicators are intended to help everyone more easily understand the importance of health promotion and disease prevention and to encourage wide participation in improving health in the next decade. Developing strategies and action plans to address one or more of these indicators can have a profound effect on increasing the quality of life and the years of healthy life and on eliminating health disparities—creating healthy people in healthy communities.

Physical Activity

Regular physical activity throughout life is important for maintaining a healthy body, enhancing psychological well-being, and preventing premature death.

In 1997, 64 percent of adolescents engaged in the recommended amount of physical activity. In the same year, only 15 percent of adults performed the recommended amount of physical activity and 40 percent of adults engaged in no leisure-time physical activity.

The objectives selected to measure progress among adolescents and adults for this Leading Health Indicator are presented below. These are only indicators and do not represent all the physical activity and fitness objectives included in Healthy People 2010.

- Increase the proportion of adolescents who engage in vigorous physical activity that promotes cardiorespiratory fitness 3 or more days per week for 20 or more minutes per occasion.

- Increase the proportion of adults who engage regularly, preferably daily, in moderate physical activity for at least 30 minutes per day.

Health Impact of Physical Activity. Regular physical activity is associated with lower death rates for adults of any age, even when only moderate levels of physical activity are performed. Regular physical activity decreases the risk of death from heart disease, lowers the risk of developing diabetes, and is associated with a decreased risk

of colon cancer. Regular physical activity helps prevent high blood pressure and helps reduce blood pressure in persons with elevated levels.
  Regular physical activity also:

- Increases muscle and bone strength

- Increases lean muscle and helps decrease body fat

- Aids in weight control and is a key part of any weight loss effort

- Enhances psychological well-being and may even reduce the risk of developing depression

- Appears to reduce symptoms of depression and anxiety and to improve mood

In addition, children and adolescents need weight-bearing exercise for normal skeletal development, and young adults need such exercise to achieve and maintain peak bone mass. Older adults can improve and maintain strength and agility with regular physical activity. This can reduce the risk of falling, helping older adults maintain an independent living status. Regular physical activity also increases the ability of people with certain chronic, disabling conditions to perform activities of daily living.

Populations with Low Rates of Physical Activity.

- Women are less active than men at all ages.

- People with lower incomes and less education are typically not as physically active as those with higher incomes and education.

- African Americans and Hispanics are generally less physically active than whites.

- Adults in northeastern and southern States tend to be less active than adults in north-central and western States.

- People with disabilities are less physically active than people without disabilities.

- By age 75, one in three men and one in two women engage in no regular physical activity.

Other Issues. The major barriers most people face when trying to increase physical activity are lack of time, access to convenient facilities, and safe environments in which to be active.

Overweight and Obesity

Overweight and obesity are major contributors to many preventable causes of death. On average, higher body weights are associated with higher death rates. The number of overweight children, adolescents, and adults has risen over the past four decades. Total costs (medical cost and lost productivity) attributable to obesity alone amounted to an estimated $99 billion in 1995.

During 1988-1994, 11 percent of children and adolescents aged 6 to 19 years were overweight or obese. During the same years, 23 percent of adults aged 20 and older were considered obese.

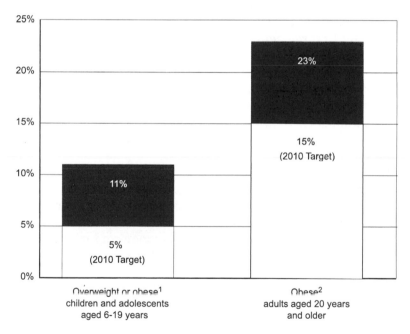

1.   In those aged 6 to 19 years, overweight or obesity is defined as at or above the sex- and age- specific 95th percentile of Body Mass Index (BMI) based on a preliminary analysis of data used to construct the year 2000 U.S. Growth Charts (provisional data).
2.   In adults, obesity is defined as a BMI of 30 kg/m² or more; overweight is a BMI of 25 kg/m² or more.

Body Mass Index (BMI) is calculated as weight in kilograms (kg) divided by the square of height in meters (m²) (BMI = weight[kg]/height[m²]). To estimate BMI using pounds (lbs) and inches (in), divide weight in pounds by the square of height in inches. Then multiply the resulting number by 704.5 (BMI = weight[lbs]/height[in²] X 704.5).

Source: Centers for Disease Control and Prevention, National Center for Health Statistics. National Health and Nutrition Examination Survey. 1988-1994.

Figure 1.10. *Overweight and obesity, United States, 1988-1994.*

The objectives selected to measure progress among children, adolescents, and adults for this Leading Health Indicator are presented below. These are only indicators and do not represent all the nutrition and overweight objectives included in Healthy People 2010.

- Reduce the proportion of children and adolescents who are overweight or obese.

- Reduce the proportion of adults who are obese.

Health Impact of Overweight and Obesity. Overweight and obesity substantially raise the risk of illness from high blood pressure; high cholesterol; Type 2 diabetes; heart disease and stroke; gallbladder disease; arthritis; sleep disturbances and problems breathing; and endometrial, breast, prostate, and colon cancers.

Obese individuals may also suffer from social stigmatization, discrimination, and lowered self-esteem.

Populations with High Rates of Overweight and Obesity. An estimated 107 million adults in the United States are overweight or obese. The proportion of adolescents from poor households who are overweight is almost twice that of adolescents from middle- and high-income households. Overweight is especially prevalent among women with lower incomes and less education. Obesity is more common among African American and Hispanic women than among white women. Among African Americans, the proportion of women who are obese is 80 percent higher than the proportion of men who are obese. This gender difference is also seen among Hispanic women and men, but the percentage of white, non-Hispanic women and men who are obese is about the same.

Reducing Overweight and Obesity. The development of obesity is a complex result of a variety of social, behavioral, cultural, environmental, physiological, and genetic factors. For example, a healthy diet and regular physical activity are both important for maintaining a healthy weight. Once overweight is established during adolescence, it is likely to remain in adulthood. For many overweight and obese individuals, substantial change in eating, shopping, exercising, and even social behaviors may be necessary to develop a healthier lifestyle.

Other Important Nutrition Issues. The quality of food consumed in terms of the proportion of calories from fat, protein, and carbohydrate sources; salt, mineral, and vitamin content; and amount of dietary fiber plays a critical role in disease prevention. The *Dietary Guidelines for Americans* recommend that, to stay healthy, one should eat a variety of foods and choose a diet that is plentiful in grain products, vegetables, and fruits; moderate in salt, sodium, and sugars; and low in fat, saturated fat, and cholesterol.

Nutritional Challenges. Although much progress has been made in making nutrition information available and in providing reduced-fat foods and other healthful food choices in supermarkets, challenges remain. One challenge is the composition of foods eaten away from home. As much as 40 percent of a family's food budget is spent in restaurants and on carry-out meals. Foods eaten away from home are generally higher in fat, saturated fat, cholesterol, and sodium and are lower in fiber and calcium than foods prepared and eaten at home.

Tobacco Use

Cigarette smoking is the single most preventable cause of disease and death in the United States. Smoking results in more deaths each year in the United States than AIDS, alcohol, cocaine, heroin, homicide, suicide, motor vehicle crashes, and fires—combined.

Tobacco-related deaths number more than 430,000 per year among U.S. adults, representing more than 5 million years of potential life lost. Direct medical costs attributable to smoking total at least $50 billion per year.

In 1997, 36 percent of adolescents were current smokers. In the same year, 24 percent of adults were current smokers.

The objectives selected to measure progress among adolescents and adults for this Leading Health Indicator are presented below. These are only indicators and do not represent all the tobacco use objectives included in Healthy People 2010.

- Reduce cigarette smoking by adolescents.
- Reduce cigarette smoking by adults.

Health Impact of Cigarette Smoking. Smoking is a major risk factor for heart disease, stroke, lung cancer, and chronic lung diseases—all leading causes of death. Smoking during pregnancy can result in miscarriages, premature delivery, and sudden infant death syndrome. Other health effects of smoking result from injuries and environmental damage caused by fires. Environmental tobacco smoke

(ETS) increases the risk of heart disease and significant lung conditions, especially asthma and bronchitis in children. ETS is responsible for an estimated 3,000 lung cancer deaths each year among adult nonsmokers.

Trends in Cigarette Smoking: Adolescents. Overall, the percentage of adolescents in grades 9 through 12 who smoked in the past month increased in the 1990s. Every day, an estimated 3,000 young persons start smoking. These trends are disturbing because the vast majority of adult smokers tried their first cigarette before age 18 years; more than half of adult smokers became daily smokers before this same age. Almost half of adolescents who continue smoking regularly will eventually die from a smoking-related illness.

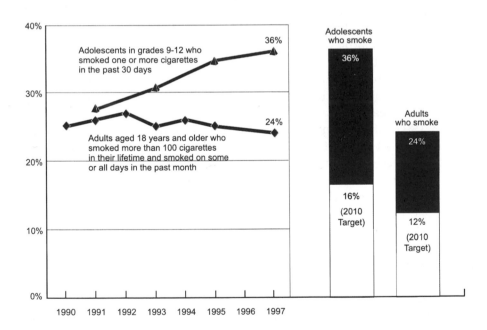

Source: Centers for Disease Control and Prevention. Youth Risk Behavior Survey. 1991-1997.
Centers for Disease Control and Prevention, National Center for Health Statistics. National Health Interview Survey. 1990-1997.

Figure 1.11. Cigarette smoking, United States, 1990-1997.

Trends in Cigarette Smoking: Adults. Following years of steady decline, rates of smoking among adults appear to have leveled off in the 1990s.

Populations with High Rates of Smoking: Adolescents. Adolescent rates of cigarette smoking have increased in the 1990s among white, African American, and Hispanic high school students after years of declining rates during the 1970s and 1980s. In 1997, 40 percent of white high school students currently smoked cigarettes compared with 34 percent for Hispanics and 23 percent for African Americans. Among African Americans in 1997 only 17 percent of high school girls, compared with 28 percent of boys, currently smoked cigarettes. Rates of smoking cigarettes in white and Hispanic high school girls and boys are not substantially different.

Populations with High Rates of Smoking: Adults. Overall, American Indians and Alaska Natives, blue-collar workers, and military personnel have the highest rates of smoking in adults. Rates of smoking in Asian and Pacific Islander men are more than four times higher than for women of the same race. Men have only somewhat higher rates of smoking than women within the total U.S. population. Low-income adults are about twice as likely to smoke as are high-income adults. The percentage of people aged 25 years and older with less than 12 years of education who are current smokers is nearly three times that for persons with 16 or more years of education.

Other Important Tobacco Issues. There is no safe tobacco alternative to cigarettes. Spit tobacco (chew) causes cancer of the mouth, inflammation of the gums, and tooth loss. Cigar smoking causes cancer of the mouth, throat, and lungs and can increase the risk of heart disease and chronic lung problems.

Substance Abuse

Alcohol and illicit drug use are associated with many of this country's most serious problems, including violence, injury, and HIV infection. The annual economic costs to the United States from alcohol abuse were estimated to be $167 billion in 1995, and the costs from drug abuse were estimated to be $110 billion.

In 1997, 77 percent of adolescents aged 12 to 17 years reported that they did not use alcohol or illicit drugs in the past month. In the same

29

year, 6 percent of adults aged 18 years and older reported using illicit drugs in the past month; 16 percent reported binge drinking in the past month, which is defined as consuming five or more drinks on one occasion.

The objectives selected to measure progress among adolescents and adults for this Leading Health Indicator are presented below. These are only indicators and do not represent all the substance abuse objectives in Healthy People 2010.

- Increase the proportion of adolescents not using alcohol or any illicit drugs during the past 30 days.

- Reduce the proportion of adults using any illicit drug during the past 30 days.

- Reduce the proportion of adults engaging in binge drinking of alcoholic beverages during the past month.

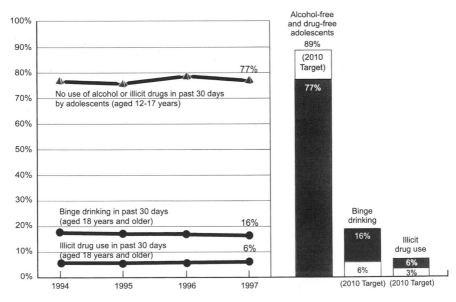

Source: Substance Abuse and Mental Health Services Administration, Office of the Assistant Secretary. National Household Survey on Drug Abuse. 1994-1997.

Figure 1.12. Use of alcohol and/or illicit drugs, United States, 1994-1997.

Health Impact of Substance Abuse. Alcohol and illicit drug use are associated with child and spousal abuse; sexually transmitted diseases, including HIV infection; teen pregnancy; school failure; motor vehicle crashes; escalation of health care costs; low worker productivity; and homelessness. Alcohol and illicit drug use also can result in substantial disruptions in family, work, and personal life.

Alcohol abuse alone is associated with motor vehicle crashes, homicides, suicides, and drowning—leading causes of death among youth. Long-term heavy drinking can lead to heart disease, cancer, alcohol-related liver disease, and pancreatitis. Alcohol use during pregnancy is known to cause fetal alcohol syndrome, a leading cause of preventable mental retardation.

Trends of Substance Abuse: Adolescents. Although the trend from 1994 to 1997 has shown some fluctuations, about 77 percent of adolescents aged 12 to 17 years report being both alcohol-free and drug-free in the past month.

Alcohol is the drug most frequently used by adolescents aged 12 to 17 years. In 1997, 21 percent of adolescents aged 12 to 17 years reported drinking alcohol in the past month. Alcohol use in the past month for this age group has remained at about 20 percent since 1992. Eight percent of this age group reported binge drinking, and 3 percent were heavy drinkers (five or more drinks on the same occasion on each of five or more days in the past 30 days).

Data from 1998 show that 10 percent of adolescents aged 12 to 17 reported using illicit drugs in the past 30 days. This rate is significantly lower than in the previous year and remains well below the all-time high of 16 percent in 1979. Current illicit drug use had nearly doubled for those aged 12 to 13 years between 1996 and 1997 but then decreased between 1997 and 1998. Youth are experimenting with a variety of illicit drugs, including marijuana, cocaine, crack, heroin, acid, inhalants, and methamphetamines, as well as misuse of prescription drugs and other "street" drugs. The younger a person becomes a habitual user of illicit drugs, the stronger the addiction becomes and the more difficult it is to stop use.

Trends of Substance Abuse: Adults. Binge drinking has remained at the same approximate level of 16 percent for all adults since 1988, with the highest current rate of 32 percent among adults aged 18 to 25 years. Illicit drug use has been near the present rate of 6 percent since 1980. Men continue to have higher rates of illicit drug use than women, and rates of illicit drug use in urban areas are higher than in rural areas.

31

Responsible Sexual Behavior

Unintended pregnancies and sexually transmitted diseases (STDs), including infection with the human immunodeficiency virus that causes AIDS, can result from unprotected sexual behaviors. Abstinence is the only method of complete protection. Condoms, if used correctly and consistently, can help prevent both unintended pregnancy and STDs.

In 1997, 85 percent of adolescents abstained from sexual intercourse or used condoms if they were sexually active. In the same year, 23 percent of sexually active adults used condoms.

The objectives selected to measure progress among adolescents and adults for this Leading Health Indicator are presented below. These are only indicators and do not represent all the responsible sexual behavior objectives in Healthy People 2010.

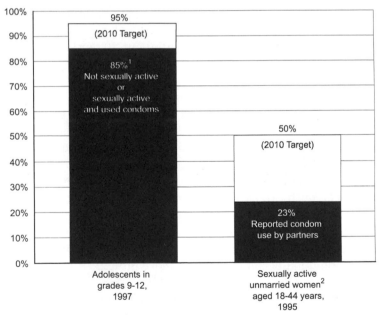

1. This 85 percent includes 52 percent of students in grades 9-12 who were not ever sexually active, 13 percent who were not sexually active in the past 3 months, and 20 percent who were sexually active but used a condom at the last intercourse.
2. Data on males aged 15-49 years will be collected in 2003.

Source: Centers for Disease Control and Prevention. Youth Risk Behavior Survey. 1997. Centers for Disease Control and Prevention, National Center for Health Statistics. National Survey of Family Growth. 1995.

Figure 1.13. Responsible sexual behavior, United States, 1995 and 1997.

- Increase the proportion of adolescents who abstain from sexual intercourse or use condoms if currently sexually active.

- Increase the proportion of sexually active persons who use condoms.

Trends in Sexual Behavior. In the past 6 years there has been both an increase in abstinence among all youth and an increase in condom use among those young people who are sexually active. Research has clearly shown that the most effective school-based programs are comprehensive ones that include a focus on abstinence and condom use. Condom use in sexually active adults has remained steady at about 25 percent.

Unintended Pregnancies. Half of all pregnancies in the United States arc unintended; that is, at the time of conception the pregnancy was not planned or not wanted. Unintended pregnancy rates in the United States have been declining. The rates remain highest among women aged 20 years or younger, women aged 40 years or older, and low-income African American women. Approximately 1 million teenage girls each year in the United States have unintended pregnancies. Nearly half of all unintended pregnancies end in abortion.

The cost to U.S. taxpayers for adolescent pregnancy is estimated at between $7 billion and $15 billion a year.

Sexually Transmitted Diseases. Sexually transmitted diseases are common in the United States, with an estimated 15 million new cases of STDs reported each year. Almost 4 million of the new cases of STDs each year occur in adolescents. Women generally suffer more serious STD complications than men, including pelvic inflammatory disease, ectopic pregnancy, infertility, chronic pelvic pain, and cervical cancer from the human papilloma virus. African Americans and Hispanics have higher rates of STDs than whites.

The total cost of the most common STDs and their complications is conservatively estimated at $17 billion annually.

HIV/AIDS. Nearly 700,000 cases of AIDS have been reported in the United States since the HIV/AIDS epidemic began in the 1980s. The latest estimates indicate that 650,000 to 900,000 people in the United States are currently infected with HIV. The lifetime cost of health care associated with HIV infection, in light of recent advances in HIV diagnostics and therapies, is $155,000 or more per person.

About one-half of all new HIV infections in the United States are among people aged 25 years and under, and the majority are infected through sexual behavior. HIV infection is the leading cause of death for African American men aged 25 to 44 years. Compelling worldwide evidence indicates that the presence of other STDs increases the likelihood of both transmitting and acquiring HIV infection.

Mental Health

Approximately 20 percent of the U.S. population are affected by mental illness during a given year; no one is immune. Of all mental illnesses, depression is the most common disorder. More than 19 million adults in the United States suffer from depression. Major depression is the leading cause of disability and is the cause of more that two-thirds of suicides each year.

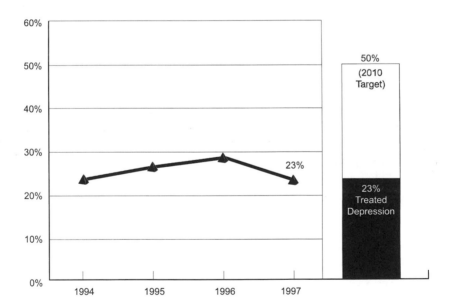

1. Depression is defined as major depressive episode in the past year.
2. Treatment is defined as treatment in the past year for psychological problems or emotional difficulties at a mental health clinic or by a mental health professional on an outpatient basis or treatment for psychological or emotional difficulties at a hospital overnight or longer.

Source: Substance Abuse and Mental Health Services Administration, Office of Applied Studies. National Household Survey on Drug Abuse. 1994-1997.

Figure 1.14. *Adults with depression (1) who received treatment, (2) United States, 1994-1997.*

In 1997, only 23 percent of adults diagnosed with depression received treatment.

The objective selected to measure progress among adults for this Leading Health Indicator is presented below. This is only an indicator and does not represent all the mental health objectives in Healthy People 2010.

- Increase the proportion of adults with recognized depression who receive treatment.

Definition of Mental Health. Mental health is sometimes thought of as simply the absence of a mental illness but is actually much broader. Mental health is a state of successful mental functioning, resulting in productive activities, fulfilling relationships, and the ability to adapt to change and cope with adversity. Mental health is indispensable to personal well-being, family and interpersonal relationships, and one's contribution to society.

Impact of Depression. A person with a depressive disorder is often unable to fulfill the daily responsibilities of being a spouse, partner, or parent. The misunderstanding of mental illness and the associated stigmatization prevent many persons with depression from seeking professional help. Many people will be incapacitated for weeks or months because their depression goes untreated.

Depression is also associated with other medical conditions, such as heart disease, cancer, and diabetes, as well as anxiety and eating disorders. Depression has also been associated with alcohol and illicit drug abuse. An estimated 8 million persons aged 15 to 54 years had coexisting mental and substance abuse disorders within the past year.

The total estimated direct and indirect cost of mental illness in the United States in 1996 was $150 billion.

Treatment of Depression. Depression is treatable. Available medications and psychological treatments, alone or in combination, can help 80 percent of those with depression. With adequate treatment, future episodes of depression can be prevented or reduced in severity. Treatment for depression can enable people to return to satisfactory, functioning lives.

Populations with High Rates of Depression. Serious mental illness clearly affects mental health and can affect children, adolescents, adults, and older adults of all ethnic and racial groups, both genders, and people at all educational and income levels.

Adults and older adults have the highest rates of depression. Major depression affects approximately twice as many women as men. Women who are poor, on welfare, less educated, unemployed, and from minority populations are more likely to experience depression. In addition, depression rates are higher among older adults with coexisting medical conditions. For example, 12 percent of older persons hospitalized for problems such as hip fracture or heart disease are diagnosed with depression. Rates of depression for older persons in nursing homes range from 15 to 25 percent.

Injury and Violence

More than 400 Americans die each day due primarily to motor vehicle crashes, firearms, poisonings, suffocation, falls, fires, and drowning. The risk of injury is so great that most persons sustain a significant injury at some time during their lives.

Motor vehicle crashes are the most common cause of serious injury. In 1997 there were 15.8 deaths from motor vehicle crashes per 100,000 persons.

Because no other crime is measured as accurately and precisely, homicide is a reliable indicator of all violent crime. In 1997, the murder rate in the United States fell to its lowest level in 3 decades, 7.2 homicides per 100,000 persons.

The objectives selected to measure progress for this Leading Health Indicator are presented below. These are only indicators and do not represent all the injury and violence prevention objectives in Healthy People 2010.

- Reduce deaths caused by motor vehicle crashes.
- Reduce homicides.

Impact of Injury and Violence. The cost of injury and violence in the United States is estimated at more than $224 billion per year, an increase of 42 percent over the last decade. These costs include direct medical care and rehabilitation as well as productivity losses to the nation's workforce. The total societal cost of motor vehicle crashes alone exceeds $150 billion annually.

Motor Vehicle Crashes. Motor vehicle crashes are often predictable and preventable. Increased use of seat belts and reductions in driving while impaired are two of the most effective means to reduce the risk of death and serious injury of occupants in motor vehicle crashes.

Death rates associated with motor vehicle traffic injuries are highest in the age group 15 to 24 years. In 1996, teenagers accounted for only 10 percent of the U.S. population but 15 percent of the deaths from motor vehicle crashes. Those aged 75 years and older had the second highest rate of motor vehicle–related deaths.

Nearly 40 percent of traffic fatalities in 1997 were alcohol-related. Each year in the United States it is estimated that more than 120 million episodes of impaired driving occur among adults. In 1996, 21 percent of traffic fatalities of children under age 14 years involved alcohol; 60 percent of the time it was the driver of the child's car who was impaired.

The highest intoxication rates in fatal crashes in 1995 were recorded for drivers aged 21 to 24 years. Young drivers who have been arrested for driving while impaired are more than four times as likely to die in future alcohol-related crashes.

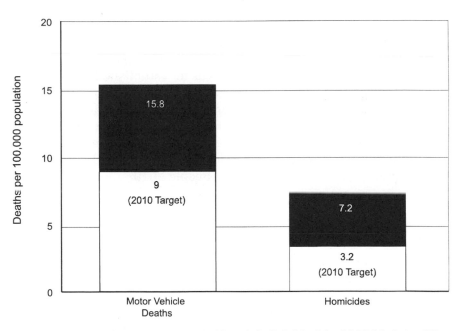

Source: Centers for Disease Control and Prevention, National Center for Health Statistics. National Vital Statistics System. 1997.

Figure 1.15. Motor vehicle deaths and homicides, United States, 1997.

Homicides. In 1997, 32,436 individuals died from firearm injuries; of this number, 42 percent were victims of homicide. In 1997, homicide was the third leading cause of death for children aged 5 to 14 years, an increasing trend in childhood violent deaths. In 1996, more than 80 percent of infant homicides were considered to be fatal child abuse.

Many factors that contribute to injuries are also closely associated with violent and abusive behavior, such as low income, discrimination, lack of education, and lack of employment opportunities.

Males are most often the victims and the perpetrators of homicides. African Americans are seven times more likely than whites to be murdered. There has been a decline in the homicide of intimates, including spouses, partners, boyfriends, and girlfriends, over the past decade, but this problem remains significant.

Environmental Quality

An estimated 25 percent of preventable illnesses worldwide can be attributed to poor environmental quality. In the United States, air pollution alone is estimated to be associated with 50,000 premature deaths and an estimated $40 billion to $50 billion in health-related costs annually. Two indicators of air quality are ozone (outdoor) and environmental tobacco smoke (indoor).

In 1997, approximately 43 percent of the U.S. population lived in areas designated as nonattainment areas for established health-based standards for ozone. During the years 1988 to 1994, 65 percent of nonsmokers were exposed to environmental tobacco smoke (ETS).

The objectives selected to measure progress among children, adolescents, and adults for this Leading Health Indicator are presented below. These are only indicators and do not represent all the environmental quality objectives in Healthy People 2010.

- Reduce the proportion of persons exposed to air that does not meet the U.S. Environmental Protection Agency's health-based standards for ozone.

- Reduce the proportion of nonsmokers exposed to environmental tobacco smoke.

Defining the Environment. Physical and social environments play major roles in the health of individuals and communities. The physical environment includes the air, water, and soil, through which exposure to chemical, biological, and physical agents may occur. The

38

social environment includes housing, transportation, urban development, land-use, industry, and agriculture and results in exposures such as work-related stress, injury, and violence.

Global Concern. Environmental quality is a global concern. Ever-increasing numbers of people and products cross national borders and may transfer health risks such as infectious diseases and chemical hazards. For example, pesticides that are not registered or are restricted for use in the United States potentially could be imported in the fruits, vegetables, and seafood produced abroad.

Health Impact of Poor Air Quality. Poor air quality contributes to respiratory illness, cardiovascular disease, and cancer. For example, asthma can be triggered or worsened by exposure to ozone and ETS. The overall death rate from asthma increased 52 percent between 1980 and 1993, and for children it increased 67 percent.

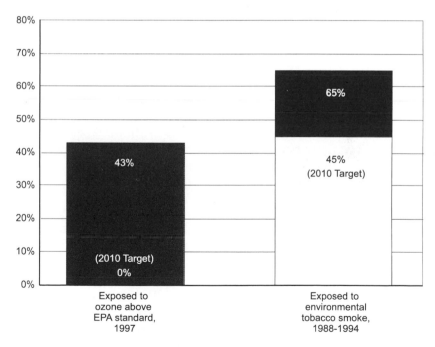

Source: U.S. Environmental Protection Agency. Aerometric Information Retrieval System. 1997.
Centers for Disease Control and Prevention, National Center for Health Statistics. National Health and Nutrition Examination Survey. 1988-94.

Figure 1.16. Ozone and environmental tobacco smoke exposure, United States, 1988-1994, 1997.

Air Pollution. Dramatic improvements in air quality in the United States have occurred over the past three decades. Between 1970 and 1997, total emissions of the six principal air pollutants decreased 31 percent. Still, million of tons of toxic pollutants are released into the air each year from automobiles, industry, and other sources. In 1997, despite continued improvements in air quality, approximately 120 million people lived in areas with unhealthy air based on established standards for one or more commonly found air pollutants, including ozone. In 1996, a disproportionate number of Hispanics and Asian and Pacific Islanders lived in areas that failed to meet these standards compared with whites, African Americans, and American Indians or Alaska Natives.

Tobacco Smoke. Exposure to ETS, or secondhand smoke, among nonsmokers is widespread. Home and workplace environments are major sources of exposure. A total of 15 million children are estimated to have been exposed to secondhand smoke in their homes in 1996. ETS increases the risk of heart disease and respiratory infections in children and is responsible for an estimated 3,000 cancer deaths of adult nonsmokers.

Improvement in Environmental Quality. In the United States, ensuring clean water, safe food, and effective waste management has contributed greatly to a declining threat from many infectious diseases; however, there is still more that can be done. Work to improve the air quality and to better understand threats such as chronic, low-level exposures to hazardous substances must also continue.

Immunization

Vaccines are among the greatest public health achievements of the 20th century. Immunizations can prevent disability and death from infectious diseases for individuals and can help control the spread of infections within communities.

In 1998, 73 percent of children received all vaccines recommended for universal administration for at least 5 years.

In 1997, influenza immunization rates were 63 percent in adults aged 65 and older, almost double the 1989 immunization rate of 33 percent. In 1997, only 43 percent of persons aged 65 and older had ever received a pneumococcal vaccine.

The objectives selected to measure progress among children and adults for this Leading Health Indicator are presented below. These are only indicators and do not represent all the immunization and infectious diseases objectives in Healthy People 2010.

- Increase the proportion of young children who receive all vaccines that have been recommended for universal administration for at least 5 years.
- Increase the proportion of noninstitutionalized adults who are vaccinated annually against influenza and ever vaccinated against pneumococcal disease.

Impact of Immunization. Many once-common vaccine-preventable diseases are now controlled. Smallpox has been eradicated, poliomyelitis has been eliminated from the Western Hemisphere, and measles cases in the United States are at a record low.

Immunizations against influenza and pneumococcal disease can prevent serious illness and death. Pneumonia and influenza deaths

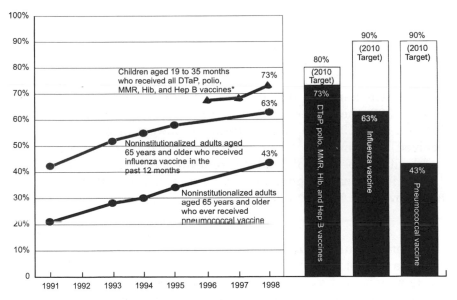

*Four or more doses of diphtheria/tetanus/acellular pertussis (DTaP) vaccine, three or more doses of polio vaccine, one or more dose measles/mumps/rubella (MMR) vaccine, three or more doses of Haemophilus influenzae type b (Hib) vacccine, and three or more doses or hepatitis B (Hep B) vaccine

Source: Centers for Disease Control and Prevention, National Center for Health Statistics and National Immunization Program. National Immunization Survey. 1996-1998. Centers for Disease Control and Prevention, National Center for Health Statistics. National Health Interview Survey. 1991-1997.

Figure 1.17. Immunization coverage, United States, 1991-1998.

41

together constitute the sixth leading cause of death in the United States. Influenza causes an average of 110,000 hospitalizations and 20,000 deaths annually; pneumococcal disease causes 10,000 to 14,000 deaths annually.

Recommended Immunizations. As of November 1, 1999, all children born in the United States (11,000 per day) should be receiving 12 to 16 doses of vaccine by age 2 years to be protected against 10 vaccine-preventable childhood diseases. This recommendation will change in the years ahead as new vaccines are developed, including combinations of current vaccines that may even reduce the number of necessary shots.

Recommended immunizations for adults aged 65 years and older include a yearly immunization against influenza (the "flu-shot") and a one-time immunization against pneumococcal disease. Most of the deaths and serious illnesses caused by influenza and pneumococcal disease occur in older adults and others at increased risk for complications of these diseases due to other risk factors or medical conditions.

Trends in Immunization. National coverage levels in children are now greater than 90 percent for each immunization recommended during the first 2 years of life, except for hepatitis B and varicella vaccines. The hepatitis B immunization rate in children was 87 percent in 1998, the highest level ever reported. In 1996, 69 percent of children aged 19 to 35 months from the lowest income households received the combined series of recommended immunizations compared with 80 percent of children from higher income households.

Both influenza and pneumococcal immunization rates are significantly lower for African American and Hispanic adults than for white adults.

Other Immunization Issues. Coverage levels for immunizations in adults are not as high as those achieved in children, yet the health effects may be just as great. Barriers to adult immunization include not knowing immunizations are needed, misconceptions about vaccines, and lack of recommendations from health care providers.

Access to Health Care

Strong predictors of access to quality health care include having health insurance, a higher income level, and a regular primary care provider or other source of ongoing health care. Use of clinical preventive services, such as early prenatal care, can serve as indicators of access to quality health care services.

In 1997, 86 percent of all individuals had health insurance, and 86 percent had a usual source of health care. Also in that year, 83 percent of pregnant women received prenatal care in the first trimester of pregnancy.

The objectives selected to measure progress for this Leading Health Indicator are presented below. These are only indicators and do not represent all the access to quality health care objectives in Healthy People 2010.

- Increase the proportion of persons with health insurance.

- Increase the proportion of persons who have a specific source of ongoing care.

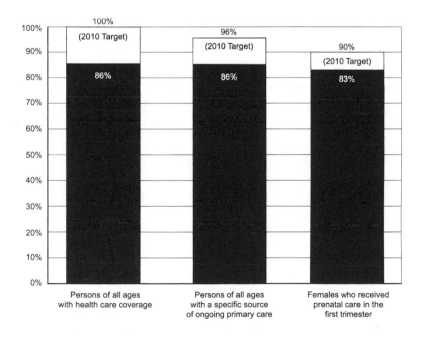

Source: Centers for Disease Control and Prevention, National Center for Health Statistics. National Health Interview Survey. 1997. Centers for Disease Control and Prevention, National Center for Health Statistics. National Vital Statistics System. 1997.

Figure 1.18. *Access to health care, United States, 1997.*

• Increase the proportion of pregnant women who begin prenatal care in the first trimester of pregnancy.

Health Insurance

Health insurance provides access to health care. Persons with health insurance are more likely to have a primary care provider and to have received appropriate preventive care such as a recent Pap test, immunization, or early prenatal care. Adults with health insurance are twice as likely to receive a routine checkup as are adults without health insurance.

More than 44 million persons in the United States do not have health insurance, including 11 million uninsured children. Over the past decade, the proportion of persons aged 65 years and under with health insurance remained steady at about 85 percent. About one-third of adults 65 years and under below the poverty level were uninsured. For persons of Hispanic origin, approximately one in three was without health insurance coverage in 1997. Mexican Americans had one of the highest uninsured rates at 38 percent.

Ongoing Sources of Primary Care. More than 40 million Americans do not have a particular doctor's office, clinic, health center, or other place where they usually go to seek health care or health-related advice. Even among privately insured persons, a significant number lacked a usual source of care or reported difficulty in accessing needed care due to financial constraints or insurance problems.

People aged 18 to 24 years were the most likely to lack a usual source of ongoing primary care. Only 76 percent of individuals below the poverty level and 74 percent of Hispanics had a usual source of ongoing primary care.

Barriers to Access. Financial, structural, and personal barriers can limit access to health care. Financial barriers include not having health insurance, not having enough health insurance to cover needed services, or not having the financial capacity to cover services outside a health plan or insurance program. Structural barriers include the lack of primary care providers, medical specialists, or other health care professionals to meet special needs or the lack of health care facilities. Personal barriers include cultural or spiritual differences, language barriers, not knowing what to do or when to seek care, or concerns about confidentiality or discrimination.

Bibliography

Introduction

McGinnis JM and Maiese DR. Defining mission, goals, and objectives. In: *Principles of Public Health Practice*. Scutchfield FD and Keck CW (eds.). Albany, NY: Delmar Publishers, 1997, pp. 140-141.

A Systematic Approach to Health Improvement: Goals

American College of Physicians. Rural primary care. *Ann Inter Med* 122(5):380-390, 1995.

American Medical Association Council Report. Health care needs of gay men and lesbians in the United States. *JAMA* 247:1354-1359, 1996.

Centers for Disease Control and Prevention. BRFSS Prevalence Data, 1998. http://ww2.cdc.gov/ nccdphp/brfss/ index.asp.

Centers for Disease Control and Prevention. Health-related quality of life and activity limitation—eight states, 1995. *MMWR* 47(7):134-140, 1998.

Centers for Disease Control and Prevention. Health-related quality-of-life measures—United States, 1993. *MMWR* 44:195-200, 1995.

Definitions: Healthy People 2010, Disability and Secondary Conditions Focus Area.

Institute of Medicine. *Improving Health in the Community*. Washington, DC: National Academy Press, 1997, pp. 48-56.

National Center for Health Statistics. *Health, United States, 1999, With Health and Aging Chartbook*. Hyattsville, MD: U.S. Department of Health and Human Services, 1999.

National Center for Health Statistics. *Healthy People 2000 Review, 1998-99*. Hyattsville, MD: Public Health Service, 1999.

Tissue T. Another look at self-rated health among the elderly. *J Gerontol* (27):91-94, 1972.

Barker WH. Prevention of disability in older persons. In: *Public Health and Preventive Medicine, Fourteenth Edition*, Wallace RB (ed.). Stamford, CT: Appleton & Lange, 1998, p. 1063.

Braden J, Beauregard K. Health Status and Access to Care of Rural and Urban Populations. AHCPR Pub. no. 94-0031. *National Medical Expenditure Survey Research Findings 18*. Rockville, MD: Public Health Service, Agency for Health Care Policy and Research, 1994.

Catalan J, Pugh K. Suicidal behaviour and HIV infection-is there a link? *AIDS Care* 7(Suppl 2):S117-S121, 1995.

Cochran SD, Mays VM. Depressive distress among homosexually active African American men and women. *Am J Psychiatry* 151:524-529, 1994.

Davidson L, Linnoila M (eds.). *Report of the Secretary's Task Force on Youth Suicide, 2: Risk Factors for Youth Suicide*. Washington, DC: U.S. Department of Health and Human Services, Public Health Service, 1989.

Frumkin H and Walker ED. Minority workers and communities. In: *Public Health and Preventive Medicine, Fourteenth Edition*, Wallace RB (ed.). Stamford, CT: Appleton & Lange, 1998, p. 685.

Hoyert DL, Kochanek KD, Murphy SL. Deaths: final data for 1997. *National Vital Statistics Reports*. Vol. 47, no. 19. Hyattsville, MD: National Center for Health Statistics, 1999.

Idler EL and Benyamini Y. Self-rated health and mortality: a review of twenty-seven community studies. *J Health Soc Behav* 38:21-37, 1997.

LaPlante MP, Rice DP, Cyril J. Health insurance coverage of people with disabilities in the U.S. Disability Statistics Abstract. *Disability Statistics Rehabilitation*. San Francisco, CA: Research and Training Center, September 1994.

Last JM. The determinants of health. In: *Principles of Public Health Practice*, Scutchfield FD and Keck CW (eds.). Albany, NY: Delmar Publishers, 1997, pp. 33-34.

Luepker RV. Heart disease. In: *Public Health and Preventive Medicine. Fourteenth Edition*, Wallace RB (ed.). Stamford, CT: Appleton & Lange, 1998, pp. 939-940.

McNeil JM. Americans with disabilities: 1994-95. *Current Population Reports*. Bureau of the Census (P70-61). Washington, DC: U.S. Department of Commerce, August 1997.

Pamuk E, Makuc D, Heck K, Reuben C, Lochner K. *Socioeconomic Status and Health Chartbook. Health, United States, 1998.* Hyattsville, MD: National Center for Health Statistics, 1998.

Pearson TA, Lewis C. Rural epidemiology: insights from a rural population laboratory. *Am J Epidemiol* 148(10):949-957, 1998.

Solarz, A (ed.). *Lesbian Health: Current Assessment and Directions for the Future.* Washington, DC: Institute of Medicine, 1997.

Syme SL and Balfour JL. Social determinants of disease. In: *Public Health and Preventive Medicine, FourteenthEdition*, Wallace RB (ed.). Stamford, CT: Appleton & Lange, 1998, pp. 800-801.

Vistnes JP and Monheit AC. *Health Insurance Status of the Civilian Noninstitutionalized Population. Medical Expenditure Panel Survey Research Findings 1.* AHCPR Pub. no. 97-0030. Rockville, MD: Agency for Health Care Policy and Research, August 1997.

A Systematic Approach to Health Improvement: Determinants of Health

Institute of Medicine. *Improving Health in the Community.* Washington, DC: National Academy Press, 1997, pp. 48-56.

McGinnis JM, Maiese DR. Defining mission, goals, and objectives. In: *Principles of Public Health Practice*, Scutchfield FD and Keck CW (eds.). Albany, NY: Delmar Publishers, 1997, pp. 136-145.

Syme SL and Balfour JL. Social determinants of disease. In: *Public Health and Preventive Medicine, Fourteenth Edition*, Wallace RB (ed.). Stamford, CT: Appleton & Lange, 1998, p. 795.

A Systematic Approach to Health Improvement: Health Status

National Center for Health Statistics. *Health, United States, 1999, With Health and Aging Chartbook.* Hyattsville, MD: U.S. Department of Health and Human Services, 1999.

Leading Health Indicators: Physical Activity

Centers for Disease Control and Prevention. Physical activity and the prevention of coronary heart disease. *MMWR* 42:669-672, 1993.

Centers for Disease Control and Prevention. Prevalence of sedentary leisure-time behavior among adults in the United States. *Health E-Stats*. Atlanta, GA: Centers for Disease Control and Prevention, National Center for Health Statistics, 1999.

National Center for Health Statistics. *Health, United States, 1999, With Health and Aging Chartbook*. Hyattsville, MD: U.S. Department of Health and Human Services, 1999.

National Center for Health Statistics. *Healthy People 2000 Review, 1998-99*. Hyattsville, MD: U.S. Department of Health and Human Services, 1999.

U.S. Department of Health and Human Services. *Physical Activity and Health: A Report of the Surgeon General*. Atlanta, GA: Centers for Disease Control and Prevention, National Center for Chronic Disease Prevention and Health Promotion, 1996.

Pamuk E, Makuc D, Heck K, Reuben C, Lochner K. *Socioeconomic Status and Health Chartbook. Health, United States, 1998*. Hyattsville, MD: National Center for Health Statistics, 1998.

Leading Health Indicators: Overweight and Obesity

Agricultural Research Service. Research News. Press Release. U.S. Department of Agriculture, Washington, DC, November 20, 1996.

National Center for Health Statistics. *Health, United States, 1999, With Health and Aging Chartbook*. Hyattsville, MD: U.S. Department of Health and Human Services, 1999.

National Center for Health Statistics. *Healthy People 2000 Review, 1998-99*. Hyattsville, MD: U.S. Department of Health and Human Services, 1999.

National Institutes of Health. *Statistics Related to Overweight and Obesity*. NIH Publication No. 96-4158. National Institute of Diabetes and Digestive and Kidney Diseases. Bethesda, MD: U.S. Department of Health and Human Services, July 1996.

U.S. Department of Agriculture/U.S. Department of Health and Human Services. *Dietary Guidelines for Americans. Fourth Edition*. USDA Home and Garden Bulletin No. 232. December 1995.

Pamuk E, Makuc D, Heck K, Reuben C, Lochner K. *Socioeconomic Status and Health Chartbook. Health, United States, 1998.* Hyattsville, MD: National Center for Health Statistics, 1998.

Lin BH and Frazao E. Nutritional quality of foods at and away from home. *FoodReview* 20(2):33-40, 1997.

Wolf AM, Colditz GA. Current estimates of the economic cost of obesity in the United States. *Obesity Research* 6(2):97-106, 1998.

Leading Health Indicators: Tobacco Use

Centers for Disease Control and Prevention. Guidelines for school health programs to prevent tobacco use and addiction. *MMWR* 43(no. RR-2):1994.

Centers for Disease Control and Prevention. Smoking-attributable mortality and years of potential life lost- United States, 1984. *MMWR* 46(20):441-451, 1997.

Centers for Disease Control and Prevention. *Targeting Tobacco Use: The Nation's Leading Cause of Death.* Atlanta, GA: U.S. Department of Health and Human Services, CDC, 1999.

Centers for Disease Control and Prevention. Youth Risk Behavior Surveillance-United States, 1997. *MMWR* 47(SS-3):1998.

National Center for Health Statistics. *Health, United States, 1999, With Health and Aging Chartbook.* Hyattsville, MD: U.S. Department of Health and Human Services, 1999.

National Cancer Institute. *Cigars: Health Effects and Trends.* Bethesda, MD: U.S. Department of Health and Human Services, National Institutes of Health, 1998.

U.S. Environmental Protection Agency. *Respiratory Health Effects of Passive Smoking: Fact Sheet.* EPA Pub. No. EPA-43-F-93-003. Washington, DC: EPA, 1993.

U.S. Department of Health and Human Services. Tobacco Use Among U.S. Racial/Ethnic Minority Groups—African Americans, American Indians and Alaska Natives, Asian Americans and Pacific Islanders, and Hispanics: A Report of the Surgeon General. Atlanta, Georgia: U.S. Department of Health and Human Services, Centers for Disease Control and Prevention, National Center for Chronic Disease Prevention and Health Promotion, Office on Smoking and Health, 1998.

Leading Health Indicators: Substance Abuse

National Clearinghouse for Alcohol and Drug Information. *Health Care Costs, the Deficit, & Alcohol, Tobacco, and Other Drugs*. Rockville, MD: NCADI Inventory Number ML007, 1995.

Substance Abuse and Mental Health Services Administration. *Summary of Findings From the 1998 National Household Survey on Drug Abuse*. Rockville, MD: U.S. Department of Health and Human Services, SAMHSA, Office of Applied Studies, 1999.

Harwood H, Fountain D, Livermore G. *The Economic Costs of Alcohol and Drug Abuse in the United States, 1992*. NIH Publication Number 98-4327. Rockville, MD: U.S. Department of Health and Human Services, National Institutes of Health, 1998.

Leading Health Indicators: Responsible Sexual Behavior

American Social Health Association. *Sexually Transmitted Diseases in America: How Many Cases and at What Cost?* Menlo Park, CA: Kaiser Family Foundation, 1998.

Centers for Disease Control and Prevention. *Fact sheet: Youth Risk Behavior Trends*. Atlanta, GA: U.S. Department of Health and Human Services, Centers for Disease Control and Prevention. National Center for Chronic Disease Prevention and Health Promotion, 1999.

Centers for Disease Control and Prevention. *From Data to Action: CDC's Public Health Surveillance for Women, Infants, and Children*. Atlanta, GA: U.S. Department of Health and Human Services, Centers for Disease Control and Prevention, National Center for Chronic Disease Prevention and Health Promotion, 1994.

Centers for Disease Control and Prevention. *HIV/AIDS Surveillance Report, Midyear edition*. Atlanta, GA: U.S. Department of Health and Human Services, Centers for Disease Control and Prevention, 1999.

Centers for Disease Control and Prevention. *PRAMS 1996 Surveillance Report*. Atlanta, GA: Centers for Disease Control and Prevention, National Center for Chronic Disease Prevention and Health Promotion, Division of Reproductive Health, 1999.

Centers for Disease Control and Prevention. Trends in sexual risk behaviors among high school students- United States, 1991-1997. *MMWR* 47(36):749-752, 1998.

Centers for Disease Control and Prevention. Young people at risk-epidemic shifts further toward young women and minorities. In: *CDC Update*. Atlanta, GA: U.S. Department of Health and Human Services, Centers for Disease Control and Prevention, National Center for HIV, TB & STD Prevention, 1999.

Division of STD Prevention. *Sexually Transmitted Disease Surveillance, 1998*. Atlanta, GA: U.S. Department of Health and Human Services, Centers for Disease Control and Prevention, September 1999.

National Center for Health Statistics. *Healthy People 2000 Review, 1998-99*. Hyattsville, MD: U.S. Department of Health and Human Services, 1999.

Holtgrave DR, Pinkerton SD. Updates of cost of illness and quality of life estimates for use in economic evaluations of HIV prevention programs. *J Acquir Immune Defic Syndr Hum Retrovirol* 16(1):54-62, 1997.

Hoyert DL, Kochanek KD, Murphy SL. Deaths: final data for 1997. *National Vital Statistics Reports*. Vol. 47, no. 19. Hyattsville, MD: National Center for Health Statistics, 1999.

Maynard RA (ed.). *Kids Having Kids; Economic Costs and Cocial Consequences of Teen Pregnancy*. Washington, DC: Urban Institute Press, 1997.

St. Louis ME, Wasserheit JN, Gayle HD. Janus considers the HIV pandemic-harnessing recent advances to enhance AIDS prevention. *Am J Public Health* 87(1):10-12, 1997.

Leading Health Indicators: Mental Health

National Center for Health Statistics. *Healthy People 2000 Review, 1998-99*. Hyattsville, MD: U.S. Department of Health and Human Services, 1999.

National Institutes of Health, Consensus Development Panel on Depression in Late Life, Diagnosis and treatment of depression in late life. *JAMA* 268:1018-1024, 1992.

National Institute of Mental Health. *Depression*. Fact sheet. http://www.nimh.nih.gov/depression/index.htm. Bethesda, MD: U.S.

Department of Health and Human Services, National Institutes of Health, 1999.

National Institute of Mental Health. *The Invisible Disease — Depression*. Fact sheet. http://www.nimh.nih.gov/ publicat/ invisible.cfm. Bethesda, MD: U.S. Department of Health and Human Services, National Institutes of Health, 1999.

Office of Applied Statistics. *Statistics Source Book, 1998*, Rouse BA (ed.). Substance Abuse and Mental Health Services Administration. Rockville, MD: U.S. Department of Health and Human Services, 1998.

Substance Abuse and Mental Health Services Administration. *Mental Health: A Report of the Surgeon General*. Rockville, MD: U.S. Department of Health and Human Services, National Institutes of Health, 1999.

Bromet EJ. Psychiatric disorders. In: *Public Health and Preventive Medicine, Fourteenth Edition*, Wallace RB (ed.). Stamford, CT: Appleton & Lange, 1998, p. 1037.

Greenberg PE, Stiglin LE, Finkelstein SN, Berndt ER. The economic burden of depression in 1990. *J Clin Psychiatry* 54:405-418, 1993.

Koenig HG and Blazer DG. Mood disorders and suicide. In: *Handbook of Mental Health and Aging, Second Edition*, Birren JE, Sloane RB, Cohen GD (eds.). San Diego, CA: Academic Press, 1992, 379-407.

Weissman MM and Klerman JK. Depression: current understanding and changing trends. *Ann Rev Public Health* 13:319-339, 1992.

Leading Health Indicators: Injury and Violence

National Center for Health Statistics. *Healthy People 2000 Review, 1998-99*. Hyattsville, MD: U.S. Department of Health and Human Services, 1999.

National Center for Injury Prevention and Control. *Impaired Driving Fact Sheet*. Atlanta, GA: U.S. Department of Health and Human Services, Centers for Disease Control and Prevention, 1999.

National Highway Traffic Safety Administration. *Traffic Safety Facts, 1998*. Washington, DC: U.S. Department of Transportation, 1998.

National Safety Council, *Accident Facts*. Washington, DC: National Safety Council, 1995.

Baker SP, O'Neill B, Ginsburg MJ, Li G. *The Injury Fact Book, 2nd Edition*, New York, NY: Oxford University Press, 1992.

Fox JA and Zawitz MW. *Homicide Trends in the United States*. U.S. Department of Justice, Bureau of Justice Statistics, 1999.

Hoyert DL, Kochanek KD, Murphy SL. Deaths: final data for 1997. *National Vital Statistics Reports.* Vol. 47, no. 19. Hyattsville, MD: National Center for Health Statistics, 1999.

Leading Health Indicators: Environmental Quality

American Lung Association. *Health Costs of Air Pollution*. Washington, DC: American Lung Association, 1990.

California Environmental Protection Agency, *Health Effects of Exposure to Environmental Tobacco Smoke*. Final Report. Sacramento, CA: California Environmental Protection Agency, Office of Environmental Health Hazard Assessment, 1997.

Centers for Disease Control and Prevention. Progress toward the elimination of tuberculosis—United States, 1998. *MMWR* 48:732-736, 1999.

Centers for Disease Control and Prevention. State-specific prevalence of cigarette smoking among adults, and children's and adolescent's exposure to environmental tobacco smoke—United States. *MMWR* 46:1038-1043, 1997.

National Center for Health Statistics. *Health, United States, 1999, With Health and Aging Chartbook*. Hyattsville, MD: U.S. Department of Health and Human Services, 1999.

U.S. Environmental Protection Agency. *National Air Quality and Trends Report*. Office of Air and Radiation. Washington, DC: EPA, 1997.

U.S. Environmental Protection Agency. *Respiratory Health Effects of Passive Smoking: Lung Cancer and Other Disorders*. EPA Pub. No. EPA/600/6-90/006F. Washington, DC: EPA, 1992.

World Health Organization. Fact Sheet 170, June 1997.

Weiss KB, Gergen PJ, Hodgson TA. An economic evaluation of asthma in the United States. *N Engl J Med* 326:862-866, 1992.

Leading Health Indicators: Immunization

Centers for Disease Control and Prevention. National Immunization Program, Immunization Services Division, Health Services Research and Evaluation Branch. Unpublished data. Atlanta, GA, 1999.

Centers for Disease Control and Prevention. National vaccination coverage levels among children aged 19-35 months—United States, 1998. *MMWR* 48:829-830, 1999.

Centers for Disease Control and Prevention. Prevention and control of influenza: recommendations of the Advisory Committee on Immunization Practices (ACIP). *MMWR* 48(no. RR-4), 1999.

Centers for Disease Control and Prevention. Prevention of pneumococcal disease: recommendations of the Advisory Committee on Immunization Practices (ACIP). *MMWR* 46(no. RR-8), 1997.

Centers for Disease Control and Prevention. Reasons reported by Medicare beneficiaries for not receiving influenza and pneumococcal vaccinations—United States, 1996. *MMWR* 48:886-890, 1999.

Centers for Disease Control and Prevention. Recommended childhood immunization schedule—United States, 1999. *MMWR* 48:12-16, 1999.

Centers for Disease Control and Prevention. Ten great public health achievements—United States, 1900-1999. *MMWR* 48:241-248, 1999.

National Center for Health Statistics. *Health, United States, 1999, With Health and Aging Chartbook*. Hyattsville, MD: U.S. Department of Health and Human Services, 1999.

Feiken DR, Schuchat A, Kolczak M, et al. Mortality from invasive pneumococcal pneumonia in the era of antibiotic resistance, 1995-1997. *Am J Public Health*, in press.

Pamuk E, Makuc D, Heck K, Reuben C, Lochner K. *Socioeconomic Status and Health Chartbook. Health, United States, 1998*. Hyattsville, MD: National Center for Health Statistics, 1998.

Leading Health Indicators: Access to Health Care

Centers for Disease Control and Prevention. Health insurance coverage and receipt of preventive health services-United States, 1993. *MMWR* 44(11):219-225, 1995.

National Center for Health Statistics. *Health, United States, 1999, With Health and Aging Chartbook*. Hyattsville, MD: U.S. Department of Health and Human Services, 1999.

U.S. General Accounting Office. *Health Insurance: Coverage Leads to Increased Health Care Access for Children*. GAO/HEHS-98-14. Washington, DC: GAO, 1998, pp. 4-20.

Acknowledgments

Healthy People 2010: Understanding and Improving Health is part of the Healthy People 2010 initiative that is sponsored by the U. S. Department of Health and Human Services. Leadership and direction were provided by David Satcher and Nicole Lurie. Development of Healthy People 2010 has been coordinated by the Office of Disease Prevention and Health Promotion under the leadership of Claude Earl Fox, Susanne A. Stoiber, Linda D. Meyers, and Randolph F. Wykoff.

Principle responsibility for Healthy People 2010: Understanding and Improving Health was carried out by Mark S. Smolinski. Critical editorial and technical support were provided by Mary Jo Deering, Matthew Guidry, Deborah R. Maiese, Linda D. Meyers, Janice T. Radak, Kelly H. Woodward, and Randolph F. Wykoff. Special thanks to David Atkins, Linda A. Bailey, Ron Davis, Kate-Louise Gottfried, James Harrell, J. Michael McGinnis, Kevin Patrick, Scott C. Ratzan, Dirk Ruwaard, Susanne Stoiber, and Tom Vischi for their ideas and support during the development of this document.

Statistical advice and data development were provided by staff of the Division of Health Promotion Statistics of the National Center for Health Statistics, Centers for Disease Control and Prevention, which included Jeanette Guyton-Krishnan, Elizabeth Jackson, Richard J. Klein, Cheryl Rose, Colleen Ryan, J. Fred Seitz, Thomas Socey, Kathleen Turczyn, Jennie Wald, and Jean Williams, under the leadership of Diane Wagener.

Research of the medical literature and other health resources was provided by the following preventive medicine residents and medical students: Madhavi Battineni, Joy L. Bottoms, Wayne Brandes, Dominic Cheung Chow, Penny Shelton-Hoffman, Robin McFee, J. Patrick Moulds, Alex Nettles, Elpidoforos Soteriades, Peter Thornquist, Edward Van Oeveren, Stephanie Weller, and Amanda Williams.

The development of the Leading Health Indicators was guided by an interagency workgroup and the Healthy People Steering Committee which included Lois Albarelli, David R. Arday, David Atkins,

Delton Atkinson, Linda A. Bailey, Olivia Carter-Pokras, Lynn Cates, Melissa H. Clarke, Marsha G. Davenport, Tuei Doong, Margaret Gilliam, Chuck Gollmar, William R. Harlan, James Harrell, Suzanne G. Haynes, Wanda K. Jones, Diane Justice, Nicole Lurie, Evelyn Kappeler, Richard J. Klein, Mary Ann MacKenzie, John Monahon, J. Henry Montes, Paul W. Nannis, Eileen Parish, Kate Rickard, Carol Roddy, Theresa Rogers, Dorita Sewell, Mary Beth Skupien, Philip B. Smith, Mark S. Smolinski, Christine G. Spain, Matthew Stagner, Irma Tetzloff, Betsy L. Thompson, Martina Vogel-Taylor, and Diane K. Wagener. Important contributions were provided by the Institute of Medicine, National Academy of Sciences Committee on Leading Health Indicators for Healthy People 2010 which included Susan Allan, Roger Bulger, Carole A. Chrvala, Donna D. Duncan, Neal Halfon, Barbara S. Hulka, Thomas J. Kean, Kelly Norsingle, Scott C. Ratzan, Stephen C. Schoenbaum, Mark Smith, Shoshanna Sofaer, Kathleen R. Stratton, and Robert B. Wallace.

Production was handled by IQ Solutions, Inc., which included Denise Avery, Ted Buxton, Eleanor Hall, Michael Huddleston, E.J. King-Carter, James R. Libbey, Josue Martinez, Craig Packer, Meredith Pond, Lisa Smith, and Karen Stroud.

Finally, a sincere debt of gratitude to all contributors to Healthy People 2010, whose efforts greatly enhanced the development of this document.

For more information about Healthy People 2010 or to access Healthy People 2010 documents online, visit: http://www.health.gov/healthypeople/ or call 1-800-367-4725

Chapter 2

Questions and Answers on the Benefits of Exercise

Television. Cars. Computers. Remote controls. Elevators. Escalators. E-mail. Leaf-blowers. Golf carts. Automatic doors. Automatic windows. Automatic toilet-flushers.

It all adds up. Little by little, we're turning into a nation of couch potatoes. And we're paying a price for it. Inactive people have a higher risk of heart disease, diabetes, colon cancer, obesity, and osteoporosis. That doesn't mean that everyone has to take up in-line skating or join a neighborhood soccer team. For many, the answer is simply to put activity back into everyday life.

Getting off the couch doesn't just ward off life-threatening illness. It may also help you function like you're 20 years younger, cut your odds of ending up in a nursing home, help you sleep better, ward off colds, and improve your outlook on life. Need any more reasons to take a hike? The following is taken from a conversation with David Nieman, author of *Exercise Testing and Prescription: A Health-Related Approach*, (Mountain View, California: Mayfield Publishing, 1999.)

Warding Off Disease

Q: What benefits of exercise are the most certain?

A: Exercise can help you live longer and make you less likely to die of heart disease and stroke. It can reduce the risk of type 2 (adult-onset)

Nutrition Action Healthletter, January 1999, vol. 26, issue 1 p. 1. © 1999 Center for Science in the Public Interest. Reprinted with permission.

diabetes and colon cancer. And almost everyone believes that an active life should prevent obesity, though that hasn't been studied in detail.

Q: How much longer would you live?

A: Regular exercise would increase average longevity by two or three years. That doesn't seem like very much, but if someone tomorrow found a magic bullet that completely cured all cancer, average longevity would increase by less than two years.

Q: If curing all cancer adds only a few years, why do we live 20 or 30 years longer than we used to?

A: Because we've prevented deaths in childhood. Only that can change average longevity dramatically.

Q: How does exercise protect the heart?

A: It lowers blood cholesterol and blood pressure. That's not the entire explanation, though, because if we factor out those variables, exercise has an independent effect. Part of it is that if you exercise regularly, your heart is a bigger, stronger, better pump. You're better able to survive your first heart attack, because you've got more heart muscle left. In addition, there are probably other as yet understood ways in which exercise reduces risk.

Q: How does exercise prevent diabetes?

A: It improves carbohydrate metabolism by increasing insulin sensitivity. In our new study, the rate of developing diabetes in unfit men was more than three times higher than in high-fit men. Fitness reduced the risk even in fit men who were overweight.

My belief is that type 2 diabetes is a disease of inactivity. It's virtually never seen in people who are highly active and have been highly active over their lifetimes. Runners just do not develop type 2 diabetes.

Q: What makes you say that exercise prevents colon cancer?

A: The documentation is really pretty consistent. Researchers see an association between inactivity and colon cancer even after they account for diet, obesity, and socioeconomic status. We've seen the association in several populations around the world for both men and women. That's why the 1996 Surgeon General's report concluded that activity protects against colon cancer.

Q: *What kind of activity?*

A: For colon cancer, we don't have a lot of data on different types or intensity. In fact, several studies measured on-the-job activity. But if you take all the studies on exercise and health, I think the single most important factor is simply the total energy expended in activity. The cells in your body don't know if you're jogging or doing aerobic dance or working hard in the fields.

Q: *So you add up the calories you burn every week or every day?*

A: Yes. If you do 1,000 calories of exercise in a week—that's walking about two miles a day for five days for a 150- or 160-pound person— I don't think the pattern, type, intensity, or duration matters. I can't say that it makes absolutely no difference, but we can be fairly confident that total work done is the most important factor.

Q: *How might exercise prevent colon cancer?*

A: One theory is that people who exercise more tend to have different bowel habits—waste moves through their systems more quickly. If colon cancer is caused by carcinogens in the fecal waste, they may not be in contact with the intestinal lining as long. Exercise also enhances immune function, so that's another possibility.

Q: *Does exercise prevent other cancers?*

A: A lot of people have high hopes for breast cancer and I hope they're right, but the studies are equivocal. Some show that active women have a lower risk, one or two show a higher risk, and several studies show no relationship. So it's just not clear what role, if any, activity may have in breast cancer.

Q: *Is it clear that exercise lowers blood pressure?*

A: Yes, in most people. And exercise prevents high blood pressure in the first place.

Q: *Is that because exercise helps prevent obesity?*

A: Not entirely. In our studies, we have an objective measure of fitness from a maximal exercise test—we see how long people can exercise on a treadmill. We look at fitness when people enter the study and then see who develops high blood pressure over time. High-fit people are much less likely to develop high blood pressure than low-fit people. That's true for men and women, the young and the old, the fat and the lean, and for those with and without a family history of high blood pressure.

Fit and Fat

Q: *So you can be fat and fit?*

A: Yes. We haven't studied this yet in our women, but in the men who are overweight or obese, but also moderately or high-fit, we don't see much increase in the risk of dying.

Q: *Is that true for more than blood pressure?*

A: Yes. Claude Bouchard and his colleagues at Laval University in Quebec had a small group of obese women exercise 90 minutes a day for 14 months—prodigious amounts of exercise. Then he had them continue the exercise and eat a low-fat diet for another 15 months. Although the women lost an average of 24 pounds, they were still obese. Yet metabolically—cholesterol, blood sugar, and so forth—they were normal. So activity is good for you whether you're obese or thin.

Q: *But most overweight people are not fit?*

A: Right. When we looked at overweight men as a group, they were less physically fit and had the highest death rate. It's only after we looked separately at the overweight men who were fit that we saw a lower death rate. Being fit lessens the harmful effects of obesity.

Q: *And the more fit, the better?*

A: Yes. We look at low-fit, moderate-fit, and high-fit individuals. Moderate fitness is what you would develop if you followed recommendations to accumulate 30 minutes of moderate-intensity activity most days. That's the advice of the American College of Sports Medicine, the Centers for Disease Control and Prevention, and a National Institutes of Health Consensus Statement. High-fit individuals do more—and probably higher-intensity—exercise.

Q: *How can you tell how fit you are?*

A: You can get a maximal exercise test at a health club or laboratory or come to the Cooper Clinic, and if the people doing the testing know about our data, they could tell you what category you fall into. But I think we should focus on the activity.

If you accumulate 30 minutes a day of moderate-intensity activity—which is briskly walking a couple of miles a day—that's certainly a sufficient dose of exercise to get almost everybody into the moderate-fit category.

High-fit is more than that—maybe 45 minutes to an hour of brisk walking and some days more vigorous exercise, like jogging or an aerobics class. Low-fit people do somewhere between less than 30 minutes a day and nothing.

Q: Is less than 30 minutes a day better than nothing?

A: Yes. Doing something is better than doing nothing at all and doing more is better still. So for 80 percent of the U.S. population, when they ask, "What should I do?" the answer is one word: more.

Better Bones

Q: Does exercise help prevent osteoporosis?

A: Yes, some clinical trials show that exercise improves bone mineral density. And there is some evidence that people who lead a fit and active life are less likely to develop osteoporosis. Their muscle strength also makes them less likely to fall and get a fracture. It's the fracture more than just the disease that we're concerned about.

Q: So exercise can help people who already have osteoporosis?

A: Right, because they'd be less likely to fall.

Q: And almost any exercise but swimming works?

A: Right. It has to be weight-bearing. Some researchers think it has to be a weight-bearing exercise with changes in direction—like dancing—to provide some stimulus for bone health. We don't know for sure about cycling. You do have some weight-bearing in the spine and you are exerting the muscles against the pedals, but it's a little unclear.

Q: Can exercise cause arthritis?

A: The evidence suggests that it doesn't, at least in the amount most people are likely to do. People who do prodigious amounts of exercise

61

can get repetitive joint injury. Jackhammer operators get arthritis of the wrist, for example. And some studies have found an increased risk in young, highly fit, healthy fighting forces, like U.S. Army Rangers or Israeli commandos. But these people get huge amounts of exercise—carrying 50-pound packs across the mountains all day. Even in runners we don't see an increased risk of arthritis. If anything, we may see a slightly reduced risk, but we can't confirm that.

Q: Can exercise cure arthritis?

A: No, but it seems to improve overall quality of life. A study at Wake Forest University in North Carolina randomly assigned elderly individuals with arthritis of the knee to do aerobic or strength-training exercise or no exercise. After a year, those who did best were in the aerobic group, but those in the strength-training group also got benefit compared to the sedentary group. They reported less pain and less disability than the non-exercise group, and their ability to walk and climb stairs and get in and out of a car improved.

Table 2.1. Exercise: Calories burned, cardiovascular fitness, and muscle strength; continued on next page.

Activity	Calories per Hour (150-lb. person)	Activity	Calories per Hour (150-lb. person)
aerobic dance (vigorous)	475	running (moderate pace, 6 mph)	680
basketball (competitive)	545	shoveling dirt or digging	580
canoeing or rowing (fast pace)	815	skating (in-line or ice)	475
cross country skiing machine	645	skiing (cross country, brisk speed)	610
cycling (fast pace)	680	skiing (downhill)	340
cycling (leisurely pace)	375	soccer (casual)	475
cycling (stationary, moderate)	475	splitting wood	410
dancing	305	stair climbing	610
gardening	340	swimming (laps, vigorous)	680
golf (walking and carrying bag)	375	swimming (moderate)	545
handball (casual)	475	tennis (competitive)	475
lawn mowing (power mower)	305	volleyball (competitive)	270
racquetball or squash (casual)	475	walking (brisk pace, 4 mph)	270
raking leaves	270	walking (slow pace, 2 mph)	170
rope jumping (moderate to hard)	680	weight training	205
running (brisk pace, 8 mph)	920	yoga	170

Table 2.1. Exercise: Calories burned, cardiovascular fitness, and muscle strength; continued from previous page.

Activity	Builds Cardiovascular Health & Burns Fat	Activity	Builds Cardiovascular Health & Burns Fat
aerobic dance (vigorous)	4	running (moderate pace, 6 mph)	5
basketball (competitive)	4	shoveling dirt or digging	4
canoeing or rowing (fast pace)	5	skating (in-line or ice)	4
cross country skiing machine	5	skiing (cross country, brisk speed)	5
cycling (fast pace)	5	skiing (downhill)	3
cycling (leisurely pace)	3	soccer (casual)	4
cycling (stationary, moderate)	4	splitting wood	4
dancing	3	stair climbing	5
gardening	3	swimming (laps, vigorous)	5
golf (walking and carrying bag)	3	swimming (moderate)	4
handball (casual)	4	tennis (competitive)	4
lawn mowing (power mower)	3	volleyball (competitive)	3
racquetball or squash (casual)	4	walking (brisk pace, 4 mph)	3
raking leaves	3	walking (slow pace, 2 mph)	2
rope jumping (moderate to hard)	5	weight training	2
running (brisk pace, 8 mph)	5	yoga	1

Rating of 5 indicates highest level of cardiovascular health and fat-burning benefits.

Activity	Builds Muscle Strength	Activity	Builds Muscle Strength
aerobic dance (vigorous)	4	running (moderate pace, 6 mph)	2
basketball (competitive)	2	shoveling dirt or digging	4
canoeing or rowing (fast pace)	4	skating (in-line or ice)	3
cross country skiing machine	4	skiing (cross country, brisk speed)	4
cycling (fast pace)	3	skiing (downhill)	3
cycling (leisurely pace)	2	soccer (casual)	3
cycling (stationary, moderate)	3	splitting wood	4
dancing	2	stair climbing	3
gardening	3	swimming (laps, vigorous)	4
golf (walking and carrying bag)	3	swimming (moderate)	3
handball (casual)	3	tennis (competitive)	3
lawn mowing (power mower)	3	volleyball (competitive)	3
racquetball or squash (casual)	3	walking (brisk pace, 4 mph)	2
raking leaves	3	walking (slow pace, 2 mph)	2
rope jumping (moderate to hard)	3	weight training	5
running (brisk pace, 8 mph)	2	yoga	2

Rating of 5 indicates highest level of strength-building benefits.

Staying Young

Q: *What's the difference between aerobic exercise and strength-training?*

A: Aerobic exercises—like brisk walking or running, swimming, and cycling—release energy by using oxygen. They're continuous and rhythmic, and they require more endurance and less power. Strength-training exercises—like weightlifting—are short and intense, and they require more power and coordination and less endurance.

Q: *Is aerobic exercise more important than strength-training for seniors?*

A: They're both important. I'm convinced that much of the disability, loss of function, and loss of independence that we see in elderly individuals is due to both low muscle and low aerobic fitness.

Studies from Tufts University make it clear that strength-training builds muscle mass and improves function even in very elderly, quite disabled individuals. Their first study was limited to people in their 90s and older. All of them had chronic disease, and on average they had five or six chronic diseases like stroke, heart attack, or emphysema. Based on the Tufts work, it's never too late to do some muscle-training and put back some muscle mass.

Q: *How does low aerobic fitness hurt older people?*

A: In our study, people with low aerobic fitness had higher rates of self-reported limitations. We asked people what they were limited in doing. We asked about everything from bathing, dressing, and feeding themselves to strenuous sports, fast walking, and jogging.

At the end of the eight-year follow-up, low-fit women and men in their forties were as likely to report limitations as high-fit men and women in their sixties. And that wasn't related to smoking, obesity, alcohol intake, or chronic disease.

Q: *So an active 65-year-old could function like an inactive 45-year-old?*

A: Yes. Unfit people start to develop limitations 20 to 25 years earlier than higher-fit people.

Not Life-or-Death

Q: Does exercise help people sleep better?

A: Yes. Abby King and colleagues at Stanford University Medical School studied middle-aged and older adults with mild sleep disorders. She randomly assigned them to an exercise or non-exercise group. Those who exercised got to sleep faster and stayed asleep longer.

Q: Can exercise reduce stress?

A: I'm not aware of well-controlled studies showing that exercise improves the ability to handle stress. That's partly because stress is difficult to define.

Now, if you asked me about my personal experience, I'd say absolutely yes. If you're having a stressful day, nothing makes you feel better than to go out for a brisk walk or to an aerobics class. I believe it in my gut, but I don't think there's much evidence from controlled studies.

Q: Does exercise prevent constipation?

A: People who are physically active have more bowel movements over the course of a week. It's possible that that's because they eat more food. We have no data on whether exercise helps people who already have constipation, but some researchers believe that it does.

Q: Can exercise help prevent colds?

A: Most researchers agree that exercise makes the immune system work better. And there is some evidence that people who exercise regularly have fewer upper respiratory infections. There's also evidence that you can do too much exercise and depress the immune system. One study found increased rates of upper respiratory infections in marathoners during the week after the marathon.

Q: Does physical activity make people happier?

A: It may. People who are active report a more positive outlook on life. They have a greater sense of well-being. There's also some data that people who are active and fit are less likely to develop depression with the passage of time. And exercise may also help treat depression.

Q: *Can exercise improve your sex life?*

A: The evidence is largely anecdotal at this point, but I wouldn't be surprised if it were true. Why do I say that? People who exercise regularly feel better. They're more fit. They have more energy. Now, I ask myself, would those things be likely to contribute to a better sex life? Yes.

Q: *How much exercise do you do every day?*

A: My exercise is running, and I've been doing it nearly every day for 30 years. I'll be 60 on my next birthday, and I'm currently running about 30 miles a week. That's not a huge amount, but it's pretty good for an old geezer like me.

Fitting Fitness In

Q: *Do you have any tips for people who have no time to exercise?*

A: That's an area of active research for us. I've been talking for years about lifestyle physical activity as opposed to structured exercise — going to the gym or going for a jog or playing a sport. If modest amounts of exercise accumulated over the course of the day provide benefits, you don't have to dress up in your leotard and go to the gym in order to burn some calories.

Q: *You can work it into your everyday life?*

A: Yes. Engineers have been very successful, especially since World War II, in cutting the need for energy expenditure. We have energy-saving devices at home, at work, and during leisure: remote controls, self-propelled vacuum cleaners, riding lawn mowers, electric windows in your car, electric doors at the mall, and on and on. A Scottish researcher estimates that in the United Kingdom, average energy expenditures have dropped by 800 calories a day just over the last 25 years.

Q: *So we're more sedentary now?*

A: Yes. I think sedentary people have three choices. They can remain sedentary and unfit and accept the risks for early death, heart disease, diabetes, etc., that go along with it. They can start what we normally think of as a structured sports program—take up rigorous sports, go to aerobics class, jog, what have you. Or, they can put more activity back into their daily lives.

Now how can you do that? Well it's not for me to say how you can do it, because there's an infinite variety of approaches. At the Cooper Institute, we're trying to give people the skills to become their own exercise advisors. We try to help people think about what they might like or be willing to do and when they could do it.

Q: *Like picking a parking place far away from the store?*

A: Yes. The most feasible approach is to look for opportunities to be on your feet and moving—to go for short walks and climb the stairs, etc. Remake your image of yourself as the kind of person who does not take elevators unless you have to go up at least five floors. I always take the stairs. It's a habit. It's who I am.

You can take the kids to the park to play. If you don't have kids, find neighbors who do and I assure you they will be delighted to have you take their kids to the park to play. Take your dog for a walk. If you don't have a dog, pretend you have a dog ... or get a dog ... or borrow a dog. I look for opportunities to walk—down the corridor to talk to my coworkers as opposed to sending an e-mail or getting on the telephone.

Bill Haskell of Stanford University calculated that an office worker who spends two minutes an hour to send e-mail to colleagues in the workplace instead of walking down the hall to speak to them, day after day, would gain the energy equivalent of 11 pounds of fat over a decade. It's a tiny amount each hour and not much each day, but it adds up.

Which Exercise?

Any kind—and any amount—of exercise is better than no exercise. Some studies suggest that as long as you burn 1,000 calories a week, you'll lower your risk of disease. The chart shown in Table 2.1 (see pages 62–63)—based on exercise specialist David Nieman's book *Exercise Testing and Prescription*—shows how many calories a 150-pound person burns by doing any of 30 common physical activities for an hour. (If you weigh more, you'll burn more calories; if you weigh less, you'll burn fewer calories.)

The chart presented in Table 2.1 shows how well each activity builds cardiovascular health, burns fat, or builds muscle strength (1 = not at all, 2 = a little, 3 = moderately, 4 = strongly, and 5 = very strongly). For muscle strength, the activity is rated high if both upper and lower body muscles are strengthened.

— by Steven Blair

Sources: David Nieman (personal communication) and *Exercise Testing and Prescription: A Health-Related Approach*, by David Nieman (Mountain View, California: Mayfield Publishing, 1999). To order, call 800-433-1279.

Chapter 3

How Fit Are You?

Aerobic capacity, strength, and flexibility all tend to decline as you get older. The simple tests described here—developed by James M. Rippe, M.D., director of the Center for Clinical and Lifestyle Research in Shrewsbury, Massachusetts—will tell you where you stand, and help you chart your progress. Note that the scoring of these tests is based on comparison with other people your age—many of whom may be in poor shape. So even if you get what's considered an "average" score, you might still benefit from more exercise. Whatever your score, you can use the tests to chart your progress if you start exercising or increase your exercise schedule.

Unless otherwise noted, start by getting the appropriate muscles ready for each test by working them briefly but briskly; then stretch the muscles.

Aerobic-Fitness Test

A good way to measure aerobic fitness—the ability to exercise without getting winded—is with a walking test. The version described here has been simplified, so you don't have to measure your pulse.

1. Find a measured track or use the odometer of your car to mark out a one-mile course along a level road.

2. Time yourself as you walk the mile as briskly as possible without experiencing signs of exhaustion, such as dizziness or breathlessness.

   Time: _____ minutes, _____ seconds.

3. Adjust your time as follows: **Men:** Add 15 seconds to your time for every 10 pounds that your weight exceeds 170 pounds, or subtract 15 seconds for every 10 pounds that you are under 170. **Women:** Make the same adjustment for every 10 pounds that your weight is above or below 125 pounds.

   Adjusted time: _____ minutes, _____ seconds.

4. Check your score against the chart in Table 3.1.

Table 3.1. Aerobic-Fitness Test *

Age	High	Above Average	Average	Below Average	Low
Women					
20-29	<13:12	13:12-14:06	14:07-15:06	15:07-16:30	>16:30
30-39	<13:42	13:42-14:36	14:37-15:36	15:37-17:00	>17:00
40-49	<14:12	14:12-15:06	15:07-16:06	16:07-17:30	>17:30
50-59	<14:42	14:42-15:36	15:37-17:00	17:01-18:06	>18:06
60-69	<15:06	15:06-16:18	16:19-17:30	17:31-19:12	>19:12
70-79	<18:18	18:18-20:00	20:01-21:48	21:49-24:06	>24:06
80-89	<21:18	21:18-23:00	23:01-24:48	24:49-27:06	>27:06
Men					
20-29	<11:54	11:54-13:00	13:01-13:42	13:43-14:30	>14:30
30-39	<12:24	12:24-13:30	13:31-14:12	14:13-15:00	>15:00
40-49	<12:54	12:54-14:00	14:01-14:42	14:43-15:30	>15:30
50-59	<13:24	13:24-14:24	14:25-15:12	15:13-16:30	>16:30
60-69	<14:06	14:06-15:12	15:13-16:18	16:19-17:18	>17:18
70-79	<15:06	15:06-15:48	15:49-18:48	18:49-20:18	>20:18
80-89	<17:06	17:06-17:48	17:49-20:48	20:49-22:18	>22:18

* Measurements in minutes and seconds.

For all fitness tests, data for ages 40 to 79 from "Fit over Forty, " by James M. Rippe, M.D. (New York., William Morrow, 1996); other data extrapolated by the author. Reprinted with author's permission.

Strength Tests

Scores on the following tests, which gauge arm and leg strength, reliably reflect strength throughout the upper and lower body, respectively. Warm up the arm or leg muscles, but don't stretch.

Upper-Body Test

1. 40 Sit in a chair with your back straight, holding a 5-pound weight in your stronger hand. (You can use either a dumbbell or a one-gallon plastic jug filled with 5 pints of water or 5 pounds of sand.)

2. Hold your arm straight down at your side, palm facing forward.

3. Keeping your upper arm stationary, do biceps curls: Bend your arm at the elbow and raise the weight to your shoulder, then lower it.

4. Count how many repetitions you can do in 30 seconds. Then check the chart in Table 3.2.

Table 3.2. Upper-Body Strength Test *

Age	Above average	Average	Below average
Women			
20-29	>32	26-32	<26
30-39	>29	23-29	<23
40-49	>27	21-27	<21
50-59	>25	20-25	<20
60-69	>22	19-22	<19
70-79	>21	18-21	<18
80-89	>19	16-19	<16
Men			
20-29	>39	35-39	<35
30-39	>36	32-36	<32
40-49	>34	30-34	<30
50-59	>33	29-33	<29
60-69	>31	26-31	<26
70-79	>28	24-28	<24
80-89	>24	20-24	<20

*Number of repetitions.

Lower-Body Test

1. Strap a 10-pound ankle weight onto the ankle of your stronger leg, or measure a total of 10 pounds of sand or small stones into two old socks and secure them to your stronger ankle.

2. Sit in a chair on enough cushions to keep your feet off the ground, or sit on a table or countertop.

3. Keeping your back straight and your thigh stationary, raise your foot by straightening the knee, then bring the foot back down.

4. Do as many repetitions as you can in 30 seconds. Then consult the "Lower-Body Strength Test" in Table 3.3.

Table 3.3. Lower-Body Strength Test *

Age	Above Average	Average	Below Average
Women			
20-29	>29	26-29	<26
30-39	>28	25-28	<25
40-49	>27	24-27	<24
50-59	>27	23-27	<23
60-69	>25	22-25	<22
70-79	>25	22-25	<22
80-89	>22	19-22	<19
Men			
20-29	>33	29-33	<29
30-39	>32	28-32	<28
40-49	>31	27-31	<27
50-59	>30	27-30	<27
60-69	>29	25-29	<25
70-79	>28	23-28	<23
80-89	>26	21-26	<21

*Number of repetitions.

Flexibility Test

Tight muscles can hamper your everyday activities, limit your athletic performance, and make you more susceptible to soreness and injury. This test evaluates how flexible the muscles are in the back of your legs, your buttocks, and your lower back. If you're stiff there, you'll probably be stiff in other parts of your body, too.

1. Tape a yardstick to the floor, then place a foot-long strip of tape perpendicular to the stick, to flag the 15-inch mark.

2. Remove your shoes and sit on the floor with the yardstick between your extended legs, the low end toward you. Keep your heels about a foot apart, on the 15-inch mark. Place one hand over the other, with middle fingers aligned.

3. Lower your head and slide your fingers forward as far as you can without bending your knees, straining, or jerking.

4. Record the farthest point where you can hold the tips of your middle fingers for two seconds. Do the test three times; then check your best score against the flexibility test chart shown in Table 3.4.

Table 3.4. Flexibility Test *

Age	Above Average	Average	Below Average
Women			
20-29	>20.5	17.5-20.5	<17.5
30-39	>19.5	16.5-19.5	<16.5
40-49	>19	14.5-19	<14.5
50-59	>17.5	14.5-17.5	<14.5
60-69	>17	14-17	<14
70-79	>16.5	13-16.5	<13
80-89	>15	12.5-15	<12.5
Men			
20-29	>17	13.5-17	<13.5
30-39	>161/2	13-16.5	<13
40-49	>16	12.5-16	<12.5
50-59	>15.5	12-15.5	<12
60-69	>14	10-14	<10
70-79	>12	9.5-12	<9.5
80-89	>10	7.5-10	<7.5

* Measurements in inches.

Balance Test

Just as strength, endurance, and flexibility tend to deteriorate as people age, so does the sense of balance. And poor balance coupled with increasing stiffness raises the risk of debilitating falls. It's preferable to have someone time you for this test, although you could time yourself. (Frail individuals should have someone stand nearby in case they start to fall.)

1. If you're age 50 or older, you'll need a stopwatch or a stopwatch feature to measure your time to a tenth of a second. Younger people can measure their time in whole seconds if they want, then round off the numbers in the chart to the nearest second (since those numbers are high enough to round off without distorting the results).

2. Raise the foot of your weaker leg and balance on the other foot, keeping your eyes open and your arms hanging limp at your sides.

3. Time how long you can keep your foot raised. Do the test three times, then check the best result against the balance test chart shown in Table 3.5.

Table 3.5. Balance Test *

Age	Above average	Average	Below average
Women			
20-29	>29.0	22.1-29.0	<22.1
30-39	>22.0	15.1-22.0	<15.1
40-49	>15.5	7.2-15.5	<7.2
50-59	>8.7	3.7-8.7	<3.7
60-69	>4.5	2.5-4.5	<2.5
70-79	>2.6	1.5-2.6	<1.5
80-89	>1.9	1.0-1.9	<1.0
Men			
0-29	>28.0	21.1-28.0	<21.1
30-39	>21.0	14.1-21.0	<1 4.1
40-49	>14.7	4.1-14.7	<4.1
50-59	>6.7	3.2-6.7	<3.2
60-69	>4.0	2.5-4.0	<2.5
70-79	>3.3	1.8-3.3	<1.8
80-89	>2.5	1.5-2.5	<1.5

*Measurements in seconds.

The sections that follow include suggestions on ways that you can increase your aerobic capacity, build strength, and improve your flexibility. To sharpen your balance, you might try practicing tai chi, a martial art that features slow, graceful movement, often while standing on one foot. Certain yoga postures can help, too. People with poor balance could also try an effective series of exercises developed by Yale researchers. For a copy of the program, send a self-addressed stamped envelope to CRH, 10 1 Truman Ave., Yonkers, N.Y. 10703-1057.

Aerobic Exercise

The old exercise prescription called for regular, vigorous, "aerobic" exercise that would boost your heart rate into its "exercise benefit zone"—60 to 85 percent of its maximum rate—for at least 20 minutes, three times a week. (Your maximum rate equals 220 minus your age.) And such vigorous exercise does indeed provide impressive benefits. It improves your wind—the ability to exercise without getting out of breath—and your endurance—the ability to exercise without getting tired. And it reduces the risk that sudden, strenuous exertion, such as running for a bus, will trigger a heart attack.

But fitness experts now recognize that you don't have to pass that "aerobic" threshold to benefit from exercise. And studies show that preventing disease depends more on how much exercise you get than on how hard you work out. So there's a more flexible approach: Get at least 30 minutes of moderate physical activity on most days, preferably every day. You can even rack that up through several brief bursts during the day.

The Benefits of Exercise "Lite"

For certain health benefits, relatively light "aerobic-style" exercise—such as brisk walking, bicycling, or even gardening—may work at least as well as strenuous exercise:

It extends your life. A number of large, lengthy studies have shown that people who exercise regularly live longer. But while that increase in lifespan continues at all fitness levels, the biggest jump lies between the most unfit people and those who are just slightly more fit. Apparently, exercise reduces mortality rates mainly by reducing the risk of cardiovascular disease, a leading cause of death.

It boosts "good" cholesterol. That's one important cardiovascular benefit, which results from even a slight increase in activity. In one study, the most common activity among people with higher HDL levels was gardening, followed by walking and bicycling.

It lowers blood pressure. Several trials have demonstrated another benefit to the heart: Low-intensity exercise—even strolling or leisurely cycling—can reduce blood pressure just as effectively as more strenuous exercise does, and possibly better.

It helps control weight. Although your body burns calories faster the harder you exercise, moderate exercise can actually help keep weight down more effectively. That's mainly because most people can sustain regular exercise longer at a moderate pace than at a strenuous pace, so they burn more calories overall. In addition, the body's metabolic rate may stay elevated longer after a lengthy, mild workout.

It may cut the risk of diabetes. The hormone insulin helps keep blood-sugar levels from climbing into the diabetic range. And physical activity appears to improve sensitivity to insulin, thus reducing the risk of developing type II diabetes. Some evidence now suggests that it doesn't take much exercise to start getting that protection. In one study, men who exercised just once a week had a 30 percent lower risk of diabetes than those who exercised less often; among women, the risk was 15 percent lower.

It may strengthen the bones. Strenuous, weight-bearing activities, such as weight lifting, jogging, and rope jumping, are the best kind of exercise for preventing osteoporosis, or fragile bones, by stopping or even reversing bone loss. But researchers are now finding that even brisk walking can be an effective alternative.

It may ease tension. Several clinical trials have shown that light-to-moderate exercise may work as well as vigorous exercise for relieving anxiety.

It may help prevent colon cancer. Exercise seems to reduce the risk of colon cancer, probably by speeding the passage of cancer-causing wastes through the colon. While studies conflict, some evidence suggests that even light-to-moderate exercise may provide a modest protective benefit.

Walk This Way

One excellent way to get light-to-moderate exercise is to take up walking. It's safe, simple, and often enjoyable—as a solitary or a social activity. All you need is a good pair of shoes. (Walking shoes should have a roomy toe box, flexible soles with good traction, and a stiff heel cup for stability.)

While even a leisurely stroll can benefit your health, the dividends naturally increase as you walk faster, farther, or more often. If you score "moderate" or below on the one-mile walking test described earlier in this chapter, you're probably a good candidate for the graduated program of light walking developed by John J. Duncan, Ph.D., for the Cooper Institute for Aerobics Research in Dallas.

If you begin the walking program and it seems too easy, skip to the next week. Or, if you've already been exercising, begin at whatever level is closest to what you're accustomed to doing. And remember that you don't have to take your walk all at once; instead, you can accumulate smaller chunks of time throughout the day, if that suits you better.

To monitor your progress, return to your one-mile test course occasionally. After a few weeks of training, you should be able to walk the mile faster, or walk it at the same pace as before without pushing your heart rate as high.

Table 3.6. Walking Program

Week	Distance (miles)	Pace* (minutes per mile)	Total time (minutes per walk)	Frequency (days per week)
1	0.5	23	11 1/2	3
2	1.0	23	23	3
3	1.5	23	34 1/2	3
4	1.5	22	33	4
5	2.0	22	44	4
6	2.0	21	42	4
7	2.5	21	52 1/2	4
8	2.5	20	50	4
9	2.5	20	50	4-5
10	3.0	20	60	4-5
11	3.0	19	57	4-5
12	3.0	18	54	4-5

*Your approximate walking speed by the end of the week.

Strength-Training Exercise

When readers of *Consumer Reports on Health* were asked about their health habits not long ago, 92 percent said they did at least some aerobic exercise, such as sustained walking. But only 44 percent said they ever did any strength training—the lowest percentage for any of the 15 health habits we surveyed. That means the majority of our readers are missing out on a number of important benefits.

What It Can Do for You

Most of the benefits of strength training can't be had from other types of exercise:

Stay strong, stay active. While aerobic exercises are good for your heart and lungs, they generally don't work the upper body, where more than half your muscles are located. Eventually, someone who doesn't exercise the upper-body muscles may start having trouble with everyday tasks such as opening windows or carrying grocery bags. Less active people, who don't even exercise their legs, may ultimately end up with bigger problems, such as trouble climbing stairs, getting up out of a chair, walking normally, or maintaining their sense of balance. As little as one strengthening workout per week can prevent much or all of that debilitating muscle loss; more frequent strength training can reverse the loss, making you far more mobile, active, and energetic than before. Stronger muscles also reduce the risk of injury to the joints as well as to the muscles themselves.

Rev up your metabolism. As people get older, their resting metabolic rate—the body's basic calorie-burning speed—tends to slow down, making it harder for them to control their weight. That slowdown stems almost entirely from loss of muscle mass, since muscle burns calories faster than fat does. Similarly, weight-loss diets tend to fail because the metabolic rate slows as the body starts consuming muscle along with the fat. The solution to both problems: Boost your body's metabolism by building muscle. Better still, combine strength training with aerobic exercise, which burns lots of calories not only during the workout itself but also for several hours afterward.

Strengthen your bones. Older people, especially women, are at risk for fractures due to thinning bones. Any kind of weight-bearing exercise, even aerobic-style exercise such as walking or running, should help reduce the risk, by stimulating bone growth when you're young and at least slowing bone loss when you're older. But strength training can help more than aerobic exercise. In studies of postmenopausal women, for example, walking only prevented bone loss in the spine, while strength training actually thickened the bones—and it did so in both the spine and the hips, the two regions most vulnerable to fractures. Equally important, strength training boosted muscle strength and improved balance; that could help prevent falls, a benefit that may cut the fracture risk as much as fortifying the bones does.

Protect your heart. While the evidence on strength training and cholesterol is mixed, one analysis of 11 clinical trials concluded that muscle-building reduces blood levels of the "bad" LDL cholesterol by an average of more than 10 percent. In contrast, aerobic exercise boosts blood levels of the "good" HDL cholesterol but generally has little effect on LDL levels. That suggests once again that a combination of strength training and aerobic exercise may be the ideal exercise regimen, not just for reducing weight but also for improving cholesterol levels. Strength training may help protect the heart in two other ways as well: It strengthens the muscles, so you don't have to strain as much when, say, shoveling snow or moving furniture; and it may even help to lower blood pressure.

Galvanize your gut. Lingering waste in the large intestine may increase the risk of developing constipation, hemorrhoids, diverticulosis, and possibly colon cancer as well. Aerobic and strength-training exercise both seem to speed waste through the intestines.

Streamlined Strengthening

If you're cringing at the thought of adding a major new obligation to your exercise program, here's good news: Reaping at least some of those benefits may take far less time and effort than previously believed. The no-frills strengthening program that follows, for example, can take as little as 15 to 20 minutes per week. Our streamlined regimen includes just six exercises, which work nearly all the major muscles. You could even skip the two lower-body exercises if you do regular aerobic workouts for the legs and have a low risk of osteoporosis. The program uses stretchable bands, which are cheaper, safer, and easier to store or transport than free weights.

How often and how intensely you train depends on your particular goals. For building muscle, boosting metabolism, and shielding the heart from overexertion, one set of each exercise seems to be just as effective as multiple sets, at least for the first few months. As for frequency, training twice a week builds three-fourths as much muscle as working out three days per week does. Even a single session per week will at least slow muscle loss and possibly stop it entirely.

A single set of each strengthening exercise can help thicken the bones; whether multiple sets would thicken them even more is not known. (The key exercises for the hips and spine are squats and, to balance the squats, hamstring curls.)

No-Frills Strength-Training Program

You can use a wide range of strength-training equipment, including weight machines, free weights (dumbbells or barbells), or a gallon jug of water. Or you can do exercises like push-ups or pull-ups, which use the resistance of your own body weight. Stretching bands are a particularly convenient option.

Latex bands are easier on the hands and come in a greater variety of resistances than elastic tubing does. One good brand is Dyna-Bands. And one low-cost supplier is Fitness Wholesale (800-537-5512), which offers a set of three different bands for $9.95 (plus shipping and handling).

For each exercise, adjust the resistance so that you can initially do only 8 to 12 repetitions. (To change the degree of resistance, grasp the band at a different point, fold it in half, switch to a different band, or use two bands at a time.) To keep building strength once you've reached 12 repetitions, increase the resistance so you can again do only around 8. For further gains, reduce the resistance after you've performed as many repetitions as you can, then push on for several more repetitions.

Seated Rows. Sit toward the front of a chair, with legs extended and heels resting on floor. Holding one end of the band in each hand, wrap band around the bottom of your feet. Seated upright, draw your elbows back, letting them flare out to the side, until your hands reach your ribs and your shoulder blades squeeze together. Keep your back straight and shoulders down.

Chest Presses. Wrap band around the middle of your back and grasp ends next to your armpits. Press your arms straight out, keeping shoulders down and chest up; stop just before elbows lock. For extra benefit, cross your hands slightly at end of maneuver.

Biceps Curl. Sit toward the front of a chair, with middle of band anchored under your feet. (if you need more slack, use only one foot.) Grasp ends of band, palms facing forward and elbows touching your waist. Seated upright, raise both hands toward your shoulders without tilting your back or moving your elbows.

Abdominal Curl. Lie on your back, with palms face down at your side. Bring knees up, keeping feet flat on floor. Slowly raise your shoulders until base of shoulder blades comes up off floor. Once you can do 12 repetitions, increase the resistance by placing your hands loosely behind your head, doing the curls on an incline, or holding a light weight on your chest.

Hamstring Curls. Tie one end of band around the middle of your foot. Holding onto the back of a chair, stand on band about 7 to 10 inches in front of tied foot. Raise tied foot behind you as high as you can by bending knee.

Squats. Stand with heels on middle of band, holding the ends. Squat down, keeping your weight on your heels, as if you were lowering yourself into a chair, until your thighs are almost parallel to floor. Don't round or arch your back or let your knees come forward, blocking your view of your toes. To work buttock muscles, contract them as you straighten up. (If squats cause knee or back pain, try them without the band or without squatting as low.)

How to Stretch Yourself

Done properly, stretching can prevent injuries that might otherwise result when a tight muscle is abruptly forced beyond its normal length. Done regularly, stretching can have many other benefits: It can improve flexibility, boost physical performance, prevent soreness, relieve aches and pains, and help you relax.

Muscles, like taffy, become more pliant when warm. So whenever you stretch, you should ideally first spend several minutes engaged in some form of easy exercise—such as walking or performing light calisthenics—that will warm your muscles without stretching them. Or if you're preparing for exercise, you can warm up by gently going through the motions; for example, lob a few tennis balls over the net, shuffle around the track, lift some light weights.

The best technique for most people is static stretching, which involves gradually extending a muscle just to the point of discomfort—

never beyond—and then holding it there for 15 to 30 seconds. Ballistic stretching—working a muscle with rapid, repeated, bouncing motions—may be appropriate for certain individuals, such as martial artists and ballet dancers, who need to develop dynamic flexibility. But it's too dangerous for most folks, since it can force a muscle to extend just as it's contracting, which can lead to pulls or tears. Two other methods—contract-relax stretching and active isolated stretching—have gained some converts of late, but offer no clear advantage over static stretching.

Ten minutes of stretching every other day or so will help you maintain overall flexibility. You should also allow a full 10 minutes for stretching if you're about to engage in an activity that requires abrupt changes in speed and direction—such as baseball, basketball, soccer, or any racquet sport. Such stop-and-go activities are most likely to cause muscle pulls. On the other hand, a couple of minutes of stretching will suffice if you're preparing for a steadier sort of activity, such as walking, jogging, hiking, bicycling, or swimming.

It's wise to take a minute to stretch now and then during physical activity as well—particularly if that activity involves periods of inactivity. Stretching during those down times helps prevent injury and muscle soreness by keeping the muscles from tightening up.

Another round of stretching after you're finished exercising will likewise help prevent muscle soreness. Follow that same 2- to 10-minute rule, depending on the nature of your workout. That's also a good time to promote overall flexibility, since your muscles will be at their warmest, allowing for maximum extension in a stretch.

All-Purpose Stretching Routine

If you're stretching to prepare for a particular sport or other form of exercise, you can concentrate on the stretches that work the muscles you'll be using most. Swimmers, for example, can concentrate on the groin and shoulder/back stretches. Bicyclists and joggers would benefit most from stretching the groin, hamstrings, calves, and quadriceps. If you're preparing for tennis or some other racquet sport, you should work on all seven of the stretches.

Move into each stretch slowly, stopping just at the point of discomfort. Hold there for 15 to 30 seconds and relax. Repeat each stretch two or three times.

Groin Stretch. Sit upright on the floor. With your knees flexed and the soles of your feet together, pull your feet toward your groin.

Place your elbows on the insides of your thighs and exhale as you slowly push your knees toward the floor.

Hamstring Stretch. Sit on the floor with one leg extended. Reach forward along that leg until you feel a gentle stretch in your hamstring, the muscles at the back of your thigh. Flex from the hips, keeping your back straight.

Calf Stretch. Place your palms against a wall at shoulder height. Step forward with one foot, bending that knee, and extend the other leg behind you, toes pointed straight ahead. Keeping both heels on the floor, lean forward until you feel the stretch in the calf of your extended leg.

Single Leg Pull. Lie on your back with one knee bent and the other leg flat on the floor. Flex both feet so your toes point upward. Grip your bent leg just behind the knee and gently pull toward your chest until you feel the stretch in your buttocks and lower back.

Triceps Stretch. Sit or stand upright with one arm flexed and raised so that the upper arm lies against the side of your head; let that hand drop down to rest on your opposite shoulder blade. Now, use the other hand to grasp that raised elbow, and exhale as you pull the elbow behind your head.

Shoulder/Back Stretch. Lock your fingers above your head, with palms facing upward. Push your arms slightly back and up until you feel the stretch in your shoulders, upper back, and arms.

Standing Quadriceps. Stand straight with knees slightly bent. Using one hand to hold the back of a chair or some other object to keep your balance, lift one leg behind you and grasp that foot with your free hand. Gently pull the foot upward toward your buttocks until you feel the stretch along your quadriceps, the muscle on the front of the thigh.

How to Start an Exercise Habit You Can Stick with

Only about 15 percent of American adults actually work out three or more times a week, according to the Centers for Disease Control and Prevention. And more than half of the people who start an exercise regimen end up quitting within just six months of when they started, usually during the first three months. That high dropout rate is not especially surprising, considering that people often approach

83

exercise in ways that are guaranteed to make it a tedious, painful, frustrating experience.

It doesn't have to be like that. Whatever regimen you choose— whether based on an aerobic-style activity such as walking, running, bicycling, cross-country skiing, or swimming; a strength-training routine using weight machines, free weights, or stretching bands; or both kinds of exercise—there are steps you can take to help you stay on track.

Build in the Motivators

In order to give yourself the best chance at long-term success, try to design the following features into your exercise program:

Find a partner. An exercise companion can make any workout more enjoyable. And you're probably less likely to skip a session—or quit entirely—when you know someone is counting on you.

Get on schedule. Mark on a calendar exactly when you plan to exercise for at least two weeks in advance. Schedule each session for the same time of day—right before your morning shower, for example, or right after you get home from work. Then make a formal commitment, perhaps in writing or to friends or family members, that you'll stick to that schedule.

Take lapses in stride. Despite that commitment, occasional lapses are nearly inevitable, due to illness, travel, boredom, or bad weather. A few missed sessions won't set you back—unless they discourage you from continuing.

Record your progress. Each time you work out, record the details on your calendar—for example, how long you exercised, how hard you pushed, how much distance you covered, or how many repetitions of a strength-training exercise you did and whether you increased the resistance since your last session.

Give yourself a boost. Periodically review your calendar record to see how much you've improved in endurance and strength. For every few weeks that you've stuck with the schedule, reward yourself by, say, going out to a fancy restaurant or buying something special.

Change your routine. After a month or two—or anytime that you start feeling bored—look for new places to work out, such as a park, a stretch of woods, an indoor mall (which may even have an organized walking program), or perhaps a local Y or health club. Better yet, you can start adding new exercises to your usual routine.

Make It All Add Up

Any kind of physical activity—from routine household chores such as sweeping or shopping to leisure pursuits such as gardening or dancing—contributes to your overall health and fitness. You can build in extra motivation to become more physically active in all areas of your life by looking at the big picture.

It helps to estimate your current level of overall activity and to track your progress in boosting that activity level. Here's a simplified version of the method developed by Steven N. Blair, P.E.D., of the Cooper Institute for Aerobics Research in Dallas.

First, figure out how much exercise you're getting now. Consult the following table to see how various activities are classified. Add up all the minutes you spend doing those activities (or similar ones) and award yourself points according to the intensity of the activity, as grouped in this table:

- **Moderate activity:** 2 points for every 10 minutes.
- **Hard activity:** 3 points for every 10 minutes.
- **Very hard activity:** 4 points for every 10 minutes.

Figure your totals for a few typical days, recording your scores on a calendar or even a graph. Then try to increase your daily totals by finding simple ways to spend more energy, using this system to record your improvement.

Where Do All the Calories Go?

Table 3.7 shows how fast various activities burn calories. Activities are grouped by degree of intensity, for purposes of the tracking method described in the preceding text. The data are based on a 128-pound woman and a 154-pound man. If you weigh more than that, you will burn more calories; if you're lighter, you'll burn fewer.

How to Play It Safe

Exercise has many benefits, but it also has its risks—including an increased chance of various ailments and injuries, especially among

Table 3.7. Calories burned.

Activity	Calories burned per 10 minutes	
	Women	Men
Moderate		
Sweeping floors	33	38
Hanging clothes to dry	34	40
Washing and waxing car	34	40
Grocery shopping	36	40
Mopping floors	36	40
Scraping paint	37	43
Mowing, power mower	38	48
Walking, brisk	38	48
Swimming, slow	38	48
Weeding garden	42	50
Painting house	45	53
Hard		
Cycling, moderate	59	71
Chopping wood	63	77
Planting garden	63	77
Scrubbing floor	63	77
Pushing hand mower	67	77
Shoveling snow	67	83
Square or folk dancing	67	77
Singles tennis	67	83
Skating	67	83
Hiking (no load)	71	83
Very hard		
Aerobic dance, high-impact	77	91
Skiing, cross-count or downhill	77	91
Soccer	77	91
Squash	77	91
Basketball	77	100
Running, slow	83	100
Rock dancing	100	111

older exercisers. You can minimize those risks by faithfully following these guidelines:

Get checked. See a physician before starting an exercise program if you're over age 45 and haven't had a checkup in more than two years; if you have high blood pressure, coronary heart disease, diabetes, or other chronic illnesses; if you're at increased risk for coronary disease; or if you're taking medications.

Warm up. To warm your muscles, march in place, do light calisthenics, or gently go through the motions of the exercise you're about to perform. Middle-aged and older people should warm up for 5 to 10 minutes; younger exercisers can get by with just 2 or 3 minutes.

Cool down. After a workout, walk slowly until your heart rate slows to just 10 or 15 beats above its resting rate. Stopping suddenly can sharply reduce blood pressure, particularly in older people, causing fainting or possibly even a heart attack.

Stretch. Finish your workout by stretching. Don't bounce or stretch beyond the point where you start feeling discomfort. (For aerobic-style workouts, stretch right after the pre-exercise warm-up as well.)

Drink up. To avoid dehydration, don't wait to get thirsty: Try to drink two 8-ounce cups of water about two hours before exercise, another cup every 20 minutes during exercise, and an additional cup or two within a half hour after the workout.

Schedule aerobics first. If you want to do aerobic-style and strength-training exercises on the same day, do the aerobic workout first, since strength training would tighten the muscles and increase the chance of injury.

Aerobic Tips

In addition to those general precautions, older exercisers in particular should follow these recommendations for aerobic-style exercise:

Don't get jarred. The shock-absorbing fat pad on the heel thins with age, the cushioning disks in the spine dry out, and the joints get weaker. So minimize high-impact activities such as running or jumping.

Take it slow. If you're just starting to exercise, you should be able to talk easily without feeling short of breath during your workouts; otherwise, you're pushing yourself too hard. You can very gradually make your workouts longer and then harder, but never so hard that you can barely get out a full sentence without gasping for air.

Strength-Training Tips

Exercisers of all ages should follow these recommendations for strength-training workouts:

Go through the motion. Move your joints through their full range of motion, but don't lock your joints.

Work slowly. Each repetition should take about six seconds—two for the first half of the maneuver, four for the return to the original position.

Don't hold your breath. Instead, exhale during the exertion phase of the maneuver. (Holding your breath can cause lightheadedness and even fainting.)

Spread out. Plan your strengthening sessions evenly over the course of the week.

How Hard Is Your Workout?

Following the traditional exercise prescription can be a bother. You need to figure your maximum heart rate (220 minus your age), shoot for a target rate (60 to 90 percent of that maximum), and then take your pulse periodically to make sure you stay within that range. Here's an easier way.

Research suggests that most exercisers can gauge the intensity of a workout well enough to stay within their target heart rate simply by assessing how hard they feel that they're working out. Exercise physiologist Rod Dishman, Ph.D., of the University of Georgia suggests following a simple technique based on a self-rating system known as the Borg scale of "perceived exertion". (Scoring is presented in Table 3.8.)

To rate your perceived exertion, notice signs such as aching muscles and breathlessness. According to Dishman, a self-rated Borg score of 11 to 16 is roughly equivalent to the traditional exercise benefit zone.

Some people exercise at the light end of the range; others prefer to push beyond the threshold of "hard exertion." By staying at a level that suits you, you'll be more likely to get a good workout and to stick with your exercise program over the long haul.

One caveat: These guidelines don't apply to people with heart or lung conditions, who often need to monitor their heart and respiration rates during exercise.

Table 3.8. The Borg scale of "perceived exertion."

Degree of exertion	Score
None	6
Very, very light	7
Very light	9
Fairly light	11
Somewhat hard	13
Hard	15
Very hard	17
Very, very hard	19
Hardest ever done	20

Chapter 4

Designing a Fitness Program

Ideally, a cardiovascular fitness program should be flexible, graduated, tailored to your individual needs, and if necessary, supervised by a fitness expert. The three key factors in designing a program are intensity, duration, and frequency of exercise.

Cardiovascular conditioning requires a sustained effort for at least 30 minutes per day, 3 days per week with your heart rate within its "target zone." This zone is between 70 and 85 percent of your maximum heart rate—the maximum number of times your pulse can beat in one minute. Maximum heart rate is calculated by subtracting your age from 220. For example, a 40-year-old's maximum heart rate is 180. The target zone is between 70 and 85 percent of the maximum heart rate, in this example, 126 to 153 beats per minute.

Exercise below 70 percent of the maximum heart rate gives the heart and lungs little conditioning; anything above 85 percent is dangerous. If you're beginning an exercise program, start at approximately 70 percent, slowly increasing to 85 percent as your conditioning improves. If you have not been exercising regularly, be careful to raise your heart rate gradually; it may take several months to raise it above 70 percent.

A simple way to determine if you are reaching your target zone is to take your pulse immediately after exercise. Simply place two or three fingers lightly over the carotid artery, located on the left and right sides of your Adam's apple, count the pulse for 10 seconds, and multiply by 6. If the pulse is below the target zone, increase the rate of exercise; if above, reduce it. Check your pulse rate once a week during the first 3 months of exercising and periodically thereafter.

Another way to assess whether you are meeting your target zone while exercising is to rate your condition on a "perceived exertion" scale of 1 to 10, in which 1 represents "not-at-all fatigued" and 10 signifies "extremely fatigued." While exercising, you should reach level 7 or 8.

Exercisers should be aware that some medications and medical conditions may affect the maximum heart rate and the target zone. For example, some medicines for hypertension lower the maximum heart rate and thus the target zone. Diabetes may also have an effect on these guidelines. If you are taking medications, be sure to consult a physician to determine whether this rate should be adjusted.

When starting an exercise program, aim to work out two to four times a week. Studies show that you need exercise only three times a week to benefit your cardiovascular system. Although the "training effect" on the body increases if you exercise more often than that, your risk of injury also increases, particularly with strenuous exercises like running. You may want to exercise more frequently if your program entails less injury-prone activities such as walking or swimming, or if weight control is one of your exercise goals.

Beginners may have trouble exercising at their target zone for all 30 minutes. If so, work out for as long as possible at the target zone, building up to 30 minutes over time. Exercising at the proper intensity, even if only for 5 or 10 minutes, can provide some training effect. On the other hand, working out at a level below the target zone, even for the full 30 minutes, won't have much of an effect, aside from burning some calories. Moderate interval training, alternating exercise of slightly increased intensity with low intensity or rest periods, is another way to begin a program.

In order to maintain the training effect, you must increase the intensity or duration of exercise as your heart becomes better conditioned. A bicycle rider, for example, may eventually have to pedal longer, faster, or cycle up hills or in a lower gear to push the heart into the target zone.

Sample Exercise Programs

Following are sample exercise programs for three individuals: a healthy 25-year-old man, a healthy 45-year-old woman, and a 65-year-old man who has had a myocardial infarction (heart attack). They are meant only as examples, not prescriptions. Before beginning your own exercise program, consult your doctor.

The 25-Year-Old Man

Running is a good and popular choice for aerobic conditioning, but be cautious if you have not been exercising regularly. Running can prove to be too strenuous for people who are out of shape. Begin a running program by alternating 3-minute walks and 3-minute jogs for 30 minutes up to three times a week. Each week, increase the jog interval by 1 minute and decrease the walk interval by 1 minute until the entire 30 minutes is spent jogging. From this point, you can add 5-minute increments every other week until the jog lasts 46 to 50 minutes. Then you can increase speed by alternating 5 minutes at a fast pace with 5 minutes at a moderate pace.

Although running offers an excellent cardiovascular workout, it does not condition the upper body (arms, shoulders, etc.). For that reason, consider supplementing a running program with workouts on a rowing machine. To start, set the rowing machine at the lowest resistance point. Then increase the setting with each 3-minute set until you reach a perceived exertion level of 7 or 8. After 2 or 3 weeks, try to begin each set at the second lowest resistance level, assuming it has become comfortable as a base level. If not, keep to the initial setting for a few more weeks.

The 45-Year-Old Woman

Aerobic dance and calisthenics performed at a fast pace are excellent aerobic activities that give the heart a thorough workout and involve most muscle groups. Whether you exercise on your own, in a class, or by following a tape, be sure to warm up and cool down with stretching exercises (often these are built into class or tape routines) every time. If you experience pain in a particular part of the body, avoid specific routines that increase the pain until it abates.

Swimming is an excellent alternate exercise. Both the crawl and the backstroke offer good conditioning. Be sure to alternate with rest periods. As you become stronger, you can add one or two laps.

The 65-Year-Old Man

Walking is an excellent aerobic exercise after a heart attack because it is versatile. It offers benefits to people who are very out of shape, but can also be intensified to keep a physically fit person in peak condition.

Before beginning or resuming any exercise program after a heart attack, it is crucial to have a symptom-limited exercise stress test (meaning the test is stopped as soon as chest pain is felt). Based on the results, the physician should set a target heart rate for you. During exercise, do regular pulse checks (a 10-second pulse multiplied by 6) to make sure you're maintaining—and not exceeding—the target rate.

See a physician immediately if you experience any recurrent chest pain, weakness, dizziness, or excessive fatigue. The doctor may want to do a repeat exercise stress test. If available, a supervised program at a YM/YWCA, YM/YWHA, or community center is preferable to individual exercise, at least for the first year following a heart attack.

Like jogging or running, walking does not usually provide upper-body conditioning. Arm calisthenics are a good alternative to walking. For a post-heart attack patient, they should first be performed with ECG monitoring. A physician should determine the appropriate frequency and number of repetitions for each exercise. Upper-body exercises can include shoulder flex-extend; elbow flex-extend; arm swing, front to back; and arm "bicycle" motion.

—by Robert Lewy

Chapter 5

Exploding Exercise Myths

Getting Americans off the couch and onto their feet could save an estimated 200,000 lives a year, says the Surgeon General. Yet most of us are either sedentary or only minimally active. Confusion may keep many couch potatoes from getting into shape. People still ask questions like: How often should I exercise? (The more, the better, but at least 30 minutes nearly every day.) Does it have to be 30 minutes straight? (No, shorter bouts are fine.) Do I need to go to the gym? (No, walking, dancing, lawn mowing, and gardening are fine, if they're intense enough.) Still, in a world where infomercials, magazines, videos, and friends may give conflicting advice, misunderstanding abounds. In this chapter, we try to clear it up.

Ten Exercise Myths

Myth #1

Strength-training will make women too muscular.

Many women are afraid that strength-training will make them bulky," says Miriam Nelson of the Jean Mayer U.S. Department of Agriculture Human Nutrition Research Center on Aging at Tufts University in Boston. "They think strength-training is only for men."

Nutrition Action Healthletter, January/February 2000, vol. 27, no. 1, p. 16.
© 2000 Center for Science in the Public Interest. Reprinted with permission.

In fact, strength-training has enormous benefits for women. In one of Nelson's studies, postmenopausal women who were sedentary were randomly assigned to do strength-training exercises twice a week or to do no additional exercise. After a year, the strength-trainers had greater bone density, muscle mass, muscle strength, and balance than the sedentary women.[1]

"Women naturally have less bone and muscle than men, so they need to take care of what they've got," says Nelson. That's why women are at greater risk of osteoporosis than men. And lost muscle puts women at greater risk of disability as they age.

"Thirty percent of middle-aged women have trouble doing physical tasks like walking a mile or carrying a few grocery bags or climbing a few flights of stairs," says Nelson. "It's pretty staggering. They're really out of shape."

And don't worry about looking like a bodybuilder. "Women don't have enough testosterone to create big, bulky muscles," says Nelson. "To become a bodybuilder, women have to do a lot of weird things that most strength-training programs don't do."

Myth #2

Light weights on your arms or legs can boost your exercise benefit.

Some people carry light (one- or two-pound) hand-held weights when they walk or run. Others strap Velcro-fastened weights around their ankles. Don't bother, says exercise physiologist Ben Hurley of the University of Maryland.

"It slows you down, so you get less benefit from aerobic exercise, and it doesn't add enough weight to give you the benefits of strength-training," he explains.

To build muscle, you have to use weights that you can lift no more than eight to 12 times in a row. "If you can go beyond the twelfth repetition, the resistance is too light to stress the muscle," says Hurley. "As your muscles get stronger, you need to add more weight—or other resistance—so you can still do only eight to 12 repetitions."

Myth #3

With the right exercise, you can get rid of trouble spots.

"Some people believe that if they exercise one area, it will cause fat to be removed from that area," says Rosemary Lindle, a University of Maryland exercise physiologist.

"In our gym the men, who tend to store their fat in their abdomens, are on the ab machines, and the women are on the total hip machines for hours," she notes. "But spot-reducing is a myth."

Abdominal and hip exercises can strengthen and tone the muscles. But those muscles are underneath the "subcutaneous" layer of fat that gives the lovely appearance of flab. Only losing weight can get rid of excess fat, and where you lose the weight depends on your genes. Losing weight around the waist is easier than losing it at the hips.

"I tell women to do some strength-training in their upper body to create a better balance between upper and lower body," says Lindle. "You can build your own natural shoulder pads."

Myth #4

Exercise burns lots of calories.

"People have the mistaken idea that exercise is a fabulous way to lose weight," says William Evans of the University of Arkansas for Medical Sciences. "But exercising doesn't burn a lot of calories."

Walking or running a mile burns about 100 calories. But sitting still for the same time burns about 50 or 60 calories. "So the extra you expend isn't huge and people get discouraged at their slow rate of weight loss."

Another misconception: You keep burning considerably more calories for a long time after you stop exercising, "Calorie expenditure is elevated for the first minute or two, but by five or six minutes the extra expenditure is pretty small, and by 40 minutes post-exercise, it's back to where you started," says Evans.

That doesn't mean dieters should give up on exercise. The more you exercise, the more fit you'll get. That means you'll burn more calories because you can walk briskly or run for five miles instead of one. So instead of burning 100 calories, you burn 500.

What's more, says Evans, "the better-conditioned you are, the more fat you burn for energy, because your muscles adapt to using an enzyme that oxidizes fat. People who are less-trained burn more carbohydrate instead."

Dieters who exercise also lose less lean body mass—that is, less muscle—than dieters who just cut calories. And physical activity can help with the toughest problem: keeping weight off.

Says Evans: "Studies show that after people lose weight, the best predictor of maintaining the weight loss is whether they exercise regularly."

Myth #5

If you don't lose weight, there's no point in exercising.

What gets most people off the couch and into their walking shoes? It's that unwanted flab that motivates most of us. It shouldn't.

"Many people don't see immediate weight loss and say it's all for naught and stop," says exercise expert William Haskell of Stanford University Medical School.

In fact, exercise has a laundry list of benefits beyond any impact on your next shopping trip Among them: "It improves the ability of insulin to enter cells, so it lowers the risk of diabetes," says Haskell. "It also lowers the risk of heart disease by improving blood clotting mechanisms, lowering triglycerides, and raising HDL ('good') cholesterol."

Exercise alters not only your risk of disease, but your quality of life, he adds. "In our studies, exercise improved sleep in people with modest sleep dysfunction," that is, people who take a long time to fall sleep or who wake up frequently at night.

"The psychological benefits of exercise are frequently overlooked," says Haskell. "Exercise isn't a panacea, but it has consistently been shown to relieve both depression and anxiety."

Myth #6

Weight gain is inevitable as you age.

Most Americans get fatter as they get older ... but they don't have to. "It's a matter of reduced physical activity levels and lower metabolic rate caused by a loss of lean body mass (muscle)," says JoAnn Manson of Harvard Medical School.

"The lifelong loss of lean body mass reduces our basal metabolic rate as we age," says Arkansas's William Evans. "It's a very subtle change that begins between ages 20 and 30. The percentage of body fat gradually increases, and it produces an ever-decreasing calorie requirement."

That's because fat cells burn fewer calories than muscle cells. And a lower metabolic rate means that unless you eat less, you'll gain weight over the decades. But exercise can mount a two-pronged attack on middle-age spread and muscle loss. Any activity makes you burn more calories (so you're less likely to wind up with an excess). And strength-training can offset the loss of muscle mass.

"Starting at age 40 in women and at 60 in men, we lose six to eight percent of our muscle per decade," says Maryland's Hurley. "However, after only two months of strength-training, women recover a decade of loss and men recover two decades."

That's with three weekly sessions that take 40 minutes each, including warm-up, rest periods, and stretching.[2] "The time spent doing the exercises that increase muscle mass is only about five minutes a session," says Hurley. Not a bad return on your time.

Myth #7

You can't be fit and fat.

"The notion that all fat people are sedentary and unfit and at high risk of disease is not true," says Steven Blair of the Cooper Clinic in Dallas, Texas. "Overweight and obese individuals who are fit do not have elevated mortality rates. We need to get off those people's backs."

But in Blair's study of 25,000 men who have come to the Cooper Clinic, ten percent of the normal-weight men—and half of the over-weight men—were unfit.

Getting all of those unfit people—fat or thin—to move more could make a difference. In Blair's study, low fitness was as strong (or stronger) a predictor of dying as other risk factors, like high cholesterol, high blood pressure, and diabetes. Yet doctors rarely test a patient's fitness as part of a checkup.

"Fitness is such an important predictor of mortality, it's inexcusable not to evaluate it as part of a person's health risk," says Blair.

It wouldn't cost much. It's just a matter of measuring your heart rate—by measuring your pulse with a wristwatch—while you cycle, walk, or run at a given speed.

"A stress test for diagnosis of coronary heart disease at a major medical center can cost several hundred dollars," he says, "but you can go down to the YMCA and get a fitness test for 25 bucks."

Myth #8

No pain, no gain.

"Many people still believe that you have to work at a very high intensity in order to get a benefit," says the Cooper Clinic's Steven Blair.

In fact, moderate-intensity exercise lowers the risk of dying just as much as high-intensity exercise. For example, says JoAnn Manson of the Harvard Medical School, "In the Nurses' Health Study, women who regularly engaged in brisk walking reduced their risk of heart disease to the same degree as women who engaged in vigorous exercise. You don't need to run a marathon."

The trick is making sure that the exercise is at least moderate-intensity—that is, equivalent to walking at a pace of three to four miles an hour.

"You can vacuum at a very low pace or at a moderately intense pace," says Blair. Running or jogging is, by definition, high-intensity. But walking, raking leaves, mowing lawns, dusting, and gardening may be either moderate- or low-intensity.

High-intensity exercise does have one advantage: it saves time. It takes less time to burn the same number of calories at higher intensity. "You can jog for 20 minutes or walk for 40 or 45," says Blair. "You pay your money and you take your choice."

Does all the heart-pounding of high-intensity exercise do anything else for you? "Some things probably respond better to high-intensity and some may respond better to moderate-intensity exercise," says Blair. "But in general, there doesn't appear to be a lot of difference as long as you expend the same number of calories."

Myth #9

If you can't exercise regularly, why bother?

It takes ten to 12 weeks of regular exercise to become "fit"—that is, to improve your performance on a treadmill (a measure of your oxygen capacity). But your health can improve after that first brisk walk or run.

"Take a 50-year-old man who is somewhat overweight and typically has moderately elevated blood sugar, triglycerides, or blood pressure," says Stanford's William Haskell. "A single bout of exercise of moderate intensity—like 30 to 40 minutes of brisk walking—will lower those numbers." And not just while you're moving. "If you exercise at, say, five o'clock in the afternoon, the improvement will be there the next morning," he adds.

That may be why postal carriers (or others who are active at work) have a lower risk of heart disease than postal clerks (or others who are sedentary at work). "There's not much difference in their fitness levels, but the carriers have lower blood sugar, triglycerides, and blood pressure," says Haskell.

People should still try to at least follow the Center for Disease Control's modest advice to get at least 30 minutes of moderate activity on most—or preferably all—days of the week, he adds. But if you can't, don't let that stop you from taking even a single walk.

"Every bout has benefits," says Haskell.

Myth #10

If you didn't exercise when you were younger, it could be dangerous to start when you're older.

Many people think they're too old to start an exercise program," says Tufts University's Miriam Nelson. "They think it's unsafe because they have heart disease or diabetes or because they're too out of shape to start."

You're never too old to start, says Nelson. And she ought to know. In one Tufts study, the participants were frail nursing-home residents whose ages ranged from 72 to 98. After just ten weeks, strength-training improved their muscle strength, ability to climb stairs, and walking speed.[3] "When they see what a difference it makes, they're thrilled," says Nelson.

The same goes for people with chronic diseases. "People say they can't exercise because they have arthritis," she adds. "But we see some of the greatest benefits in people with arthritis. Exercise reduces pain and increases range of motion, strength, and mobility."

That doesn't mean that anyone can plunge into a bout of vigorous exercise, regardless of health history. In a recent study, ordinarily inactive people—especially men who had high cholesterol or angina or were smokers or obese—were ten times more likely to have a heart attack within an hour of exerting themselves (usually by jogging or heavy lifting) than at other times.[4] Anyone with multiple risk factors for heart disease should check with a physician and start slowly.

As for the all-too-common "I don't have time to exercise," Nelson responds, "somehow, you've got to make the time, or you're going to have medical problems like heart disease, diabetes, or osteoporosis. And it will take a lot more time to deal with them than it takes to exercise."

[1] *J. Amer. Med. Assoc.* 272:1909, 1994.
[2] *J. Appl. Physiol.* 86:195, 1999.
[3] *N. Eng. J. Med.* 330: 1769, 1994.
[4] *J. Amer. Med. Assoc.* 282:1731, 1999.

A Dozen Other Reasons to Exercise

The promise of thinner thighs or a slimmer midsection is what gets most people off the couch. And exercise can help you lose fat, preserve muscle, and keep off the excess weight you manage to lose. But if that's your only reason for moving, you're missing a lot. Here are a dozen others, including some concrete findings from selected studies. For more information, check out the *1996 Surgeon General's Report on Physical Activity and Health* at www.cdc.gov/nccdphp/sgr/sgr.htm.

Sleep

A 16-week exercise program (30 to 40 minutes of brisk walking or low-impact aerobics four times a week) improved the quality, duration, and ease of falling asleep in healthy older adults.[1] Exercise may improve sleep by relaxing muscles, reducing stress, or warming the body.

[1] *J. Amer. Med. Assoc.* 277: 32, 1997.

Gallstones

Active women are 30 percent less likely to have gallstone surgery than sedentary women. In one study, women who spent more than 60 hours a week sitting at work or driving were twice as likely to have gallstone surgery as women who sat for less than 40 hours a week.[1]

[1] *N. Eng. 1. Med.* 34 7: 777, 1999.

Colon Cancer

The most active people have a lower risk of colon cancer—in two studies half the risk—compared to the least active people.[1,2] Exercise may lower levels of prostaglandins that accelerate colon cell proliferation and raise levels of prostaglandins that increase intestinal motility. Increased motility may speed the movement of carcinogens through the colon.

[1] *Nat. Cancer Inst.* 89: 948, 1997.
[2] *Ann. Intem. Med.* 122: 327, 1995.

Diverticular Disease

In one of the few studies that have been done, the most active men had a 37 percent lower risk of symptomatic diverticular disease than the least active men. [1] Most of the protection against diverticular disease—pockets in the wall of the colon that can become inflamed—was due to vigorous activities like jogging and running, rather than moderate activities like walking.

[1] *Gut* 36: 276, 1995.

Arthritis

Regular moderate exercise, whether aerobic or strength-training, can reduce joint swelling and pain in people with arthritis.[1]

[1] *Amer. Med. Assoc.* 277: 25, 1997.

Anxiety and Depression

Getting people with anxiety or depression to do aerobic exercises like brisk walking or running curbs their symptoms, possibly by releasing natural opiates.[1,2]

[1] *J. Psychosom. Res.* 33: 537, 1989.
[2] *Arch. Intern. Med.* 759: 2349, 1999.

Heart Disease

In one study, men with low fitness who became fit had a lower risk of heart disease than men who stayed unfit.[1] In another, women who walked the equivalent of three or more hours per week at a brisk pace had a 35 percent lower risk of heart disease than women who walked infrequently.[2] Exercise boosts the supply of oxygen to the heart muscle by expanding existing arteries and creating tiny new blood vessels. It may also prevent blood clots or promote their breakdown.

[1] *Amer. Med, Assoc.* 273: 1093, 1995.
[2] *N. Eng. J. Med.* 341: 650, 1999.

Blood Pressure

If your blood pressure is already high or high-normal, low- or moderate-intensity aerobic exercise—three times a week—can lower it.[1] If your blood pressure isn't high, regular exercise helps keep it that way

[1] *J. Clin. Epidem.* 4S: 439, 1992.

Diabetes

The more you move, the lower your risk of diabetes, especially if you're already at risk because of excess weight, high blood pressure, or parents with diabetes. In one study, women who walked at least three hours a week had about a 40 percent lower risk of diabetes than sedentary women.[1]

[1] *J. Am. Med. Assoc* 282: 1433, 1999.

Falls and Fractures

Older women assigned to a home-based (strength- and balance-training) exercise program had fewer falls than women who didn't exercise.[1] Exercise may prevent falls and broken bones by improving muscle strength, gait, balance, and reaction time.

[1] *Brit. Med. J.* 315: 1065, 1997.

Enlarged Prostate, (Men Only)

In one study, men who walked two to three hours a week had a 25 percent lower risk of benign prostatic hyperplasia (enlarged prostate) than men who seldom walked.[1]

[1] *Arch. Intern. Med.* 158: 2349, 1998.

Osteoporosis

Exercise, especially strength-training, can increase bone density in middle-aged and older people.[1] Bonus: postmenopausal women who take estrogen gain more bone density if they exercise.

[1] *J. Bone Min. Res.* 17: 218, 1996.

—by Bonnie Liebman

Chapter 6

Get Fit, Get Recognized: The Presidential Sports Award

Q. *What is the Presidential Sports Award Program?*

A. The Presidential Sports Award Program was developed by the President's Council on Physical Fitness and Sports in 1972 as a means to motivate all Americans to be active throughout life, and emphasizes regular exercise rather than outstanding performance. It is a non-profit program that runs entirely from participant fees and is administered by the Amateur Athletic Union.

Q. *How does the program work?*

A. Participants age 6 and older can earn an award in any one or more of the 66 sports and fitness activities included in the program. Participants should 1) select a category, 2) fulfill the requirements for that category, and 3) mail the completed and signed fitness log with $8.00 per award to the Amateur Athletic Union for fulfillment.

NOTE: The cost per award is $10.00 in Canada and $15.00 in all other countries.

Q. *What does the recipient receive?*

A. A recipient of the Presidential Sports Award receives:

Information in this chapter is from the President's Council on Physical Fitness and Sports, Washington, DC. The Presidential Sports Award is a program of the President's Council on Physical Fitness and Sports, administered by the Amateur Athletic Union.

1. A personalized certificate of achievement with facsimile signature of the current President of the United States.

2. Letter of congratulations from the Executive Director of the President's Council on Physical Fitness and Sports.

3. A blazer patch (embroidered emblem) signifying the sport/activity in which the award was earned.

4. A magnetic wipe-off memo board.

Qualifying Standards

(Now available for ages 6 and up)

1. For maximum benefit, the criteria for each activity should be fulfilled within a four-month period. Exceptions will be made only for such things as (but not limited to) injury, illness, change of season, or individual medical history, and must be briefly explained when the participant applies to receive an award.

2. Individuals who participate in a variety of categories within a four-month period, but not enough to earn an award in any one category, should log their activity under either the Cross-Training or Sports/Fitness categories. If requested, those who meet the requirements for Sports/Fitness can choose to receive an award for the category in which the majority of the 50 hours is accumulated.

Aerobic Dance

1. Participate a minimum of 50 hours of aerobics, aerobic dance, step aerobics, dance exercise, or a similar activity.

2. Credit only 1 hour each day/4 hours per week.

3. Recommendation: One hour of activity includes 5-10 minute warm up, 20-30 minutes aerobic activity within the target heart rate range, 10-15 minutes strengthening exercises and 5-10 minutes cool down.

Archery

1. Shoot a minimum of 3,000 arrows; no more than 90 arrows credited daily.

2. Minimum target distance of 15 yards. In field, roving archery, should include 14 different targets, each at 15 or more yards.

Backpacking

1. Backpack a minimum of 50 hours; no more than three (3) hours credited daily.

2. Pack must weigh at least 10% body weight.

Badminton

1. Play badminton a minimum of 50 hours; no more than two (2) hours credited daily.

2. Play must include a minimum of 125 total games; no more than five (5) games credited daily.

Baseball

1. Play and/or practice baseball skills a minimum of 50 hours; no more than 1 hour credited daily.

2. At least 15 of 50 hours must be played in organized league or baseball competition.

Basketball

1. Play and/ or practice basketball skills a minimum of 50 hours; no more than 1 hour credited daily.

2. At least 15 of 50 hours must be in an organized league or basketball competition.

Baton Twirling

1. Practice twirling skills and/or compete in baton twirling a minimum of 50 hours; no more than two (2) hours credited daily.

2. Practice must include work in a minimum of two of the recognized events (1 baton, 2 baton, 3 baton, strut, dance twirl, group twirling).

3. Participate in a minimum of three (3) organized competitions.

Bicycling

1. On bicycle with more than five gears, bicycle a minimum of 600 miles; no more than 12 miles credited daily.

2. On bicycle with five or fewer gears, bicycle a minimum of 400 miles with no more than eight (8) miles credited daily.

3. On stationary bicycle, bicycle a minimum of 25 hours; no more than 30 minutes bicycling within target heart rate range credited daily.

Bowling

1. Bowl a minimum of 150 games; no more than six (6) games credited to daily total.

2. Total of 150 games must be bowled on fewer than 34 different days.

Canoe-Kakak

1. Paddle a minimum of 200 miles with no more than seven (7) miles credited to daily total.

Cheerleading

1. Cheerlead/practice a minimum of 50 hours; no more than one (1) hour credited daily.

2. A minimum of 15 of 50 hours must be accumulated during organized games/ competition.

Cross-Training

1. Simultaneously complete a minimum of one-half requirements of two different award program categories.

2. Activities should develop cardio-respiratory endurance, muscle strength, endurance, and flexibility.

Dance

1. Dance a minimum of 50 hours: Ballroom, Square, Folk, Round, Pattern, Clogging, Country Western or dance combination; no more than 1½ hours credited daily.

Disc Sports

1. Practice flying disc skills a minimum of 50 hours; no more than two (2) hours credited daily.

2. Practice must include work in a minimum of three recognized events: distance, accuracy, self-caught flight, double disc court, golf, freestyle, discathon, ultimate or guts.

Double Dutch

1. Complete a minimum of 50 hours Double Dutch activity (jump between ropes or turn ropes) with no more than 1 hour credited daily.

2. Include a minimum of one organized Double Dutch competition (Speed, Compulsory and Freestyle) as part of 50 hour requirement.

Equitation

1. Ride horseback or train horses a minimum of 50 hours with no more than one and one-half (1½) hours credited daily.

Fencing

1. Practice fencing skills a minimum of 50 hours; no more than two (2) hours credited daily.

2. At least 30 of 50 hours must be under supervision of instructor or competition.

Field Hockey

1. Play and/or practice field hockey skills a minimum of 50 hours; no more than one (1) hour credited daily.

2. At least 15 or 50 hours must be in organized league or tournament play.

Figure Skating

1. Skate a minimum of 50 hours; no more than 1½ hours credited daily.

2. Skating should include at least one of following: a) figure-eight (patch), b) free skating, c) ice dancing d) precision skating.

Fitstart

1. Participate in a minimum of 30 hours of light to moderate physical activity, starting with no less than 10 consecutive minutes and no more than 40 minutes of activity credited to the total per day.

2. Activities may include walking, aerobics, aquadynamics, calisthenics, exercise or conditioning classes, fitness dancing, workouts on fitness apparatus including cycling, rowing, stepping and treadmills, or a combination of any or all of these activities.

Football

1. Play football and/or practice football skills a minimum of 50 hours; no more than one (1) hour credited to daily total.

2. At least 15 of 50 hours must be in organized league or competition football.

Golf

1. Play/practice golf a minimum of 100 hours; no more than three (3) hours credited daily.

2. No motorized carts may be used.

3. At least 15 rounds (18 holes) must be played as part of the 100-hour requirement.

Gymnastics

1. Practice gymnastic skills and/or compete a minimum of 50 hours; no more than two (2) hours credited daily.

2. Practice must include work in at least one-half of the recognized events (two of four for women and girls; three of six for men/ boys)

Handball

1. Play handball a minimum of 50 hours; no more than 1½ hours credited daily.

2. Total must include at least 25 matches (2 of 3 games) of singles and/or doubles.

Horseshoe Pitching

1. Pitch horseshoes a minimum of 50 hours; no more than two (2) hours credited daily.

2. Sanctioned league or tournament games may be used; 100 sanctioned games required.

3. If combination practice and official games are used, credit one half (½) hour per sanctioned game (more than two hours can be credited for sanctioned tournament participation).

Ice Hockey

1. Play/practice ice hockey skills a minimum of 50 hours; no more than one hour credited daily.

2. At least 15 of 50 hours must be in organized ice hockey league or competition.

Ice Skating

1. Skate a minimum of 50 hours; no more than one and one-half (1½) hours credited daily.

Jogging

1. Jog a minimum of 125 miles with no more than two and one-half (2½) miles credited daily.

Judo

1. Practice judo skills a minimum of 50 hours; no more than one (1) hour credited daily.

2. At last 30 of 50 hours must be under supervision of qualified instructor.

Karate

1. Practice karate skills a minimum of 50 hours; no more than one (1) hour credited daily.

2. At least 30 of 50 hours must be under supervision of qualified instructor.

Lacrosse

1. Play/practice lacrosse a minimum of 50 hours; no more than one hour credited daily.

2. At least 15 of 50 hours must be in organized league/ tournament play.

Lawn Bowling

1. Participate in a minimum of 40 games in social, interclub or division events, no more than three (3) games credited daily.

2. These games may be singles (18 points), pairs, triples, fours, (games of no less than 23 ends).

3. These games must be played in no less than 45 days and within a maximum of 120 days.

Marathon

1. Run a minimum of 40 miles per week for at least two months.

2. Weekly mileage should not be increased more than 10% over the previous week. At least every 10 days a longer training run must be done at a minimum 15-mile distance for two months once mileage level reaches 40 miles per week.

3. At end of four-month cycle, must complete TAC-sanctioned marathon of 26.2 miles.

Martial Arts

For all martial arts other than Judo, Karate, and Tae Kwon Do:

1. Practice martial arts skills a minimum of 50 hours with no more than 1 hour credited to the total per day.

2. At least 30 of the 50 hours must be under the supervision of a qualified instructor.

Racquetball

1. Play racquetball a minimum of 50 hours; no more than 1½ hours credited daily.

2. Total must include at least 25 matches (2 or 3 games) of singles and/or doubles.

Roller/Inline Skating

1. Roller or Inline skate a minimum of 50 hours; no more than one and one-half (1½) hours credited daily.

Rope Skipping

1. Skip rope a minimum of 25 hours; no more than 30 minutes credited daily.

2. May be done in single or Double Dutch ropes.

Rowing

1. Boat-Row a minimum of 50 miles; no more than 1½ miles credited daily.

2. Wherry-Row a minimum of 100 miles; no more than three (3) miles credited daily.

3. Shell-Row a minimum of 120 miles; no more than 3½ miles credited daily.

Rugby

1. Play and practice rugby skills or conditioning a minimum of 50 hours; no more than 2 hours of rugby or 1 hour conditioning credited daily.

Running

1. Run a minimum of 200 miles.

2. Run continuously at least 3 miles during each outing. No more than 5 miles maybe credited daily (miles counted toward 200-mile total must spread over at least 40 outings).

3. Average time must be 9 minutes or less per mile (i.e., 27 minutes for 3 miles, 45 minutes for 5 miles)

Please note exceptions due to injury or age.

Sailing

1. Sail (practice/competition) a minimum of 50 hours; no more 2½ hours credited daily.

Scuba-Skin Diving

1. Skin or scuba dive, or train for diving, a minimum of 50 hours; no more than three (3) hours of total diving time credited daily.

2. Total time must include at least 15 logged dives on 15 separate dates under Safe Diving Standards of one of following: National Association Skin Diving Schools, National Association Underwater Instructors, National YMCA, Professional Association Diving Instructors, Underwater Society of America.

Skeet-Trap

1. Fire at a minimum of 800 standard trap or skeet targets or sporting clays with no more than 50 targets credited daily.

2. All shooting events must be under safe, regulated conditions.

Skiing, Alpine

1. Ski, or train for skiing a minimum of 50 hours; no more than 3 hours skiing or 30 minutes on ski-training apparatus credited daily.

Skiing, Nordic

1. Ski a minimum of 150 miles; no more than 10 miles credited daily.

2. Comparable mileage accumulated on workout apparatus may be credited daily.

Skiing, Water

1. Water ski a minimum of 50 hours; no more than three (3) hours skiing activity credited daily.

Snowshoeing

1. Snowshoe a minimum of 50 hours; no more than 4 hours per outing credited daily.

Soccer

1. Play/practice soccer skills a minimum of 50 hours with no more than one (1) hour credited daily.

2. At least 15 of 50 hours must be in organized league or soccer competition.

Softball

1. Play/practice softball skills a minimum of 50 hours; no more than 1 hour credited daily.

2. At least 15 of 50 hours must be in organized league or softball competition.

Sports/Fitness

1. Participate in a minimum of 50 hours exercise activities, or combination of exercise/sports; no more than 1 hour credited daily.

2. Exercise activity may consist of aerobics; aquadynamics; calisthenics; exercise or conditioning classes; fitness dancing; rope jumping; apparatus workout, including stationary bicycles, rowing machines, treadmills; or combination of these activities.

3. Sports activity may include participation in one or more of sports in which Presidential Sports Award is offered, or other sports, such as diving, water polo.

Squash

1. Play squash a minimum of 50 hours; no more than 1½ hours credited daily.

2. Total must include at least 25 matches (3 or 5 games) singles and/or doubles.

Swimming

1. Swim a minimum of 25 miles (44,000 yards); no more than 3/4 of mile (1,320 yards) daily.

T'ai Chi

1. Participate in a minimum of 50 hours of T'ai Chi Chuan following standards set by American T'ai Chi Association.

2. Credit no more than 1 hour per day, 5 hours per week to total.

3. Recommendation: one hour of activity include: 10-15 minutes (flexibility, strengthening) warm-up, 20-30 minutes T'ai Chi within target heart-rate range, 15-minute cool down.

Table Tennis

1. Play table tennis a minimum of 50 hours; no more than 1½ hours credited daily.

2. At least 10 of 50 hours must be in league, tournament, club, ladder, round-robin play.

Tae Kwon Do

1. Practice Tae Kwon Do skills a minimum of 50 hours; no more than one (1) hour credited daily.

2. At least 30 of 50 hours must be under supervision of qualified instructor.

Tennis

1. Play tennis a minimum of 50 hours; no more than 1½ hours credited daily.

2. Total must include at least 25 sets of singles and/or doubles (tie-break rules may apply).

Track and Field

1. Compete in/practice track and field events a minimum of 50 hours; no more than one (1) hour credited daily.

2. At least 10 of 50 hours must be accumulated during organized meets.

Triathalon

1. Run a minimum of 10 miles per week for at least two months. Participants must run minimum three days per week.

2. Bike a minimum of 35 miles per week for at least two months. Individuals must bike minimum of two days per week.

3. Swim a minimum of 1 mile per week for at least two months. Individuals must swim minimum of two days per week.

4. Add no more than 10% to distances for each sport each week. Individual should complete three times distance in their training mileage per week as the spring distance event in which they intend to compete up to one week prior to the event. One week prior to the event, training would be reduced to 1 time the distance of event athlete intends to compete (called tapering).

5. Minimum of 1, maximum of 2 sports should be practiced at least four days per week. One to two days of rest each week is recommended for recovery time.

6. At least one workout per week should include swim/bike or bike/run workout that includes performing sports back-to-back, but would include practicing transition of going from one sport to another (called a "brick").

7. At end of the four-month period, compete in Triathlon Federation/ USA sanctioned sprint distance event (approximately a ½-mile swim, 12-mile bike, and 3.1-mile run).

Volkssports

1. Train for or participate in, a minimum of 50 hours in organized volkssports or volksmarch events; no more than 2 hours credited daily.

2. Exercise activity may consist of running, walking, cycling, climbing, hiking, skiing or any combination of similar activities that promote healthful physical activity.

3. For longer duration events, additional hours may be credited toward other awards.

Volleyball

1. Play/practice volleyball skills, or condition for volleyball a minimum of of 50 hours; no more than two (2) hours of volleyball or one (1) hour conditioning credited daily.

2. Conditioning may include participation in any eligible activity of this program, or in any of the exercise activities listed under Sports/Fitness category.

Walking, Endurance

1. Walk a minimum of 225 miles, combining training walks and endurance walks.

2. Training walks must be a minimum of 1-hour duration. At least three must be completed each week, and the mileage should be credited to the 225-mile total.

3. Walks must be continuous for at least 5 miles. At least five of outings must be 10 miles long and one must be 15 miles long during the time the 225 miles is being completed. No more than one 10-mile, or one 15-mile walk can be credited to the total each week.

Walking, Fitness

1. Walk a minimum of 125 miles; no more than 2 ½ miles credited daily.

2. Each walk must be continuous, without pauses for rest and the pace must be at least four (4) mph (15 minutes per mile).

Walking, Race

1. Race walk a minimum of 200 miles.

2. Race walk continuously at least 3 miles each outing. credit no more than 5 miles daily toward total. Miles total must be spread over at least 40 outings.

3. Must average 12 minutes or less per mile.

4. Follow basic race walking rules: one foot on ground at all times; supporting leg straight as it comes under body.

5. At least two outings must be judged events.

Water Exercise

1. Participate in a minimum of 50 hours of water exercise.

2. Credit no more than one (1) hour per day and four (4) hours per week to total.

3. Recommendation: one hour activity include 5-10 minute warm-up, 20-30 minutes activity within target heart-rate range, 10-15 minutes strengthening exercise 5-10 minute cool down.

Weight Training

1. Train with weights a minimum of 50 hours; no more than one (1) hour credited daily.

2. Workout must include at least eight separate weight/strength training exercises. Workouts should be balanced so that each body part is exercised during each cycle (daily, weekly, etc.). Each exercise to be performed in multiple sets, six to 15 times.

Wrestling

1. Wrestle or practice wrestling skills a minimum of 50 hours; no more than 1 hour credited daily.

2. At least 15 of 50 hours must be in an organized league or wrestling competition.

Personal Fitness Log

NOTE: To order a free copy of the Presidential Sports Award entry personal fitness log, call (407) 934-7200 or write to:

Presidential Sports Award/AAU
c/o Walt Disney World Resort
P.O. Box 10,000
Lake Buena Vista, FL 32830-1000

Chapter 7

Stretching: Key to Avoiding Athletic Injuries

"No pain, no gain" has been a credo of some coaches and athletes regarding warm-up stretches. Here are better words to keep in mind while you stretch: "No pain, no pain."

"You can do a disservice to yourself when you stretch past the point of pain," said Edward R. Laskowski, M.D., co-director of the Mayo Clinic Sports Medicine Center, Rochester, Minnesota. "We always say you should never hold a painful stretch. You should back off just to where it's not painful, and that's what you want to hold during the duration of the stretch."

The goal of routine stretching exercises is to improve flexibility. Flexibility, aerobic conditioning and strength training are the three broad objectives to focus on as you maintain your body for the rigors and enjoyment of sports. Proper stretching actually lengthens the muscle tissue, making it less "tight" and therefore less prone to trauma and tears. A stretching routine also feels good and can be a relaxing period of your day.

Don't Stretch These Rules

Dr. Laskowski advises the following to get the most out of your stretching program:

- *Everybody's different*—We all aren't gymnasts. Focus on maintaining adequate flexibility for your sports and activity level.

Reprinted with permission from Mayo Foundation for Medical Education and Research, Rochester, MN 55905.

- *Be sport-specific*—Different sports emphasize different muscle groups. Concentrate on the ranges of motion and the muscle groups that you're likely to use in your sport.

- *Start slowly*—Example: A ballet dancer begins slowly, with one hand on the bar, before beginning high kicks out on the floor.

- *Hold your stretch*—It takes time to lengthen tissue safely. Hold your stretches at least 30 seconds, and up to a minute with a particularly tight muscle or problem area.

- *Stretch "heated" muscles*—Stretching a cold muscle can strain and irritate the tissue. Warm up first. Walk before you jog, jog before you run, etc. It's most beneficial to stretch after you exercise, when the muscle is heated by blood flow and is more accommodating of a stretch.

- *Do not bounce!*—Bouncing can cause microtrauma in the muscle, which must heal itself with scar tissue. The scar tissue tightens the muscle, making you less flexible and more prone to pain.

- *Think equality*—Strive for balance in flexibility on each side of your body. For example, if one hamstring is tighter than the other, you may be more prone to injury.

- *Don't be afraid to ask*—A sports medicine specialist, athletic trainer, physical therapist, or health-club advisor may help improve your stretching technique.

New Research

Mayo sports medicine doctors are researching whether total relaxation of a muscle may be an important part of achieving flexibility, perhaps apart from or in combination with stretching. Anecdotally, they've observed a high degree of flexibility in "tight" people while they are under general anesthesia—even though their muscles are structurally the same as when they are awake. Although it's too early to draw conclusions, the theory behind this new research is that stimulation from the central nervous system influences the flexibility of muscles, and that relaxing a muscle may be a viable method of enhancing flexibility.

Chapter 8

Pump Fiction: Tips for Buying Exercise Equipment

Looking for a way to shape up? Keep fit? Stay limber? A diet of regular exercise can help. Different types of exercise benefit the body in different ways: some improve flexibility; some improve muscular strength. Others enhance physical endurance, and still others improve cardiovascular and respiratory efficiency. The benefits of exercise are widely known, but the keys to maintaining an exercise program can be elusive. Unfortunately, relatively few consumers stick with their programs: basements, rec rooms, and yard sales are stocked with costly stationary cycles, treadmills, and rowing machines that have been underused, neglected, or turned into clothes hangers. Good intentions are no match for stretching, walking, lifting, swimming—or any other regular physical activity.

Which Exercise Is Best?

The one you're really going to do. Buying fitness equipment for home workouts can represent a sizable financial commitment as well as a lifestyle change. The Federal Trade Commission advises workout "wannabes" to exercise good judgment when evaluating advertising claims for fitness products. Before you buy, the FTC suggests you ask yourself the following questions:

What are your goals? Whether you want to build strength, increase flexibility, improve endurance, or enhance your health, look for

From Federal Trade Commission (FTC) brochure, "Tips for Buying Exercise Equipment," July 1997.

a program that meets your personal goals. Remember that the best route to overall fitness and health is one that incorporates a variety of physical activities as part of a daily routine.

Will you really use exercise equipment? In theory, exercising at home sounds great. But if you don't use a piece of equipment regularly, it can burn a hole in your pocket without burning off any calories. Before you buy, prove to yourself that you're ready to stick to an ongoing fitness program. Set aside some time in your day for physical activity—and then do it.

Can exercise equipment help you spot reduce? No. No exercise device can burn fat off a particular part of your body. To lose the proverbial spare tire or trim your hips, you must combine sensible eating with regular exercise that works the whole body. The reason: Everything you eat has calories and everything you do uses calories. Your weight depends on the number of calories you eat and use each day. Increasing your daily physical activity will burn extra calories.

Can you see through outrageous claims? Exercising regularly can help you shape up. But some companies claim that you can get results by using their equipment for three or four minutes a day, three times a week. Sounds fabulous, right? But realistic? Not really. Here's how you can spot the fantasies when you're sizing up claims by equipment manufacturers:

- Any ads that promise "easy" or "effortless" results are false. Many ads that make big promises about the number of calories you'll burn also may be deceptive. Indeed, some of the claims are true only for athletes who already are in top physical condition; others may not be true for anyone.

- Claims that one machine can help you burn more calories or lose weight faster than others can be tough to evaluate—especially when you can't read the "scientific studies" mentioned in the ads. For these claims, apply two rules:

  1. Equipment that works the whole body, or major portions of it, probably will burn more calories than devices that work one part of the body.

  2. The more you use your equipment, the more calories you'll burn. That's why it's important to select equipment that

suits you and your lifestyle. A study might show that a different device burns more calories an hour, but if it's uncomfortable or difficult to use, chances are it will gather dust rather than help you burn calories.

Have you checked the fine print? Look for tip-offs that getting the advertised results requires more than just using the machine. Sometimes the fine print mentions a diet or "program" that must be used in conjunction with the equipment. Even if it doesn't, remember that diet and exercise together are much more effective for weight loss than either diet or exercise alone. Many ads also feature dramatic testimonials or before-and-after pictures from satisfied customers. These stories may not be typical. Just because one person has had success doesn't mean you'll get the same results. And endorsements—whether they're from consumers, celebrities, or star athletes—don't mean the equipment is right for you.

Can you try the equipment before you buy? Before you buy any exercise equipment, try it out. A few minutes at a sporting goods store while you're wearing street clothes isn't very helpful. Test different types of equipment at a local gym or recreation center. Better still, go to the store dressed for exercise and give the equipment a full workout.

Have you shopped around? Before you buy, check out articles in consumer or fitness magazines that rate the exercise equipment on the market. Much of the equipment advertised on television or in magazines also is available at local sporting goods, department, or discount stores. That makes it easier to shop for the best price. Don't be fooled by companies that advertise "three easy payments of ..." or "just $49.95 a month." Before you buy any product, find out the total cost, including shipping and handling, sales tax, delivery, and set-up fees. Get the details on warranties, guarantees, and return policies: A "30-day money back guarantee" may not sound so good if you have to ante up a hefty fee to return a bulky piece of equipment you've bought through the mail. Check out the company's customer service and support, too. Who can you call if the machine breaks down or you need replacement parts? Try any toll-free numbers to see whether help really is accessible.

Occasionally, you can get a great deal on a piece of fitness equipment from a second-hand store, a consignment shop, a yard sale, or the classifieds in your local newspaper. But buy wisely. Items bought second-hand usually aren't returnable and don't have the warranties of new equipment.

You can file a complaint with the FTC by contacting the Consumer Response Center by phone: toll-free 1-877-FTC-HELP (382-4357); TDD: (202) 326-2502; by mail: Consumer Response Center, Federal Trade Commission, 600 Pennsylvania Ave, NW, Washington, DC 20580; or through the Internet (www.ftc.gov), using the online complaint form. Although the Commission cannot resolve individual problems for consumers, it can act against a company if it sees a pattern of possible law violations. The FTC publishes free brochures on many consumer issues. For a complete list of publications, write for Best Sellers, Consumer Response Center, Federal Trade Commission, 600 Pennsylvania Ave, NW, Washington, DC 20580; or call toll-free 1-877-FTC-HELP (382-4357); TDD: (202) 326-2502.

Part Two

Fitness and Your Diet

Chapter 9

Questions Most Frequently Asked about Sports Nutrition

What is the best diet for an athlete?

It's important that an athlete's diet provides the right amount of energy, the 50-plus nutrients the body needs and adequate water. No single food or supplement can do this. A variety of foods are needed every day. But, just as there is more than one way to achieve a goal, there is more than one way to follow a nutritious diet.

Do the nutritional needs of athletes differ from non-athletes?

Competitive athletes, sedentary individuals and people who exercise for health and fitness all need the same nutrients. However, because of the intensity of their sport or training program, some athletes have higher calorie and fluid requirements. Eating a variety of foods to meet increased caloric needs helps to ensure that the athlete's diet contains appropriate amounts of carbohydrate, protein, vitamins and minerals.

Are there certain dietary guidelines athletes should follow?

Health and nutrition professionals recommend that 55 to 60% of the calories in our diet come from carbohydrates, no more than 30%

Information provided by The President's Council on Physical Fitness and Sports, reviewed by the American Academy of Family Physicians Foundation, and produced as a public service by the Sugar Association, Inc., P.O. Box 2033 Annapolis Junction, MD 20701, www.sugar.org.

from fat and the remaining 10 to 15% from protein. While the exact percentages may vary slightly for some athletes based on their sport or training program, these guidelines will promote health and serve as the basis for a diet that will maximize performance.

How many calories do I need a day?

This depends on your age, body size, sport and training program. For example, a 250-pound weight lifter needs more calories than a 98-pound gymnast. Exercise or training may increase calorie needs by as much as 1,000 to 1,500 calories a day.

The best way to determine if you're getting too few or too many calories is to monitor your weight. Keeping within your ideal competitive weight range means that you are getting the right amount of calories.

Which is better for replacing fluids—water or sports drinks?

Depending on how muscular you are, 55 to 70% of your body weight is water. Being "hydrated" means maintaining your body's fluid level. When you sweat, you lose water, which must be replaced if you want to perform your best. You need to drink fluids before, during and after all workouts and events.

Whether you drink water or a sports drink is a matter of choice. However, if your workout or event lasts for more than 90 minutes, you may benefit from the carbohydrates provided by sports drinks. A sports drink that contains 15 to 18 grams of carbohydrate in every 8 ounces of fluid should be used. Drinks with a higher carbohydrate content will delay the absorption of water and may cause dehydration, cramps, nausea or diarrhea. There are a variety of sports drinks on the market. Be sure to experiment with sports drinks during practice instead of trying them for the first time the day of an event.

What are electrolytes?

Electrolytes are nutrients that affect fluid balance in the body and are necessary for our nerves and muscles to function. Sodium and potassium are the two electrolytes most often added to sports drinks. Generally, electrolyte replacement is not needed during short bursts of exercise since sweat is approximately 99% water and less than 1% electrolytes. Water, in combination with a well-balanced diet, will restore normal fluid and electrolyte levels in the body. However, replacing electrolytes may be beneficial during continuous activity of longer than 2 hours, especially in a hot environment.

What do muscles use for energy during exercise?

Most activities use a combination of fat and carbohydrate as energy sources. How hard and how long you work out, your level of fitness and your diet will affect the type of fuel your body uses. For short-term, high-intensity activities like sprinting, athletes rely mostly on carbohydrate for energy. During low-intensity exercises like walking, the body uses more fat for energy.

What are carbohydrates?

Carbohydrates are sugars and starches found in foods like breads, cereals, fruits, vegetables, pasta, milk, honey, syrups, and table sugar. Carbohydrates are the preferred source of energy for your body. Regardless of origin, your body breaks down carbohydrates into glucose that your blood carries to cells to be used for energy. Carbohydrates provide 4 calories per gram, while fat provides 9 calories per gram. Your body cannot differentiate between glucose that comes from starches or sugars. Glucose from either source provides energy or working muscles.

Is it true that athletes should eat a lot of carbohydrates?

When you are training or competing, your muscles need energy to perform. One source of energy for working muscles is glycogen, which is made from carbohydrates and stored in your muscles. Every time you work out, you use some of your glycogen. If you don't consume enough carbohydrates, your glycogen stores become depleted, which can result in fatigue. Both sugars and starches are effective in replenishing glycogen stores.

When and what should I eat before I compete?

Performance depends largely on the foods consumed during the days and weeks leading up to an event. If you regularly eat a varied, carbohydrate-rich diet you are in good standing and probably have ample glycogen stores to fuel activity. The purpose of the precompetition meal is to prevent hunger and to provide the water and additional energy the athlete will need during competition. Most athletes eat 2 to 4 hours before their event. However, some athletes perform their best if they eat a small amount 30 minutes before competing, while others eat nothing for 6 hours beforehand. For many athletes, carbohydrates-rich foods serve as the basis of the meal. However, there is no magic pre-event diet. Simply choose foods and beverages that you enjoy and that don't bother your stomach. Experiment during the weeks before an event to see which foods work best for you.

Will eating sugary foods before an event hurt my performance?

In the past, athletes were warned that eating sugary foods before exercise could hurt performance by causing a drop in blood glucose levels. Recent studies, however, have shown that consuming sugar up to 30 minutes before an event does not diminish performance. In fact, evidence suggests that a sugar-containing pre-competition beverage or snack may improve performance during endurance workouts and events.

What is carbohydrate loading?

Carbohydrate loading is a technique used to increase the amount of glycogen in muscles. For five to seven days before an event, the athlete eats 10-12 grams of carbohydrate per kilogram body weight and gradually reduces the intensity of the workouts. (To find out how much you weigh in kilograms, simply divide your weight in pounds by 2.2.) The day before the event, the athlete rests and eats the same high-carbohydrate diet. Although carbohydrate loading may be beneficial for athletes participating in endurance sports that require 90 minutes or more of non-stop effort, most athletes needn't worry about carbohydrate loading. Simply eating a diet that derives more than half of its calories from carbohydrates will do.

As an athlete, don't I need to take extra vitamins and minerals?

Athletes need to eat about 1,800 calories a day to get the vitamins and minerals they need for good health and optimal performance. Since most athletes eat more than this amount, vitamin and mineral supplements are needed only in special situations. Athletes who follow vegetarian diets or who avoid an entire group of foods (for example, never drink milk) may need a supplement to make up for the vitamins and minerals not being supplied by food. A multivitamin-mineral pill that supplies 100% of the Recommended Dietary Allowance (RDA) will provide the nutrients needed. An athlete who frequently cuts back on calories, especially below the 1,800 calorie level, is not only at risk for inadequate vitamin and mineral intake, but also may not be getting enough carbohydrate. Since vitamins and minerals do not provide energy, they cannot replace the energy provided by carbohydrates.

Will extra protein help build muscle mass?

Many athletes, especially those on strength-training programs or who participate in power sports, are told that eating a ton of protein or taking protein supplements will help them gain muscle weight. However, the true secret to building muscle is training hard and consuming enough calories. While some extra protein is needed to build muscle, most American diets provide more than enough protein. Between 1.0 and 1.5 grams of protein per kilogram body weight per day is sufficient if your calorie intake is adequate and you're eating a variety of foods. For a 150-pound athlete, that represents 68-102 grams of protein a day.

Why is iron so important?

Hemoglobin, which contains iron, is the part of red blood cells that carries oxygen from the lungs to all parts of the body, including muscles. Since your muscles need oxygen to produce energy, if you have low iron levels in your blood, you may tire quickly. Symptoms of iron deficiency include fatigue, irritability, dizziness, headaches and lack of appetite. Many times, however, there are no symptoms at all. A blood test is the best way to find out if your iron level is low. It is recommended that athletes have their hemoglobin level checked once a year.

The RDA for iron is 15 milligrams a day for women and 10 milligrams a day for men. Red meat is the richest source of iron, but fish and poultry also are good sources. Fortified breakfast cereals, beans and green leafy vegetables also contain iron. Our bodies absorb the iron found in animal products best.

Should I take an iron supplement?

Taking iron supplements will not improve performance unless an athlete is truly iron deficient. Too much iron can cause constipation, diarrhea, nausea and may interfere with the absorption of other nutrients such as copper and zinc. Therefore, iron supplements should not be taken without proper medical supervision.

Why is calcium so important?

Calcium is needed for strong bones and proper muscle function. Dairy foods are the best source of calcium. However, studies show that many females athletes who are trying to lose weight cut back on dairy products. Female athletes who don't get enough calcium may be at risk for stress fractures and, when they're older, osteoporosis. Young women between the ages of 9 and 18 need about 1,300 milligrams of calcium a day. Adults aged 19 through 50 need 1,000 milligrams daily, while those 51 and older should aim for 1,200 milligrams. Low-fat dairy products are a rich source of calcium and also are low in fat and calories.

Table 9.1 presents a list of popular foods rich in carbohydrates (CHO), protein, iron and/or calcium. The nutrient analysis for each food was obtained using The Food Processor II computer program.

Sources of information for this article include: *Haymes, E. M.: Vitamin and Mineral Supplementation to Athletes. (1991). International Journal for Sports Nutrition. 1, 146-169; Sherman, W. M. (1991). Carbohydrate Feedings Before and After Exercise. In D.R. Lamb & M. H. Williams (Eds.), Perspectives in Exercise Science and Sports Medicine: Vol. 4. Ergogenics—Enhancement of Performance in Exercise and Sport. (pp. 1-34). Indianapolis, Indiana: Brown & Benchmark; Sherman, W.M., et. al. (1989). Effects of 4h Preexercise Carbohydrate Feedings on Cycling Performance. Medical Science Sports Exercise 21, 598-604; Tarnopolsky, M. A. (1993). Protein, Caffeine and Sports. Physician and Sports Medicine. 21, 137-149.*

Reviewed by Ann Grandjean, Ed. D., Director, International Center for Sports Nutrition; Chief Nutrition Consultant, United States Olympic Committee.

Table 9.1. Nutrient Content of Selected Foods.

Food	Serving Size	Energy (kcal)	Protein (g)	CHO (g)	Fat (g)	Calcium (mg)	Iron (mg)
Lean Beef	3 ounces	189	27	0	8	4	2.9
Hamburger	3 ounces	246	20	0	18	9	2.1
Lean Pork, Broiled	3 ounces	196	27	0	9	4	.8
Chicken, Breast	3 ounces	167	25	0	7	12	.9
Egg, Hard-Boiled	1 whole	77	6	1	5	25	.6
Peanut Butter	2 tablespoons	190	8	7	16	11	.5
Roasted Peanuts	1 ounce	104	7	5	14	24	5
Navy Beans, Cooked	1/2 cup	129	8	24	0	64	2.2
Salmon, Broiled/Baked	3 ounces	183	23	0	9	6	.5
Salmon, Canned with Bones	3 ounces	118	17	0	5	182	.7
Milk, Whole	1 cup	150	8	11	8	291	.1
2% Low-Fat	1 cup	121	8	12	5	297	.1
1% Low-Fat	1 cup	102	8	12	3	300	.1
Skim	1 cup	86	8	12	0	302	.1
Yogurt, Low-Fat	1 cup	193	11	31	3	388	.2
Cheddar Cheese	1.5 ounces	171	11	0	14	305	.3
Cottage Cheese, 2%	1/2 cup	102	16	4	2	78	.2
Ice Cream, Vanilla	1/2 cup	134	2	16	7	88	.1
Bread, White/Wheat	1 slice	72	3	13	1	35	1.0
Bran Flakes, Fortified	1 ounces	91	4	25	0	14	8.1
Muffin, Bran	1 whole	125	3	19	6	60	1.4
Cookie, Choc. Chip	3 whole	139	2	19	8	8	.8
Baked Potato	1 whole	220	5	51	0	20	2.8
Spaghetti	1/2 cup	98	3	20	0	5	1.0
Green Peas	1/2 cup	63	4	11	0	19	1.2
Broccoli, Cooked	1/2 cup	22	2	4	0	36	.7
Banana	1 whole	105	1	28	0	7	.1
Orange	1 whole	60	1	15	0	52	.1
Butter	1 tablespoon	102	0	0	12	3	0
Margarine	1 tablespoon	102	0	0	11	4	0
Table Sugar	1 teaspoon	16	0	4	0	0	0
Jelly	1 teaspoon	16	0	4	0	1	0

Chapter 10

Do You Drink Enough Water?

A well-conditioned NBA rookie. A 34-year-old businesswoman. A 58-year old executive, recently retired. Each complained of the same symptoms: muscle cramps, headaches, and fatigue, especially near the end of the day. In each case, Susan Kleiner, Ph.D., a registered dietitian in Seattle, suspected the same problem: too little water. "They were all somewhat dehydrated—just dehydrated enough to make their days a little miserable." In each case, a simple water prescription cured the problem.

Those cases are hardly unique: In fact, most people consume less than the optimal amount of water—and a significant number of them do experience symptoms. Moreover, a skimpy water intake may cause more than just symptoms. It clearly contributes to constipation and increases the risk of heat exhaustion or heat stroke. It probably helps cause or worsen asthma, dental disease, kidney stones, and urinary-tract infections. It may even increase the risk of colds and cancer.

Insufficient water intake is a particular concern for older people, because aging, certain drugs (notably sedatives and tranquilizers), and certain diseases (such as diabetes and stroke) may all weaken the sense of thirst. In fact, dehydration is one of the top ten reasons why older people are hospitalized.

Young or old, you need to know whether your body requires more water—and whether wetting your whistle more could really help your health.

Water Shortage

The body is constantly losing water via the breath, skin, urine, and feces; the more you weigh, the more water you lose. On a cool, inactive day, the average man loses about 12 eight-ounce cups of water, but takes in only about 9 cups (about half of that from the water in fruits, vegetables, and other solid foods). The deficit eventually triggers enough thirst to restore water equilibrium, but the average man still spends most days slightly dehydrated.

The average woman experiences a somewhat smaller deficit: about 9 cups lost on a cool, quiet day, but only about 7½ cups consumed. However, that 1½-cup shortfall matters more for women, since they generally weigh less than men.

The Damage from Dryness

Severe dehydration—a net water loss of as little as 4 percent of body weight—can make blood volume and blood pressure plummet, potentially causing muscle spasms, dimmed vision, delirium, fainting, or even a heart attack

Such drastic problems are relatively rare, since thirst typically kicks in when water loss hits about 2 percent of body weight. But some people may start feeling symptoms of mild dehydration—including headache, fatigue, lightheadedness, muscle cramps, and slightly dulled thinking—after just a 1 percent loss. And the average man's daily water deficit does reduce body weight by about that much; some women with a slightly higher-than-average deficit may also feel the effects of their water shortage.

In addition, some evidence suggests that consuming an ample amount of water may provide more important health benefits—possibly including protection against a common killer.

Reduced cancer risk. Consuming plenty of fluids can speed the elimination of feces from the colon and urine from the bladder, thereby helping to prevent and treat constipation and urinary-tract infection. Researchers now suspect that getting enough fluid might cut the risk of cancer, mainly by flushing out or diluting carcinogens in the bladder and colon.

While that notion is still just theoretical, observational studies do lend some support. In the largest one, a ten-year Harvard study of some 50,000 men, published last May in *The New England Journal of Medicine*, those who consumed the most fluid had roughly half the bladder-cancer risk of those who consumed the least. Two smaller, earlier observational studies linked a low fluid intake with an increased risk of bladder or urinary-tract cancer; another suggested that drinking at least five glasses of water a day might cut the risk of colon cancer. One very small study even linked consumption of water, but not that of other beverages, with a reduced likelihood of breast cancer, possibly because water may help wash away or dilute carcinogens not only in the bladder and colon but also in individual cells throughout the body.

Less chance of kidney stones. Stones form when calcium, uric acid, and other substances in the urine become sufficiently concentrated to form crystals. Drinking lots of liquids helps prevent stones, presumably by keeping those concentrations low. People who've already had kidney stones need as much as two extra quarts of water a day, according to some research, to prevent recurrence.

Fewer asthma attacks. Researchers have long known that people with asthma have more trouble breathing when it's dry outside, presumably because parched airways don't function properly. Researchers from the University of Buffalo recently showed that lung function declines when asthmatic individuals get dehydrated, increasing the chance of asthma symptoms even in humid weather. (Dehydration similarly dries the mucus membranes in the nose and throat, reducing their ability to trap airborne bacteria and viruses. So dehydration just might increase susceptibility to colds and other respiratory infections.)

Better oral health. Saliva helps neutralize the cavity-causing acids in the mouth, wash away food particles and sugars, and inhibit the growth of microorganisms that cause gum disease and other oral problems. Even slight dehydration can reduce saliva. Some people try to moisten their mouth by chewing gum or sucking candy or lozenges rather than by drinking more. But unless you're using sugar-free products, such sugary items compound the risk of cavities—and, of course, they still leave you dehydrated.

Reduced weight. In theory, drinking more water, especially with meals, may help curb the appetite by making you feel fuller. While there's no supporting evidence, that simple step is certainly worth trying if you want to slim down.

In addition, some people tend to eat rather than drink when they're thirsty, for two possible reasons. Many foods make you feel less thirsty, since they contain some water and relieve dryness in the mouth by stimulating salivation. And some people simply confuse thirst with hunger. Deliberately drinking more can rectify the problem.

How Much Water Do You Need?

To calculate the minimum daily amount of water you should be getting from all sources, follow these steps:

1. Enter your weight: _____ pounds
2. Multiply line one by .04: _____ pounds of water lost
3. Multiply line two by 2: _____ cups of water needed

The following factors help determine the amount of water you should consume:

Exercise. In cool weather and for ordinary exercise like walking, drink one cup—8 ounce—of water beforehand, an additional 4 ounces every 20 minutes or so during the activity, and another 8 ounces within a half-hour after the workout. Step up your intake when you're exercising harder or the weather's hot. And drink more than you need to satisfy your thirst after the workout.

Height, heat and humidity. The reduced humidity at high elevations and in dry weather increases the amount of water you lose through respiration and perspiration. And you obviously sweat more when it's hot out. To compensate, consume an additional one or two cups of water a day when the elevation exceeds 5,000 feet, the temperature exceeds 80 degrees Fahrenheit or so, or the humidity is unusually low. Note that indoor air can be quite dry, due to heating in winter or air conditioning in summer.

Pregnancy and breastfeeding. Pregnant women need at least one extra cup of water a day. Breastfeeding mothers need an additional three to four cups.

Caffeine and alcohol Those substances may pull as much water out of you as they put in, or possibly even more. To be on the safe side, consume an extra half-cup of water for every cup of caffeinated or alcoholic beverages you drink.

Diarrhea or fever. Try to consume an additional 2 to 3 quarts of water per day when you have diarrhea, and an extra cup for every degree of fever.

Water, Water, Everywhere

Getting more than the minimum amount of water you need each day may possibly provide additional benefits. In general, the only people who may be harmed by consuming too much fluid are those whose bodies retain water due to congestive heart failure, hypothyroidism, or long-term use of certain medications, notably nonsteroidal anti-inflammatory drugs (NSAIDs), such as ibuprofen, ketoprofen, and naproxen. In addition, men with an enlarged prostate should weigh the possible benefits of ample hydration against the likely inconvenience. But while all those people should avoid drinking excessive amounts of water, they should still try to consume the recommended amount. Nor do people who take diuretics need to worry that the recommended intake of water will interfere with their medication.

You can get your water from a combination of beverages and solid foods. But it probably makes sense to get at least five 8-ounce cups from water itself, partly because it's cheap and calorie-free, and partly because some of the cancer evidence suggests greater protection from water than from other drinks. Other good sources include healthful beverages such as 100 percent fruit juice and low-fat milk or soup. Non-caffeinated soft drinks and fruit drinks also count toward your total, but they're loaded with sugar. And caffeinated or alcoholic drinks don't count at all, since caffeine and alcohol are diuretics—they boost urine output and could leave you more dehydrated than before.

Fruits and vegetables are the best food sources of fluid: Each serving of produce typically provides about one-third of a cup of water. A serving of red meat, poultry, or fish usually provides about one-fourth of a cup; a serving of grain provides about one-sixth of a cup.

Because you may start feeling symptoms of dehydration before you start feeling thirsty, particularly if you're older, don't rely on thirst to guide your water intake. Instead, drink steadily over the course of the day. You can tell you're getting enough fluid if your urine is clear

Table 10.1. Water Content of Selected Foods

Food	Percent water[1]	Water per serving (oz)
FRUITS		
Apple, 1	84	3.9
Orange, 1	87	3.9
Banana, 1	74	2.9
Watermelon, ½ cup	92	2.5
Cantaloupe, ½ cup	90	2.4
Grapes, ½ cup	81	2.2
VEGETABLES (raw unless otherwise specified)		
Tomato, 1	93	3.9
Cucumber, 1/3	96	3.2
Potatoes (mashed), ½ cup cooked	76	2.7
Broccoli, ½ cup cooked	91	2.4
Carrot, 1	88	2.1
Iceberg lettuce, 1 cup	96	1.8
MEAT, FISH, AND SEAFOOD (3 oz cooked)		
Shrimp	77	2.2
Flounder	73	2.1
Chicken breast, no skin	65	1.9
Sirloin steak	62	1.8
Salmon	60	1.7
Hamburger	54	1.5
GRAIN		
Rice, ½ cup cooked	69	2.4
Spaghetti, ½ cup cooked	66	1.6
Whole-wheat bread, 1 slice	38	0.4

[1]Foods with a high water percentage do not necessarily supply more water per serving than foods with a lower percentage, because the serving sizes may be different.

or very pale yellow and virtually odorless; dark-yellow, strong-smelling urine means you need to drink more.

Summing Up

Most people, particularly men, don't consume enough water. The evidence that the resulting deficit may keep you from feeling your best or may help promote or worsen various health problems—including constipation, urinary-tract infection, kidney stones, asthma, dental disease, and possibly even colds and cancer—is not conclusive. But boosting your fluid intake is so cheap and simple that even a slight possibility of payoffs make that step a good idea for most people.

Try to consume at least 9 to 12 cups of fluid a day, depending on how much you weigh. Drink extra water when you exercise, when it's hot or dry inside or outside, and in the other special situations described in "How Much Water Do You Need?" Aim to get at least half your quota from water itself, the rest from healthful beverages or solid foods, especially fruits and vegetables.

Eat Your Water

Most people actually get about as much water from solid foods as they do from beverages. And the body treats the water from both sources the same. Fruits and vegetables supply the most water, providing one more reason to eat plenty of produce (see Table 10.1).

Chapter 11

Carbohydrates, Protein, and Performance

Great workouts can give you more strength, more muscle, more speed, more endurance. But so can watching TV, sleeping, and washing the car. That's right—you can build muscle, burn fat, and increase endurance even in your downtime.

Simply eating the right stuff between weight-lifting sessions can make a 15 to 25 percent difference in how much strength you gain, how much muscle you put on, and how much fat you take off, says Marcus Elliott, M.D., a sports-conditioning specialist.

For men who do a lot of cardiovascular exercise, the time off between workouts can be even more crucial. Eating before a long run or ride can increase endurance by more than 50 percent. And giving your body enough R and R between sessions can keep you on the road and off the DL.

The following nutrition and recuperation tips blaze the trail from your last workout to your next one. They'll show you what to eat, when to eat it, how long to wait, and what you'll gain, all without moving an extra muscle. And you'll notice the results almost immediately.

Add Muscle before You Go to the Gym

The miracle of muscle growth—getting bigger and stronger after a workout—actually begins several hours before you pick up your first barbell. A study in the *Journal of Applied Physiology* found that your

From *Men's Health*, June 1999, vol. 14, issue 5, p. 78. © 1999 Rodale Press Inc. Reprinted with permission.

body's production of growth hormone, an important tool for muscle making, increases significantly when you eat a combination of carbohydrates and protein 2 hours before a hard workout and immediately after it.

Eating too soon before a workout might be a problem, though. A UCLA study found that working out with undigested food in your gut can inhibit your body's production of growth hormone by up to 54 percent. If you must eat within 2 hours of starting your workout, it's better to eat carbohydrates than fat. But even eating carbohydrates can cut your growth-hormone release by 24 percent. "If your primary goal is to build or rebuild muscle, stop eating a few hours before you work out," Dr. Elliott says.

Right after exercise, your body enters what researchers call the "rapid phase of recovery." You call it "so hungry I could eat roadkill." It's time to chug down a shake or a sports drink that contains carbohydrates and protein, preferably in a 4-to-1 ratio, says exercise physiologist Edmund Burke, Ph.D., author of *Optimal Muscle Recovery*. Here's how this combination builds muscle.

- The protein helps repair damaged muscles after the workout; it helps your body build the tiny filaments that actually make your muscles bigger.

- The fluid in the sports drink floats nutrients to your muscles and carries away the garbage that makes your muscles sore— the lactic acid and carbon dioxide.

- The carbohydrates help your muscles refuel for the next workout.

- Together, the carbohydrates and protein create a surge in the hormone insulin, which injects your muscles with nutrients.

Eat a full meal 30 minutes to 2 hours after your workout. Go ahead and have the hunk of meat you crave, but add a baked potato, three slices of French bread, and a bowl of light ice cream for dessert. This will create a second wave of insulin to carry more nutrients to your muscles.

How much time between workouts: The object of weight training is to shock your muscles so much that they're scared to lift the same weights again. They'll grow bigger and stronger, so the next time you work out it'll be easier. But muscles need time to pull off this trick. Here's how much.

- If you're doing total-body workouts, rest 48 hours between sessions.

- If you're over 40, give yourself 3 days of rest between full-body sessions.

- If you're doing split routines (working different muscle groups on different days), give each muscle group at least 2 days' rest between workouts. Many men see results by waiting even longer—up to 4 or 5 days.

Burn Fat

Caffeine loosens up your body's fat, which you can use for energy during a workout. But the fat won't burn without some carbohydrates for lighter fluid. So knock down two cups of coffee an hour before exercise, along with half a bagel, and you'll incinerate your flab, according to Jacqueline Berning, Ph.D., a nutritionist at the University of Colorado.

After your workout, eating the wrong kind of carbohydrates can block your progress. Fast-acting energy foods, which your body burns almost immediately, create an insulin surge. This temporarily prevents your body from using fat for energy. So if you're trying to lose fat, eat slow-acting, low-octane carbohydrates at your post-workout meal: Your body will take a while to burn them. Examples: milk, yogurt, apples, oranges, pasta, and beans.

Another fat-burning trick: Eat some fat between workouts. "A low-fat diet, below 20 percent, lowers testosterone levels," Dr. Elliott says. Most active men need 25 percent fat. Lower testosterone means you build less muscle during your workouts, and that equals a missed opportunity to burn additional calories throughout the day, since adding muscle mass cranks up your metabolic rate.

How much time between workouts: To really burn fat, you'll need to do some type of exercise almost every day. Just don't do the same type of workout 2 days in a row. That way, your body will recover from weight lifting while you run, and recover from running while you lift.

Eat Breakfast, Increase Endurance

How much you benefit depends on how long you exercise, so eat the right foods before you hit the road. A recent study in *Medicine and*

Science in Sports and Exercise found that trained cyclists who ate a meal of slow-acting carbohydrates (All-Bran cereal, an apple, and unsweetened yogurt) 30 minutes before exercise were able to pedal 59 percent longer than those who ate a meal of fast-acting carbohydrates (corn-flakes, a banana, and low-fat milk).

As a general rule, if performance is your goal, you don't want much protein or fat in your stomach before running, cycling, or swimming. "Carbohydrates have the nutrients that you're going to digest most rapidly," says nutritionist Susan M. Kleiner, Ph.D., author of *Power Eating*.

After exercise, you want to load your muscles with carbohydrates, to refuel them for the next big push. Eat or drink a mix of fast-acting carbohydrates and protein to create an insulin surge, which will quickly replenish supplies of energy and nutrients.

How much time between workouts: Go for a run before breakfast, and by dinner your heart and lungs will already be in better shape. But you may need longer than that to refuel, and your muscles and joints may need extra time to repair themselves. Dr. Elliott suggests that if you've run, cycled, or swum one-quarter to one-half of your maximum distance, you can do it again 24 hours later. If you go more than 50 percent of your maximum, you need 48 hours to refuel fully. Your back, knees, ankles, and feet will repay you for the extra rest.

Many endurance athletes work out the day after a hard session, but if you do, make sure it's something different: a shorter run, weight lifting, or another type of cardiovascular activity.

You're Fueling Yourself

The glycemic index shows what kind of boost you can expect from which foods. Eat the right food at the right time and you can build your muscles, help your body burn fat, and get a huge energy jolt. Here's what to put in your tank when.

Low-Octane Foods. Eat low-index foods before exercise to increase endurance, and eat them after exercise to help your body burn fat.

- All-Bran cereal
- Baked beans
- Chocolate
- Apples
- Cherries
- Dried apricots

- Flavored yogurt
- Grapes
- Milk
- Oranges
- Pears
- Sponge cake
- Unripe bananas
- Grapefruit
- Kidney beans
- Mixed-grain bread
- Pasta
- Rice-bran cereal
- Tomato soup

Medium-Octane Foods. Eat medium-index foods throughout the day for fuel.

- Back-bean soup
- Cheese pizza
- Green peas
- Mangoes
- 1-minute oats
- Popcorn
- Ripe bananas
- Sweet potatoes
- Cantaloupe
- Fresh apricots
- Ice cream
- Muffins (cake-style)
- Orange juice
- Raisins
- Soft drinks
- Table sugar (sucrose)

High-Octane Foods. Eat high-index foods right after exercise to build muscle or increase endurance.

- Baked potatoes
- Cornflakes
- Instant mashed potatoes
- Rice cakes
- Sports drinks
- Watermelon
- Whole wheat bread
- Carrots
- Honey
- Pretzels
- Shredded Wheat
- Waffles
- White bread

—by Ethan Boldt

Chapter 12

Nutrition Supplements: Science vs. Hype

Nutrition supplements are a lucrative business in the United States. According to the Council for Responsible Nutrition[1], the retail sale of dietary supplements generated $3.3 billion in 1990, and revenues increase each year. This enormous expenditure is largely the result of aggressive advertising aimed at high school, college, and recreational athletes, all eager for anabolic-steroid-like gains through dietary aids. Riding the crest of the fitness wave, nutrition supplements appeal to millions of consumers willing to pay billions of dollars for alleged benefits that are too good to be true.

Unfortunately, these supplements are subject to little regulation by the US Food and Drug Administration (FDA). Advertised claims to the contrary, many supplements have not been subjected to the scientific scrutiny required of prescription drugs. Furthermore, given the size and continued growth of the supplement industry, the FDA will probably never be able to monitor its products effectively. The resulting lack of regulation can lead to unscrupulous advertising, impurities in manufacturing, and potentially dangerous reactions among supplement users.

Such potential outcomes obligate physicians to learn about current nutrition supplements so they can educate patients about the effects and risks of supplement use. Team physicians in particular can advise athletes, coaches, and administrators in these matters. Competing with slick advertisements and exaggerated claims can be difficult,

From *The Physician and Sportsmedicine*, vol. 25, no. 6, June 1997. © 1997 The McGraw-Hill Companies. Reproduced with permission of McGraw-Hill, Inc.

but by using recent scientific research on commonly used supplements, their mechanisms of action, and possible adverse reactions, physicians can offer sound recommendations to patients who are either users or interested in trying these aids.

Creatine Monohydrate

Creatine, or methylguanidine-acetic acid, is an amino acid that was first identified in 1835 by Chevreul. It is synthesized from arginine and glycine in the liver, pancreas, and kidneys and is also available in meats and fish.[2] Creatine was first introduced as a potential ergogenic aid in 1993 as creatine monohydrate and is currently being used extensively by athletes throughout the United States. A National Collegiate Athletic Association (NCAA) study, publication pending, revealed that 13% of intercollegiate athletes have used creatine monohydrate in the past 12 months (Frank Uryasz, personal communication, February 1997).

According to current theory, creatine supplementation increases the bioavailability of phosphocreatine (PCr) in skeletal muscle cells. This increase is thought to enhance muscle performance in two ways. First, more available PCr allows faster resynthesis of adenosine triphosphate (ATP) to provide energy for brief, high-intensity exercise, like sprinting, jumping, or weight lifting. Second, PCr buffers the intracellular hydrogen ions associated with lactate production and muscle fatigue during exercise. Therefore, creatine supplementation may provide an ergogenic effect by increasing the force of muscular contraction and prolonging anaerobic exercise[3].

Numerous well-designed studies have demonstrated that creatine supplementation has an ergogenic potential. Greenhaff et al[4] showed that 5-day oral dosages of 20 g/day increased muscle creatine availability by 20% and significantly accelerated PCr regeneration after intense muscle contraction. Birch et al[5] and Harris et al,[6] in laboratory and field studies, demonstrated significant performance enhancement in male athletes, in both brief, high-intensity work and total time to exhaustion, using creatine supplementation of 20 to 30 g/day. Recent data reveal that the mean creatine concentration in human skeletal muscle is 125 mmole/kg-dm (dry muscle), with a normal range between 90 and 160 mmole/kg-dm.[7] This wide spectrum of creatine concentration may explain why some of the published studies have not demonstrated significant ergogenic effects. In a study by Greenhaff[7], approximately half of the tested athletic subjects exhibited concentrations lower than 125 mmole/kg-dm, with strict vegetarians substantially lower. These individuals exhibited the most significant increases in muscle creatine concentration, PCr regeneration, and performance enhancement with the use of creatine. On the other hand, athletes with elevated baseline levels of creatine showed little or no ergogenic effect when tested after ingesting creatine.

While creatine use has skyrocketed, no serious side effects have been scientifically verified in subjects using relatively brief (less than 4 weeks) creatine regimens. However, there are anecdotal reports of a dramatic increase in muscle cramping associated with the use of creatine monohydrate (J. Kinderknecht, MD, personal communication, June 1996). Future research will, we hope, clarify whether these adverse reactions are caused by creatine supplementation.

Chromium Picolinate

Chromium is an essential trace mineral present in various foods, such as mushrooms, prunes, nuts, whole grain breads, and cereals[8]. A normal American diet contains 50% to 60% of the recommended daily allowance (RDA) of chromium. It has an extremely low gastrointestinal absorption rate, so supplement manufacturers have bound chromium with picolinate (CrPic) to increase the absorption and bioavailability.

Chromium supplementation became popular after it was found that exercise increases chromium loss, raising the concern that chromium deficiency may be common among athletes[9]. Chromium seems to function as a co-factor that enhances the action of insulin, especially in carbohydrate, fat, and protein metabolism. Promoters of CrPic claim it increases glycogen synthesis, improves glucose tolerance and lipid profiles, and increases amino acid incorporation in muscle.

CrPic supplementation gained scientific credence in the early 1980s when researchers demonstrated anabolic-steroid-like effects with dosages of 200 micrograms/day. Evans[10,11] and Hasten et al[12] demonstrated a decreased percentage of body fat and increased lean mass among college athletes and students who took CrPic supplements and performed resistance exercise training. However, critical analysis of these studies reveals that imprecise measurement techniques, rather than CrPic supplementation, may account for these "ergogenic" results. More recent studies by Clancy et al[13] and Hallmark et al[14], using more precise measurement techniques, failed to demonstrate any significant improvement in percent body fat, lean body mass, or strength. Most studies of CrPic supplementation reveal no side effects except gastrointestinal intolerance with dosages of 50 to 200 micrograms/day for less than 1 month. However, anecdotal reports of serious adverse effects, including anemia[15], cognitive impairment[16], chromosome damage [17], and interstitial nephritis[18] have been reported with CrPic ingestion in increased dosages and/or durations. Therefore, the use of chromium picolinate supplementation as an ergogenic aid should be strongly discouraged and considered potentially dangerous.

Amino Acids

Amino acids are the basic structural units of proteins, and one might expect that the more amino acids ingested, the greater the potential for building skeletal muscle. According to the 1989 RDA, an average adult must ingest 0.8 g/kg lean body mass/day of protein in order to fulfill the body's protein requirements. Athletes, however, have traditionally been assumed to need significantly more protein than the average individual, so they commonly use various protein supplements.

Theories suggest that increasing the bioavailability of amino acids promotes protein synthesis and attenuates the muscle loss that occurs during both strength and endurance exercise. These theories have gained support through scientific experimentation in protein metabolism. Fern et al[19] and Lemon et al[20] demonstrated that strength trainers increased protein synthesis with substantially increased protein ingestion during 4 weeks of resistance training. By tracking the nitrogen balance of these athletes, a new daily protein requirement (1.4 to 1.8 g/kg lean mass/day) was developed for strength athletes.

Amino acid supplementation also plays a role in endurance athletes. Lemon[21] and Gontzen et al[22] demonstrated that endurance athletes who train at moderate intensity (55% to 65% of VO2 max) and high intensity (80% of VO2 max) for more than 100 minutes significantly increase protein breakdown unless their protein intake equals 1.2 to 1.4 g/kg lean mass/day.

Several factors make the amount of amino acids that athletes need less clear. Although all of the cited studies demonstrate the advisability of protein intakes higher than the current RDA, no well-designed study has yet shown that amino acid supplementation enhances performance. In addition, no scientific evidence supports protein supplementation in dosages greater than 2 g/kg lean mass/day. Finally, the improved conditioning that occurs over a 4- to 8-week training period may decrease protein breakdown, which may result in a maintenance protein requirement much closer to the current RDA.

L-Carnitine

Carnitine is a quaternary amine whose physiologically active form is beta-hydroxy-gamma-trimethylammonium butyrate. This is found in meats and dairy products and is synthesized in the human liver and kidneys from two essential amino acids, lysine and methionine. L-carnitine is thought to be ergogenic in two ways. First, by increasing free fatty acid transport across mitochondrial membranes, carnitine may increase fatty acid oxidation and utilization for energy, thus sparing muscle glycogen. Second, by buffering pyruvate, and thus reducing muscle lactate accumulation associated with fatigue, carnitine may prolong exercise.

Early studies by Gorostiaga et al[23], Wyss et al[24], and Natalie et al[25] indirectly demonstrated an ergogenic effect of this compound. These studies showed a decreased respiratory exchange ratio (RER) with L-carnitine supplementation (2 to 6 g/day) during exercise, suggesting that fatty acids rather than carbohydrates were used for energy. However, these studies had several problems in methodology, including the use of the RER as the sole measure of enhanced fatty acid oxidation. The RER is an indirect measure of lipid utilization that is influenced by many factors, such as preexercise diet, fitness level, and exercise intensity and duration[26]. These confounders were not controlled and may have influenced the results.

A more controlled study by Vuchovich et al[27] avoided these problems by directly measuring muscle glycogen and lactate levels through biopsy and serum analysis. This study failed to demonstrate any glycogen-sparing effect or reductions in lactate levels while supplementing with 6 g/day of L-carnitine. Furthermore, no study to date has confirmed performance enhancement with carnitine supplementation. Finally, many currently available supplements actually contain D-carnitine, which is physiologically inactive in humans but may cause significant muscle weakness through mechanisms that deplete L-carnitine in tissues. Therefore, carnitine should not be advocated as an ergogenic supplement.

L-Tryptophan

L-tryptophan, an essential amino acid, is not commercially available in its pure form but is found in many combination supplement products and reportedly remedies insomnia, depression, anxiety, and premenstrual tension.[28] Athletes in the past decade have taken L-tryptophan because of its advertised ergogenic effects. The theoretical mechanism for these effects is an increase in serotonin levels in the brain; these increases produce analgesia and reduce the discomfort of prolonged muscular effort, thereby delaying fatigue. This theoretical model gained scientific credence in 1988 when Segura and Ventura[29] demonstrated a 49% increase in total exercise time to exhaustion when subjects ingested a total of 1.2 g of L-tryptophan (four 300-mg doses within 24 hours of exercise) vs placebo. Such a profound improvement in performance is difficult to imagine, and these results have never been replicated. Two larger, well-designed studies by Seltzer et al[30] and Stensrud et al[31] failed to demonstrate any improvement in subjective or objective outcome measures when supplementing with 1.2 g of L-tryptophan vs placebo. The results of these two studies are more consistent with current research data on exercise.

Physicians should be aware of two other developments that argue against supplementing with L-tryptophan. Its use has declined among elite athletes, possibly suggesting that they are recognizing its minimal ergogenic effects. More important, L-tryptophan ingestion was linked to multiple cases of eosinophilia myalgia syndrome and 32 deaths.[28] Though these cases were probably due to contamination of L-tryptophan produced by one Japanese manufacturer, and not to the amino acid itself, they illustrate the quality and purity questions regarding unregulated supplements.

Beta-Hydroxy-Beta-Methylbutyrate

One of the most recent additions to the nutrition supplement market is beta-hydroxy-beta-methylbutyrate (HMB). It is a metabolite of the essential branched-chain amino acid leucine and is produced in small amounts endogenously. HMB is also found in catfish, citrus fruits, and breast milk. In the early 1980s, researchers at Iowa State University hypothesized that HMB was the bioactive component in leucine metabolism that regulates protein metabolism. The exact mechanism of this process is unknown, but promoters hypothesize that HMB regulates the enzymes responsible for protein breakdown. They propose that high HMB levels decrease protein catabolism, thereby creating a net anabolic effect. Research in livestock[32-36] and humans seems to suggest that supplementation with HMB may increase muscle mass and strength. Nissen conducted two randomized, double-blind, placebo-controlled studies[37,38] to evaluate the ergogenic potential of HMB in exercising men. In the first study, 41 untrained subjects participated in a 4-week resistance training program. The subjects, whose diets were controlled, were given either HMB supplements of 1.5 or 3 g/day or a placebo. Those receiving HMB supplements showed significant improvements in muscle mass and strength as well as significant decreases in muscle breakdown products (3-methylhistidine and creatine phosphokinase) when compared with placebo subjects. The second study evaluated trained and untrained male subjects in a similarly designed weight training program. Relative to a placebo group, the subjects supplementing with 3 g/day demonstrated significant increases in muscle mass and one-repetition maximum bench press as well as decreases in percent body fat.

Further studies of HMB may continue to support the supplement's anabolic effects and elucidate its role in protein metabolism. No side effects of HMB supplementation have been reported, but the safety of this agent is still unknown. Therefore, it is premature to recommend its use as a safe and effective ergogenic aid.

Dehydroepiandrosterone

Attention focused on dehydroepiandrosterone (DHEA) in 1996 when the FDA banned its sale and distribution for therapeutic uses until its safety and value could be reviewed. The ensuing media attention popularized this supplement, and manufacturers began selling it as a nutritional aid rather than a therapeutic drug.

DHEA was identified in 1934 as an androgen produced in the adrenal glands. It is a precursor to the endogenous production of both androgens and estrogens in primates.[39] It is also available in wild yams, which are sold in many health food stores as a source of DHEA. As a precursor to androgenic steroids, DHEA may increase the production of testosterone and provide an anabolic steroid effect. Promoters claim that this compound slows the aging process and accordingly advertise it as the "fountain of youth."

Only a few randomized, double-blind, placebo-controlled studies on the effects of DHEA supplementation have been published. Two have demonstrated significant increases in androgenic steroid plasma levels, along with subjective improvements in physical and psychological well-being, while supplementing with 50 mg/day for 6 months[40] or 100 mg/day for up to 12 months.[41] Whether DHEA has any effect on body composition or fat distribution is still unclear. Its effect on healthy individuals younger than 40 years old is also virtually unstudied.

DHEA users have reported few adverse effects from the supplement, but one is irreversible virilization in women, including hair loss, hirsutism, and voice deepening.[42] In addition, men have reported irreversible gynecomastia, which may result from an elevation in estrogen levels. Because this supplement is so new, long-term adverse effects are unknown. Unlike most other nutrition supplements, DHEA may substantially increase the risk of uterine and prostate cancer that accompanies prolonged elevation in the levels of unopposed estrogen and testosterone. Therefore, the safety of this supplement must be questioned.

Of particular interest to competitive athletes is the effect that DHEA supplementation may have on the test used by the International Olympic Committee and NCAA in their screening for exogenous testosterone use. Using DHEA could alter the testosterone-epitestosterone ratio so it exceeds the 6:1 limit set by both groups (personal communication, Don Catlin, MD, 1997); thus DHEA users could risk disqualification from international competition. Given the lack of evidence that DHEA enhances athletic performance and its potentially devastating adverse effects, DHEA supplementation is not recommended.

Purity, Cost, and Final Thoughts

Although some of the supplements discussed here may have benefits, physicians should remain skeptical about the use of any supplement. The purity of agents available to consumers is in doubt, as we have seen with L-tryptophan. The Medical Letter, for example, analyzed several commercial preparations of melatonin and found unidentifiable impurities in four of six samples (43). The supplements used for the research reported in this review were pure, but consumers in the largely unregulated marketplace cannot be assured of that same purity in the products they buy.

There is also the issue of cost (Tables 12.1 and 12.2). At current rates, doses of the supplements discussed range as high as $7.20/day, the cost of a loading dose of creatine (20 to 30 g/day). It makes little sense to invest in supplements that offer minimal or no benefit, especially for athletic departments in this era of shrinking budgets.

The key word in nutrition supplements is nutrition. NCAA guidelines state that "there are no shortcuts to sound nutrition, and the use of suspected or advertised ergogenic aids may be detrimental and will, in most instances, provide no competitive advantage."[44] Physicians need to educate athletes, parents, coaches, trainers, and athletic administrators in sound dietary practices or see to it that a nutrition professional does so. Then nutrition supplements can be put in proper perspective, and decisions regarding their use can be based on proper scientific study and proven benefit to the individual.

Table 12.1. Daily Dose Costs of Various Nutrition Supplements Used by Athletes

Creatine

- 20-30 g/day (loading dose): $7.20/day for one week
- 10-15 g/day (maintenance dose): $3.60/day

Chromium

- 200 mg/day: $0.43/day

L-Carnitine

- 2.0 g/day: $2.67/day

Beta-Hydroxy-Beta-Methylbutyrate

- 13 g/day: $3.48/day
- 11.5 g/day: $1.74/day

Dehydroepiandrosterone

- 150 mg/day: $0.67/day
- 1100 mg/day: $1.34/day

L-Tryptophan

- Currently unavailable in pure form due to federal regulation

Sources: National Supplement Association and General Nutrition Centers

Table 12.2. Protein Supplements Cost Comparison: Daily Cost of 2 g Protein/kg for a 70-kg Individual

Brand name protein powder:

- $9.80/day ($0.07/g protein)

Generic Protein Powder:

- $2.80/day ($0.02/g protein)

Tuna:

- $2.80/day ($0.02/g protein)

Source: National Supplement Association

References

1. Cowart VS: Dietary supplements: alternatives to anabolic steroids? *Phys Sportsmed* 1992;20(3):189-198.

2. Walker JB: Creatine: biosynthesis, regulation and function. *Adv Enzymol Relat Areas Mol Med* 1979;50:177-242.

3. Maughan RJ: Creatine supplementation and exercise performance. *Int J Sport Nutr* 1995;5(2):94-101.

4. Greenhaff PL, Bodin K, Soderlund K, et al: The effect of oral creatine supplementation on skeletal muscle phosphocreatine resynthesis. *Am J Physiol* 1994;266(5 pt 1):E725-E730.

5. Birch R, Noble D, Greenhaff GL: The influence of dietary creatine supplementation on performance during repeated bouts of maximal isokinetic cycling in man. *Eur J Appl Phys* 1994;69(3):268-276.

6. Harris RC, Soderlund K, Hultman E: Elevation of creatine in resting and exercised muscle of normal subjects by creatine supplementation. *Clin Sci* 1992;83(3):367-374.

7. Greenhaff PL: Creatine and its application as an ergogenic aid. *Int J Sport Nutr* 1995;5(suppl):S100-S110.

8. Clarkson PM: Do athletes require mineral supplements? *Sports Med Digest* 1994;16(4):1-3.

9. Campbell WW, Anderson RA: Effects of aerobic exercise and training on trace minerals chromium, zinc, and copper. *Sports Med* 1987;4(1):9-18.

10. Evans GW: The role of picolinic acid in metal metabolism. *Life Chem Reports* 1982;1:57-67.

11. Evans GW: The effect of chromium picolinate on insulin controlled parameters in humans. *Int J Biosocial Med* 1989;11:163-180.

12. Hasten DL, Rome EP, Franks ED, et al: Effects of chromium picolinate on beginning weight training students. *Int J Sport Nutr* 1994;2(4):343-350.

13. Clancy SP, Clarkson PM, DeCheke ME, et al: Effects of chromium picolinate supplementation on body composition,

strength, and urinary chromium loss in football players. *Int J Sport Nutr* 1994;4(2):142-153.

14. Hallmark MA, Reynolds TH, DeSouza CA, et al: Effects of chromium and resistive training on muscle strength and body composition. *Med Sci Sports Exerc* 1996;28(1):139-144.

15. Lefavi RG: Sizing up a few supplements. *Phys Sportsmed* 1992;20(3):190-191.

16. Huszonek J: Over-the-counter chromium picolinate. [Letter] *Am J Psychiatry* 1993;150(10):1560-1561.

17. Stearns DM, Wise JP, Patierno SR, et al: Chromium picolinate produces chromosome damage in Chinese hamster ovary cells. *FASEB* 1995;9(15):1643-1648.

18. Wasser WG, Feldman NS: Chronic renal failure after ingestion of over-the-counter chromium picolinate. [Letter] *Ann Int Med* 1997;126(5):410.

19. Fern EB, Bielinski RN, Schultz Y: Effects of exaggerated amino acid and protein supply in man. *Experimentia* 1991;47(2):168-172.

20. Lemon PW, Tarnopolsky MA, MacDougall JD, et al: Protein requirements, muscle mass/strength changes during intensive training in novice bodybuilders. *J Appl Physiol* 1992;73(2):767-775.

21. Lemon PW: Effect of exercise on protein requirements. *J Sports Sci* 1991;9(special):53-70.

22. Gontzen I, Sutzecu P, Dumitrache S: The influence of muscular activity on the nitrogen balance and on the need of man for proteins. *Nutr Rep Int* 1974;10:35-43.

23. Gorostiaga EM, Maurer CA, Eclache JP: Decrease in respiratory quotient during exercise following L-carnitine supplementation. *Int J Sports Med* 1989;10(3):169-174.

24. Wyss V, Ganzit GP, Rienzi A: Effects of L-carnitine administration on VO2 max and the aerobic-anaerobic threshold in normoxia and acute hypoxia. *Eur J Appl Physiol* 1990;60(1):1-6.

25. Natalie A, Santoro D, Brandi LS, et al: Effects of acute hypercarnitinemia during increased fatty substrate oxidation in man. *Metabolism* 1993;42(5):594-600.

26. Krogh A, Lindhard J: The relative value of fat and carbohydrate as sources of muscular energy. *Biochem J* 1920;14(July):290-363.

27. Vuchovich MD, Costill DL, Fink WJ: Carnitine supplementation: effect on muscle carnitine and glycogen content during exercise. *Med Sci Sports Exerc* 1994;26(9):1122-1129.

28. Teman AJ, Hainline B: Eosinophilia-myalgia syndrome. *Phys Sportsmed* 1991;19(2):81-86.

29. Segura R, Ventura JL: Effect of L-tryptophan supplementation on exercise performance. *Int J Sports Med* 1988;9(5):301-305.

30. Seltzer S, Stoch R, Marcus R, et al: Alterations of human pain thresholds by nutritional manipulation of L-tryptophan supplementation. *Pain* 1982;13(4):385-393.

31. Stensrud T, Ingjer F, Holm H, et al: L-tryptophan supplementation does not improve running performance. *Int J Sports Med* 1992;13(6):481-485.

32. Gatnau R, Zimmerman DR, Nissen SL, et al: Effect of excess dietary leucine and leucine catabolites on growth and immune response in weanling pigs. *J Animal Sci* 1995;73(1):159-165.

33. Nissen SL, Fuller JC, Sell J, et al: The effect of ß-hydroxy ß-methylbutyrate on growth, mortality, and carcass qualities of broiler chickens. *Poultry Sci* 1994;73(1):137-155.

34. Nissen SL, Morrical D, Fuller JC: The effects of the leucine catabolite ß-hydroxy ß-methylbutyrate on the growth and health of growing lambs. *J Animal Sci* 1992;77(suppl 1):243.

35. Ostaszewski P, Kostiuk S, Balasinska B, et al: The effect of the leucine metabolite ß-hydroxy ß-methylbutyrate (HMB) on muscle protein synthesis and protein breakdown in chick and rat muscle. *J Animal Sci* 1996;74(suppl):138.

36. Van Koevering MT, Dolezal HG, Gill DR, et al: Effects of ß-hydroxy ß-methylbutyrate on performance and carcass quality of feedlot steers. *J Anim Sci* 1994;72(8):1927-1935.

37. Nissen SL, Sharp R, Ray M, et al: The effect of the leucine metabolite beta-hydroxy beta-methylbutyrate on muscle metabolism during resistance-exercise training. *J Appl Physiol* 1996;81(5):2095-2104.

38. Nissen SL, Panton J, Wilhelm R, et al: The effect of beta-hydroxy beta-methylbutyrate (HMB) supplementation on strength and body composition of trained and untrained males undergoing intense resistance training. *FASEB J* 1996;10(3):A287.

39. Hardman JG, Limdird LE (eds): *Goodman and Gillman's The Pharmacologic Basis of Therapeutics, ed 9.* New York City, McGraw-Hill, 1996, p 1413.

40. Morales AJ, Nolan JJ, Nelson JC, et al: Effects of replacement dose dehydroepiandrosterone in men and women of advancing age. *J Clin Endocrinol Metab* 1994;78(6):1360-1367.

41. Yen SS, Morales AJ, Khorram O: Replacement of DHEA in aging men and women: potential remedial effects. *Ann NY Acad Sci* 1995;774(Dec 29):128-142.

42. Abramowicz M (ed): Dehydroepiandrosterone (DHEA). *The Medical Letter On Drugs and Therapeutics* 1996;38(985):91-92.

43. Abramowicz M (ed): Melatonin. *The Medical Letter On Drugs and Therapeutics* 1995;37(962):111-112.

44. Benson MT (ed): *NCAA Sports Medicine Handbook 1994-95, ed 7.* Overland Park, Kansas, National Collegiate Athletic Association, 1994, p 30.

— by Thomas D. Armsey Jr, MD and Gary A.Green, MD.

Dr Armsey is a clinical instructor and sports medicine fellow, and Dr. Green is a clinical associate professor in the Department of Family Medicine at the University of California, Los Angeles, Medical Center. Address correspondence to Gary A. Green, MD, University of California, Los Angeles, Medical Center, Box 951683, Los Angeles, CA 90095-1683.

Chapter 13

Exercise and Diet: Weight Loss for Life

Who should lose weight? Health experts generally agree that adults can benefit from weight loss if they are moderately to severely overweight. Health experts also agree that adults who are overweight and have weight-related medical problems or a family history of such problems can benefit from weight loss. Some weight-related health problems include diabetes, heart disease, high blood pressure, high cholesterol levels, or high blood sugar levels. Even a small weight loss of 10 to 20 pounds can improve your health, for example, by lowering your blood pressure and cholesterol levels. You do not need to lose weight if your weight is within the healthy range on the weight-for-height chart, if you have gained less than 10 pounds since you reached your adult height, and if you are otherwise healthy.

How We Lose Weight

Your body weight is controlled by the number of calories you eat and the number of calories you use each day. So, to lose weight you need to take in fewer calories than you use. You can do this by becoming more physically active or by eating less. Following a weight-loss program that helps you to become more physically active and decrease the number of calories that you eat is most likely to lead to successful weight loss. The weight-loss program should also help you keep the weight off by making changes in your physical activity

WIN (Weight-Control Information Network), U.S. Department of Health and Human Services, NIH Publication #98-3700, January 1998.

and eating habits that you will be able to follow for the rest of your life.

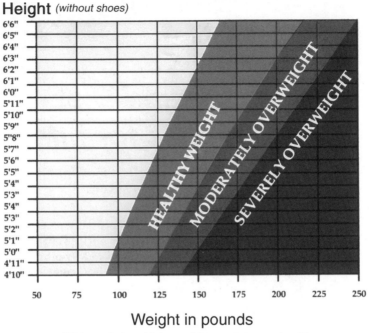

Height *(without shoes)*

Weight in pounds

(Without clothes. Higher weights apply to people with more muscle and bone, such as many men.)

Figure 13.1. *Weight-for-Height Chart.*

Types of Weight-Loss Programs

To lose weight and keep it off, you should be aware of the different types of programs available and the important parts of a good program. Knowing this information should help you select or design a weight-loss program that will work for you. The three types of weight-loss programs include: do-it-yourself programs, non-clinical programs, and clinical programs.

Do-It-Yourself Programs

Any effort to lose weight by yourself or with a group of like-minded others through support groups, worksite or community-based programs fits in the "do-it-yourself" category. Individuals using a do-it-yourself program rely on their own judgment, group support, and products such as diet books for advice (Note: Not all diet books are reliable sources of weight-loss information).

Non-Clinical Programs

These programs may or may not be commercially operated, such as through a privately owned, weight-loss chain. They often use books and pamphlets that are prepared by health-care providers. These programs use counselors (who usually are not health-care providers and may or may not have training) to provide services to you. Some programs require participants to use the program's food or supplements.

Clinical Programs

This type of program may or may not be commercially owned. Services are provided in a health-care setting, such as a hospital, by licensed health professionals, such as physicians, nurses, dietitians, and/or psychologists. In some clinical programs, a health professional works alone; in others, a group of health professionals works together to provide services to patients. Clinical programs may offer you services such as nutrition education, medical care, behavior change therapy, and physical activity.

Clinical programs may also use other weight-loss methods, such as very low-calorie diets, prescription weight-loss drugs, and surgery, to treat severely overweight patients. These treatments are described below:

- **Very low-calorie diets** (VLCDs) are commercially prepared formulas that provide no more than 800 calories per day and replace all usual food intake. VLCDs help individuals lose weight more quickly than is usually possible with low-calorie diets. Because VLCDs can cause side effects, obesity experts recommend that only people who are severely overweight use these diets, and only with proper medical care. A fact sheet on VLCDs is available from the Weight-Control Information Network (WIN).

- **Prescribed weight-loss drugs** should be used only if you are likely to have health problems caused by your weight. You should not use drugs to improve your appearance. Prescribed weight-loss drugs, when combined with a healthy diet and regular physical activity, may help some obese adults lose weight. However, before these medications can be widely recommended, more research is needed to determine their long-term safety and effectiveness. Whatever the results, prescription weight-loss drugs should be used only as part of an overall program that includes long-term changes in your eating and physical activity habits. A fact sheet on prescription medications for the treatment of obesity is available from WIN.

- You may consider **gastric surgery** to promote weight loss if you are more than 80 pounds overweight. The surgery, sometimes called bariatric surgery, causes weight loss in one of two ways: 1) by limiting the amount of food your stomach can hold by closing off or removing parts of the stomach or 2) by causing food to be poorly digested by bypassing the stomach or part of the intestines. After surgery, patients usually lose weight quickly. While some weight is often regained, many patients are successful in keeping off most of their weight. In some cases, the surgery can lead to problems that require follow-up operations. Surgery may also reduce the amount of vitamins and minerals in your body and cause gallstones. For additional information, a fact sheet on gastric surgery is available from WIN.

- If you are considering a weight-loss program and you have medical problems, or if you are severely overweight, **programs run by trained health professionals** may be best for you. These professionals are more likely to monitor you for possible side effects of weight loss and to talk to your doctor when necessary.

Whether you decide to use the do-it-yourself, non-clinical, or clinical approach, the program should help you lose weight and keep it off by teaching you healthy eating and physical activity habits that you will be able to follow for the rest of your life.

Diet

The word "diet" probably brings to mind meals of lettuce and cottage cheese. By definition, "diet" refers to what a person eats or drinks during the course of a day. A diet that limits portions to a very small size or that excludes certain foods entirely to promote weight loss may not be effective over the long term. Rather, you are likely to miss certain foods and find it difficult to follow this type of diet for a long time.

Instead, it is often helpful to gradually change the types and amounts of food you eat and maintain these changes for the rest of your life. The ideal diet is one that takes into account your likes and dislikes and includes a wide variety of foods with enough calories and nutrients for good health.

How much you eat and what you eat play a major role in how much you weigh. So when planning your diet, you should consider: What calorie level is appropriate? Is the diet you are considering nutritionally balanced? Will the diet be practical and easy to follow? Will you be able to maintain this eating plan for the rest of your life? The following information will help you answer these questions.

Calorie Level

Low-calorie diets. Most weight-loss diets provide 1,000 to 1,500 calories per day. However, the number of calories that is right for you depends on your weight and activity level. At these calorie levels, diets are referred to as low-calorie diets. Self-help diet books and clinical and non-clinical weight-loss programs often include low-calorie diet plans. The calorie level of your diet should allow for a weight loss of no more than 1 pound per week (after the first week or two when weight loss may be more rapid because of initial water loss). If you can estimate how many calories you eat in a day, you can design a diet plan that will help you lose no more than 1 pound per week. You may need to work with a trained health professional, such as a registered dietitian. Or you can use a standardized low-calorie diet plan with a fixed calorie level. The selected calorie level, however, may not produce the recommended rate of weight loss, and you may need to eat more or less.

Good Nutrition

Make sure that your diet contains all the essential nutrients for good health. Using the Food Guide Pyramid (see Figure 13.2) and the Nutrition Facts Label that is found on most processed food products can help you choose a healthful diet. The Pyramid shows you the kinds and amounts of food that you need each day for good health. The Nutrition Facts Label will help you select foods that meet your daily nutritional needs. A healthful diet should include:

Adequate vitamins and minerals. Eating a wide variety of foods from all the food groups on the Food Guide Pyramid will help you get the vitamins and minerals you need. If you eat less than 1,200 calories per day, you may benefit from taking a daily vitamin and mineral supplement.

Adequate protein. The average woman 25 years of age and older should get 50 grams of protein each day, and the average man 25 years of age and older should get 63 grams of protein each day. Adequate protein is important because it prevents muscle tissue from breaking down and repairs all body tissues such as skin and teeth. To get adequate protein in your diet, make sure you eat 2-3 servings from the Meat, Poultry, Fish, Dry Beans, Eggs, and Nuts Group on the Food Guide Pyramid every day. These foods are all good sources of protein.

Adequate carbohydrates. At least 100 grams of carbohydrates per day are needed to prevent fatigue and dangerous fluid imbalances. To make sure you get enough carbohydrates, eat 6-11 servings from the Bread, Cereal, Rice, and Pasta Group on the Food Guide Pyramid every day.

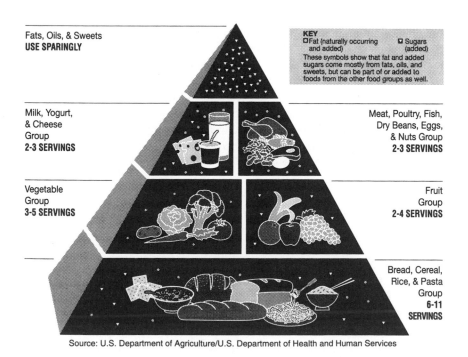

Source: U.S. Department of Agriculture/U.S. Department of Health and Human Services

Figure 13.2. The Food Guide Pyramid.

A daily fiber intake of 20 to 30 grams. Adequate fiber helps with proper bowel function. If you were to eat 1 cup of bran cereal, ½ cup of carrots, ½ cup of kidney beans, a medium-sized pear, and a medium-sized apple together in 1 day, you would get about 30 grams of fiber.

No more than 30 percent of calories, on average, from fat per day, with less than 10 percent of calories from saturated fat (such as fat from meat, butter, and eggs). Limiting fat to these levels reduces your risk for heart disease and may help you lose weight. In addition, you should limit the amount of cholesterol in your diet. Cholesterol is a fat-like substance found in animal products such as meat and eggs. Your diet should include no more than 300 milligrams of cholesterol per day (one egg contains about 215 milligrams of cholesterol, and 3.5 ounces of cooked hamburger contain 100 milligrams of cholesterol).

At least 8 to 10 glasses, 8 ounces each, of water or water-based beverages, per day. You need more water if you exercise a lot.

These nutrients should come from a variety of low-calorie, nutrient-rich foods. One way to get variety and, with it, an enjoyable and nutritious diet, is to choose foods each day from the Food Guide Pyramid.

One Serving Equals

Bread, Cereal, Rice and Pasta Group

> 1 slice of bread
> 1 ounce of ready-to-eat cereal
> ½ cup of cooked cereal, rice, or pasta

Vegetable Group

> 1 cup of raw leafy vegetables
> ½ cup of other vegetables-cooked or chopped raw
> 3/4 cup of vegetable juice

Fruit Group

> 1 medium apple, banana, or orange
> ½ cup of chopped, cooked, or canned fruit
> 3/4 cup of fruit juice

Milk, Yogurt and Cheese Group

1 cup of milk or yogurt
1 ½ ounces of natural cheese
2 ounces of processed cheese

Meat, Poultry, Fish, Dry Beans, Eggs and Nuts Group

2-3 ounces of cooked lean meat, poultry, or fish
½ cup of cooked dry beans or 1 egg counts as 1 ounce of lean
meat. Two tablespoons of peanut butter or 1/3 cup of nuts count
as 1 ounce of meat.

NOTE: A range of servings is given for each food group. The smaller
number is for people who consume about 1,600 calories a day, such
as sedentary women. The larger number is for those who consume
about 2,800 calories a day, such as active men.

Types of Diets

Fixed-menu diet. A fixed-menu diet provides a list of all the foods
you will eat. This kind of diet can be easy to follow because the foods
are selected for you. But, you get very few different food choices, which
may make the diet boring and hard to follow away from home. In
addition, fixed-menu diets do not teach the food selection skills necessary for keeping weight off. If you start with a fixed-menu diet, you
should switch eventually to a plan that helps you learn to make meal
choices on your own, such as an exchange-type diet.

Exchange-type diet. An exchange-type diet is a meal plan with
a set number of servings from each of several food groups. Within each
group, foods are about equal in calories and can be interchanged as
you wish. For example, the "starch" category could include one slice
of bread or ½ cup of oatmeal; each is about equal in nutritional value
and calories. If your meal plan calls for two starch choices at breakfast, you could choose to eat two slices of bread, or one slice of bread
and ½ cup of oatmeal. With the exchange-type diet plans, you have
more day-to-day variety and you can easily follow the diet away from
home. The most important advantage is that exchange-type diet plans
teach the food selection skills you need to keep your weight off.

Prepackaged-meal diet. These diets require you to buy prepack-
aged meals. Such meals may help you learn appropriate portion sizes.
However, they can be costly. Before beginning this type of program,

find out whether you will need to buy the meals and how much the meals cost. You should also find out whether the program will teach you how to select and prepare food, skills that are needed to sustain weight loss.

Formula diet. Formula diets are weight-loss plans that replace one or more meals with a liquid formula. Most formula diets are balanced diets containing a mix of protein, carbohydrate, and usually a small amount of fat. Formula diets are usually sold as liquid or a powder to be mixed with liquid. Although formula diets are easy to use and do promote short-term weight loss, most people regain the weight as soon as they stop using the formula. In addition, formula diets do not teach you how to make healthy food choices, a necessary skill for keeping your weight off.

Questionable diets. You should avoid any diet that suggests you eat a certain nutrient, food, or combination of foods to promote easy weight loss. Some of these diets may work in the short term because they are low in calories. However, they are often not well-balanced and may cause nutrient deficiencies. In addition, they do not teach eating habits that are important for long-term weight management.

Flexible diets. Some programs or books suggest monitoring fat only, calories only, or a combination of the two, with the individual making the choice of both the type and amount of food eaten. This flexible type of approach works well for many people, and teaches them how to control what they eat. One drawback of flexible diets is that some don't consider the total diet. For example, programs that monitor fat only often allow people to take in unlimited amounts of excess calories from sugars, and therefore don't lead to weight loss.

It is important to choose an eating plan that you can live with. The plan should also teach you how to select and prepare healthy foods, as well as how to maintain your new weight. Remember that many people tend to regain lost weight. Eating a healthful and nutritious diet to maintain your new weight, combined with regular physical activity, helps to prevent weight regain.

Physical Activity

Regular physical activity is important to help you lose weight and build an overall healthy lifestyle. Physical activity increases the number of calories your body uses and promotes the loss of body fat instead of muscle and other nonfat tissue. Research shows that people who include physical activity in their weight-loss programs are more likely to keep their weight off than people who only change their diet. In addition to promoting weight control, physical activity improves your strength and flexibility, lowers your risk of heart disease, helps control blood pressure and diabetes, can promote a sense of well-being, and can decrease stress.

Any type of physical activity you choose to do—vigorous activities such as running or aerobic dancing or moderate-intensity activities such as walking or household work—will increase the number of calories your body uses. The key to successful weight control and improved overall health is making physical activity a part of your daily life.

For the greatest overall health benefits, experts recommend that you do 20 to 30 minutes of vigorous physical activity three or more times a week and some type of muscle strengthening activity, such as weight resistance, and stretching at least twice a week. However, if you are unable to do this level of activity, you can improve your health by performing 30 minutes or more of moderate-intensity physical activity over the course of a day, at least five times a week. When including physical activity in your weight-loss program, you should choose a variety of activities that can be done regularly and are enjoyable for you. Also, if you have not been physically active, you should see your doctor before you start, especially if you are older than 40 years of age, very overweight, or have medical problems. A fact sheet on physical activity and weight control is available from WIN.

Vigorous Activities

- aerobic dancing
- running
- brisk walking
- cycling
- swimming

Moderate-Intensity Activities

- walking up the stairs instead of taking the elevator
- walking part or all of the way to work
- using a push mower to cut the grass
- playing actively with children

Behavior Change

Behavior change focuses on learning eating and physical activity behaviors that will help you lose weight and keep it off. The first step is to look at your eating and physical activity habits, thus uncovering behaviors (such as television watching) that lead you to overeat or be inactive. Next you'll need to learn how to change those behaviors.

Getting support from others is a good way to help you maintain your new eating and physical activity habits. Changing your eating and physical activity behaviors increases your chances of losing weight and keeping it off. For additional information on behavior change, you may wish to ask a weight-loss counselor or refer to books on this topic, which are available in local libraries.

What Works for You?

A variety of options exists to help you lose weight and keep it off. The key to successful weight loss is making changes in your eating and physical activity habits that you will be able to maintain for the rest of your life.

Additional Reading

"Binge-Eating Disorder." NIH Publication No. 94-3589. This fact sheet describes the symptoms, causes, complications, and treatment of binge-eating disorder, along with a profile of those at risk for the disorder. 1993. Available from WIN.

"Dieting and Gallstones." NIH Publication No. 94-3677. This fact sheet describes what gallstones are, how weight loss may cause them, and how to lessen the risk of developing them. 1993. Available from WIN.

"Gastric Surgery for Severe Obesity." NIH Publication No. 96-4006. This fact sheet describes the different types of surgery available to treat severe obesity. It explains how gastric surgery promotes weight loss and the benefits and risks of each procedure. 1996. Available from WIN.

"Physical Activity and Weight Control." NIH Publication No. 964031. This fact sheet explains how physical activity helps promote weight control and other ways it benefits one's health. It also describes the different types of physical activity and provides tips on how to become more physically active. 1996. Available from WIN.

"Prescription Medications for the Treatment of Obesity." NIH Publication No. 97-4191. This fact sheet presents information on appetite suppressant medications. These medications may help some obese patients lose more weight than with non-drug treatments. The types of medications and the risks and benefits associated with the use of these medications are described. Revised 1997. Available from WIN.

"Very Low-Calorie Diets." NIH Publication No. 95-3894. Information on who should use a very low-calorie diet (VLCD) and the health benefits and possible adverse effects of VLCDs is provided in this fact sheet. 1995. Available from WIN.

"Weight Cycling." NIH Publication No. 95-3901. Based on research, this fact sheet describes the health effects of weight cycling, also known as "yo-yo" dieting, and how it affects obese individuals' future weight-loss efforts. 1995. Available from WIN.

"Are You Eating Right?" *Consumer Reports*. October 1992, pp. 644-55. This article summarizes advice from 68 nutrition experts, including a discussion on weight control and health risks of obesity. Available from WIN.

"Losing Weight: What Works. What Doesn't" and "Rating the Diets." *Consumer Reports*. June 1993, pp. 347-57. These articles report on a survey of readers' experiences with weight-loss diets, discuss research related to weight control, and outline pros and cons of different diet programs. Available in public libraries.

"The Facts About Weight-Loss Products and Programs." DHHS Publication No. (FDA) 92-1189. This pamphlet provides basic facts about the weight-loss industry and what the consumer should expect from a diet program and/or product. Available from the Food and Drug Administration, Office of Consumer Affairs, HFE-88, Rockville, MD 20857.

Nutrition and Your Health: Dietary Guidelines for Americans, Fourth Edition. Home and Garden Bulletin No. 232. 1995. This booklet answers some of the basic questions about healthy eating and the link between poor nutrition and disease. It stresses the importance of a balanced diet and a healthy lifestyle. Available from WIN.

A Report of the Surgeon General: Physical Activity and Health. 1996. Produced by the Centers for Disease Control and Prevention, this report compiles decades of research concerning physical activity and health. It addresses the nationwide health problems associated with physical inactivity and outlines the benefits of becoming more physically active. Available for $19.00 from the U.S. Government Printing Office, Superintendent of Documents, Washington, DC 20402; (202) 512-1800. Stock Number 017-023-00196-5.

Weight-Control Information Network

The Weight-Control Information Network (WIN) is a service of the National Institute of Diabetes and Digestive and Kidney Diseases, part of the National Institutes of Health, under the U.S. Public Health Service. Authorized by Congress (Public Law 103-43), WIN assembles and disseminates to health professionals and the general public information on weight control, obesity, and nutritional disorders. WIN responds to requests for information; develops, reviews, and distributes publications; and develops communication strategies to encourage individuals to achieve and maintain a healthy weight.

Publications produced by WIN are reviewed for scientific accuracy, content, and readability. Materials produced by other sources are also reviewed for scientific accuracy and are distributed, along with WIN publications, to answer requests.

Weight-control Information Network
1 WIN Way
Bethesda, MD 20892-3665
(202) 828-1025
FAX: (202) 828-1028
Website: http://www.niddk.nih.gov/health/nutrit/win.htm
Toll-free number: (877) 946-4627

Part Three

Fitness for Specific Groups of People

Chapter 14

Physical Activity and Well-Being at Different Life Stages

Regular physical activity is important throughout the life cycle, from childhood to old age. In the young child, the main effects are upon attitudes and habit formation. During adolescence, intensity often increases, which results in more physical risks but also counters developing cardiac risk factors. In adult life, benefits shift to the prevention of work loss and premature death from chronic disease. Finally, in old age, exercise conserves function and improves the quality of life.

Childhood (5-12 Years)

Quality physical education programs should expose the child to a good balance of sports and individual activities, including pursuits that involve the family. Curtailment of the academic timetable to allow a daily hour of required physical education does not have an adverse effect upon learning, at least in primary school (Shephard, Lavallee, Voilc, LaBarre, & Beaucage, 1994). Indeed, an enhancement of self-image and a relief of boredom may enhance classroom performance.

Aerobic power, expressed in milliliters per kilogram per minute, often deteriorates over the course of schooling (Bailey, 1974). Older

From *Research Quarterly for Exercise and Sport*, December 1995, vol. 66, no. 4, p. 298(5).© 1995 American Alliance for Health, Physical Education, Recreation and Dance. Reprinted with permission of *Research Quarterly for Exercise and Sport*.

children may also show a number of cardiac risk factors. These can be reversed immediately by vigorous activity, but it is less certain how far such benefits track from childhood to adult life (Despres, Bouchard, & Malina, 1990; Raitakari et al., 1994). The main arguments for encouraging children to engage in regular physical activity are the establishment of good health habits (Godin, Valois, Shephard, & Desharnais, 1987) and the avoidance of smoking and drug abuse (Verschuur, 1987). Potential adverse consequences of required physical education and structured sport include (a) the creation of negative attitudes through poor teaching or lack of success in competition (Ilmarinen & Rutenfranz, 1980); (b) traumatic and overuse injuries involving the epiphyses (Grogan & Bobechko, 1984; Torg, 1995); and (c) very rarely, deaths due to injury or undetected cardiovascular disease (Mueller & Cantu, 1990).

Adolescence (13-19 Years)

For those who continue to participate, the intensity of physical activity is commonly higher for an adolescent than it is for a child, and there is a correspondingly greater tendency for reductions in cardiac risk factors to persist and track into adult life (Kemper, Storm van-Essen, & Verschuur, 1989). However, growing freedom and lack of experience increase the dangers of the more adventurous activities. Although participation in physical activity can lead to character development (Shields & Bredemeier, 1995), abuse of performance-enhancing drugs (Radakovich, Broderick, & Pickell, 1993) and a philosophy of "winning at all costs" can have a negative effect on ethical development. Attempts to induce substantial weight loss in wrestlers (Webster, Rutt, & Weltman, 1990) and the preparation for competitions that are judged partly on physical appearance (Slavin, 1985) sometimes progress to dangerous anorexia and/or bulimia. Excessive physical activity and a negative energy balance can also cause a reduction of bone calcium content that is hard to correct later in life (Drinkwater, 1994). Further, excessive time demands of athletic training can lead to a rapid rejection of both physical activity and a healthy lifestyle once high-level competition ceases (Astrand et al., 1963).

Adolescence shifts motivation for an active lifestyle from the parent or coach to the individual's peer group. Immediate stimuli and social benefits of exercise are valued, but long-term health gains are of little concern. There is need for further study of the long-term motivational effects of structured sport and physical education. Sometimes the influence is positive, but interest in activity can be lost once physical education is no longer a required subject (Ilmarinen & Rutenfranz, 1980). Motivation of the adolescent may be helped by linking physical activity to personal interests or to pursuits that can be followed as a family over the entire life span (Telama, 1991).

Adult Life (20-65 Years)

The health benefits of regular physical activity become more apparent upon entering adult life (Bouchard, Shephard, & Stephens, 1994). Self-reported data describe an immediate enhancement of work performance (Shephard, 1986, 1995), and psychometric measurements show a tendency toward relief of anxiety and enhancement of mood state, most obvious in the person who is initially depressed or anxious (Biddle, 1995; North, McCullagh, & Tran, 1990).

Regular physical activity also offers an effective long-term control of moderate obesity and plasma lipids. It elevates mood and conserves lean tissue relative to dieting alone (Shephard, 1994), although an excessive energy expenditure can itself cause lean tissue depletion. Further, the rise of core temperature and the secretion of catecholamines stimulate energy consumption postexercise, countering the depression of metabolism normally associated with a negative energy balance. Atherogenic lipoprotein levels are usually reduced, and high-density lipoprotein cholesterol levels are increased, provided that the training volume is adequate (for most people, the equivalent of a walking distance of 18-20 km/week; Williams, Wood, Haskell, & Vranizan, 1982). Further, the improved lipid profile is obtained without the complications that accompany some drug treatments, such as an increase in suicides and cancer deaths (Muldoon, Bonci, Rodriguez, Kaplan, & Manuck, 1994).

Vigorous exercise increases the immediate risk of sudden death, particularly if physical or emotional preparation for exercise is poor (Vuori, 1995b), but the person who is regularly active shows a 2- to 3-fold net reduction in the risk of both illness and premature death from cardiovascular disease (Powell, Thompson, Caspersen, & Kendrick, 1987). Regular exercise also reduces daytime blood pressures, both systolic and diastolic, by 5-10 mmHg (Tipton, 1991), although nighttime readings puzzlingly show little change. The daytime response matches that achieved by many drug regimens, with fewer complications. There may be an associated reduction in strokes (Kohl & McKenzie, 1994) and renal disease (Goldberg & Harter, 1994) among regular exercisers.

The control of obesity and exercise-induced increases in glucose metabolism decrease the risk of developing Type II diabetes mellitus and reduce insulin needs in established cases (Gudat, Berger, & Lefebvre, 1994). Nevertheless, if the diabetes is advanced, peripheral neuropathy, skin lesions, and possible detachment of the retina require a cautious approach to exercise. The risk of certain types of cancer (particularly tumors of the transverse and descending colon) is substantially reduced in regular exercisers (Lee, 1995; Shephard, 1993). Possible cancer-preventing mechanisms include increased colonic motility, suppression of estrogen production, the control of obesity, and enhanced immune function. Regular resisted or weight-bearing exercise also increases bone density, reducing the risk of osteoporotic fractures in older adults (Drinkwater, 1994; Vuori, 1995a).

The impact of exercise upon other facets of lifestyle is smaller than is sometimes claimed, although involvement in endurance running sometimes helps to cure a cigarette addiction (Shephard, 1989). Finally, the adult who has little subcutaneous fat and above average aerobic power is a good surgical risk (Christensen, 1994).

In addition to the small risk that vigorous exercise will provoke myocardial infarction or sudden death, very heavy training can suppress natural killer cell activity, causing a temporary increase in vulnerability to infection (Brenner, Shek, & Shephard, 1994). The pursuit of adventurous forms of sport also carries continuing risks of severe injury and death. Other costs of exercise include investments in clothing, equipment, facilities, and leisure time (Shephard, 1986).

Old Age (65 Years and Greater)

Exercise programs for older adults must be matched to the initial capacity of the individual. Three categories of biological age are recognized: the young-old (typically aged 65-75 years), the middle-old (aged 75-85 years), and the very old (aged > 85 years; Shephard, 1987). Continuing involvement in regular exercise protects the older individual against most of the chronic diseases where benefit was noted earlier in adult life (Shephard, 1987). However, physical activity now has particular importance in preserving a sufficient margin of function to undertake the activities of daily living, thus conserving independence and avoiding institutionalization (Shephard, 1991). The reasons for institutionalization vary, but regular exercise can often temper this risk. Sometimes, regular training can reverse deteriorating mental function (Tomporowski & Ellis, 1986), although it is unclear whether the mechanism is an improvement of cerebral circulation, an avoidance of small strokes, or merely a maintenance of an overall interest in life. In other individuals, dependency is secondary to a medical catastrophe, such as the sudden onset of blindness or a major stroke. Again, exercise can sometimes avoid such incidents; for example, by protecting against diabetes or hypertension (Bouchard et al., 1994). Another cause of institutionalization is the sudden loss of a domestic caregiver, such as a spouse or child. Again, involvement in a group exercise program may provide the social support that will allow a person to cope with such a change in personal circumstances (Shephard, 1987).

Perhaps the most common basis for loss of independence is a simple deterioration of physical condition (Shephard, 1991). Maximal oxygen intake may have deteriorated to a level where simple aerobic tasks occupy an unacceptable fraction of aerobic power, leading to intolerable breathlessness. Quadriceps strength may be insufficient to lift the body mass from an armchair or a toilet seat. Flexibility may be insufficient to allow negotiation of steps, climbing into a car or a bath, or even dressing without assistance. Increased body sway and a loss of righting reflexes may lead to an increasing number of falls. And in all of these situations, regular exercise can enhance function to the point that a person can sustain independence for a further 10-20 years, with a substantial improvement in the quality of life, and thus the quality-adjusted life expectancy (Shephard, 1991).

Although regular physical activity protects against premature mortality, it has little influence upon unadjusted life expectancy in the middle-old and very old. The survival curves for active and sedentary individuals appear to converge around 80 years of age (Pekkanen et al., 1987) and, in the oldest age categories, the active person may have a slightly shorter life expectancy than someone who is sedentary. Thus, an active lifestyle helps a person to avoid the final 8-10 years of partial disability and 1 year of total dependency that seem the norm for a sedentary individual (Health & Welfare, Canada, 1982). Despite substantial information on the physiological benefits of physical activity for the middle-old and very old, there remains an urgent need to determine the most effective methods of encouraging exercise in those who are over 65 years of age.

Discussion

Too little attention has been given to the potential of exercise to replace or serve as an adjuvant to hormone replacement therapy in many of the conditions that develop or are exacerbated in the perimenopausal years: obesity, diabetes mellitus, depression, and osteoporosis. Physical activity programs also have particular importance in protecting the health of citizens in countries and subpopulations that are undergoing rapid modernization. In such situations, there has been a dramatic decline in habitual physical activity with the rapid appearance of diabetes mellitus and cardiovascular disease. There is currently an urgent need to introduce culturally appropriate voluntary activity programs to match the daily energy expenditures that formerly ensured the health of such populations (Rode & Shephard, 1995).

Physicians see most of their patients at least annually and see older adults on a more regular basis. They are thus an important potential vehicle for exercise promotion. But perhaps because of shortcomings in the medical curriculum, the average physician is not very familiar with techniques of prescribing exercise. Often this task is delegated to a specifically trained exercise physiologist. The physician rarely sees the successes of exercise therapy because such individuals remain well; medical advice is sought only for occasional complications, such as a traumatic fracture or an exercise-induced myocardial infarction. The physician thus gains a distorted view of the ratio of costs to benefits and may either neglect to offer advice on exercising or be excessively cautious about prescribing exercise.

Any therapeutic recommendation carries risks as well as benefits. A physician or surgeon usually has a personal stake in major surgery or a complicated pharmaceutical regimen. He or she thus gives considerable weight to the occasional "miracle" cure and tends to downplay the complications of such treatment. Further, too little attention is directed to the quality of any extension of life span that is achieved by conventional medical therapy. For example, the drug treatment for hyperlipidemia that is advocated by many nutritionists reduces the likelihood of sudden (and relatively "pleasant") cardiac deaths, but in some instances has replaced this outcome by suicidal depression or cancer, with no change in overall life expectancy, and a substantial deterioration in quality-adjusted life expectancy.

There remains an urgent need to complete detailed cost-effectiveness and cost-utility analyses where exercise prescription is compared with surgery and with drug therapy. Drug treatment and surgery have the tactical advantage of targeting the person who has advanced disease, but it seems likely that formal economic analyses will lead future generations of medical practitioners to learn more about exercise and to incorporate it more fully into their treatment plans.

Conclusions

1. Regular physical activity is important at all stages in the life cycle, from childhood to extreme old age.

2. School programs should include an adequate time allocation to quality programs of physical activity. Such initiatives are particularly important under the special conditions of developing urbanization in the Third World. Daily exercise can be incorporated into school curricula without compromising academic success. Habits are a potent determinant of future behavior, and although improved lifestyle does not always track from childhood to adult life, such programs have the potential to develop habits that will have a positive influence on adult lifestyle.

3. Regular exercise can enhance fitness and correct developing cardiac risk factors in adolescents. Steroid abuse, drastic weight loss, excessive training, and "winning at all costs" are concerns in organized sport programs for adolescents. Interventions should stress a diversity of activity experiences suitable for continuation in adult life.

4. Exercise programs enhance the work performance of adults and reduce the overall risk of many chronic diseases, particularly ischemic heart disease, hypertension, hyperlipidemia, obesity, maturity-onset diabetes, osteoporosis, and certain types of cancer. The risk of premature death is diminished by exercising, but excessive activity can cause injuries and predispose individuals to acute infections.

5. Exercise can be an effective alternative or adjuvant to hormone replacement therapy in treating such menopausal problems as obesity, diabetes mellitus, osteoporosis, and depression.

6. In old age, exercise does not extend the life span, but it does increase function, with major effects on biological age and thus on quality-adjusted life expectancy.

7. Physicians are an important potential vehicle for encouraging exercise, and they should be encouraged to include appropriate activity prescriptions in their treatment plans. This will require changes in medical curricula. Many physicians currently know little about exercise and are more familiar with its complications than with its benefits. Research is needed that compares cost-benefit ratios for exercise therapy relative to conventional medical and/or surgical treatment.

References

Astrand, P. O., Engstrom, L., Eriksson, B., Karlberg P., Nylander, I., Saltin, B., & Thoren, C. (1963). Girl swimmers, with particular reference to respiratory and circulatory adaptation and gynecological and psychiatric aspects. *Acta Paediatrica Scandinavica*, 147(Suppl.), 1-75.

Bailey, D. A. (1974). Exercise, fitness, and physical education for the growing child. In W. A. R. Orban (Ed.), *Proceedings of the National Conference on Fitness and Health* (pp. 13-22). Ottawa, Ontario, Canada: Health & Welfare, Canada.

Biddle, S. (1995). Exercise and psychosocial health. *Research Quarterly for Exercise and Sport*, 66, 292-297.

Bouchard, C., Shephard, R. J., & Stephens, T. (Eds.). (1994). *Physical activity, fitness, and health*. Champaign, IL: Human Kinetics.

Brenner, I., Shek, P. N., & Shephard, R. J. (1994). Infection in athletes. *Sports Medicine*, 17, 86-107.

Christensen, T. (1994). Physical activity, fitness, and recovery from surgical trauma. In C. Bouchard, R. J. Shephard, & T. Stephens (Eds.), *Physical activity, fitness, and health* (pp. 832-839). Champaign, IL: Human Kinetics.

Despres, J.P., Bouchard, C., & Malina, R. (1990). Physical activity and coronary heart disease risk factors during childhood and adolescence. *Exercise and Sport Sciences Reviews*, 18, 243-261.

Drinkwater, B. (1994). Physical activity, fitness and osteoporosis. In C. Bouchard, R. J. Shephard, & T. Stephens (Eds.), *Physical activity, fitness, and health* (pp. 724-736). Champaign; IL: Human Kinetics.

Godin, G., Valois, P., Shephard, R. J., & Desharnais, R. (1987). Prediction of leisure-time exercise behavior: A path analysis (LISREL V model). *Journal of Behavioral Medicine*, 10, 145-158.

Goldberg, A. P., & Harter, H. R. (1994). Physical activity, fitness, and kidney disease. In C. Bouchard, R. J. Shephard, & T. Stephens (Eds.), *Physical activity, fitness, and health* (pp. 762-773). Champaign, IL: Human Kinetics.

Grogan, D. P., & Bobechko, W. P. (1984). Pathogenesis of a fracture of the distal femoral epiphysis [Case report]. *Journal of Bone and Joint Surgery*, 66A, 621-622.

Gudat, U., Berger, M., & Lefebvre, P. (1994). Physical activity, fitness, and non-insulin dependent (Type II) diabetes mellitus. In C. Bouchard, R. J. Shephard, & T. Stephens (Eds.), *Physical activity, fitness, and health* (pp. 669-683). Champaign, IL: Human Kinetics.

Health & Welfare, Canada. (1982). *Canada Health Survey*. Ottawa, Ontario, Canada: Author.

Ilmarinen, J., & Rutenfranz, J. (1980). Longitudinal studies of the changes in habitual activity of schoolchildren and working adolescents. In K. Berg & B. O. Eriksson (Eds.), *Children and exercise IX* (pp. 149-159). Baltimore: University Park Press.

Kemper, H., Storm-van Essen, L., & Verschuur, R. (1989). Tracking of risk indicators for coronary heart disease from teenager to adult: The Amsterdam growth and health study. In S. Oseid & H. K. Carlsen (Eds.), *Children and exercise XIII* (pp. 235-245). Champaign, IL: Human Kinetics.

Kohl, H. W., & McKenzie, J. D. (1994). Physical activity, fitness, and stroke. In C. Bouchard, R. J. Shephard, & T. Stephens (Eds.), *Physical activity, fitness, and health* (pp. 609-621). Champaign, IL: Human Kinetics.

Lee, I.M. (1995). Exercise and physical health: Cancer and immune function. *Research Quarterly for Exercise and Sport*, 66, 286-291.

Mueller, F. O., & Cantu, R. C. (1990). Catastrophic injuries in high school and college sports, Fall 1982–Spring 1988. *Medicine and Science in Sports and Exercise*, 22, 737-741.

Muldoon, M. F., Bonci, L. J., Rodriguez, V., Kaplan, J. R., & Manuck, S. B. (1994). Health effects of serum cholesterol reduction: The potential for good and the potential for harm. *Medicine, Exercise, Nutrition, and Health*, 3, 74-90.

North, T. C., McCullagh, P., & Tran, Z. V. (1990). Effect of exercise on depression. *Exercise and Sport Sciences Reviews*, 18, 379-415.

Pekkanen, J., Marti, B., Nissinen, A., Tuomilehto, J., Punsar, S., & Karvonen, M. (1987). Reduction of premature mortality by high physical activity: A 20-year follow-up of middle-aged Finnish men. *Lancet*, i, 1473-1477.

Powell, K. E., Thompson, P. D., Caspersen, C. J., & Kendrick, J. S. (1987). Physical activity and the incidence of coronary heart disease. *Annual Reviews of Public Health*, 8, 253-287.

Radakovich, J., Broderick, P., & Pickell, G. (1993). Rate of anabolic-androgenic steroid use among students in junior high school. *Journal of the American Board of Family Practitioners*, 6, 341-345.

Raitakari, O. T., Parkka, K. V. K., Taimela, S., Telama, R., Rasanen, L., & Viikari, J. S. A. (1994). Effects of persistent physical activity and inactivity on coronary risk factors. *American Journal of Epidemiology*, 140, 195-205.

Rode, A., & Shephard, R. J. (1995). *"Modernization" and the health of the circumpolar peoples*. London: Cambridge University Press.

Shephard, R. J. (1986). *Economic benefits of enhanced physical activity*. Champaign, IL: Human Kinetics.

Shephard, R. J. (1987). *Physical activity and aging (2nd ed.)*. London: Croom Helm.

Shephard, R. J. (1989). Exercise and lifestyle change. *British Journal of Sports Medicine*, 23, 11-22.

Shephard, R. J. (1991). Fitness and aging. In C. Blais (Ed.), *Aging into the twenty first century* (pp. 22-35). North York, Ontario, Canada: Captus Publications.

Shephard, R. J. (1993). Exercise in the prevention and treatment of cancer: An update. *Sports Medicine*, 15, 258-280.

Shephard, R. J. (1994). Physical activity and reduction of health risks. How far are the benefits independent of fat loss? *Journal of Sports Medicine and Physical Fitness*, 34, 91-98.

Shephard, R. J. (1995). Worksite health promotion and productivity. In R. Kaman (Ed.), *Worksite health promotion economics* (pp. 147-173). Champaign, IL: Human Kinetics.

Shephard, R. J., Lavallee, H., Volle, M., LaBarre, R., & Beaucage, C. (1994). Academic skills and required physical education: The Trois Rivieres experience. *CAHPER Research Supplement*, 1(1), 1-12.

Shields, D. L. L., & Bredemeier, B. J. L. (1995). *Character development and physical activity*. Champaign, IL: Human Kinetics.

Slavin, J. L. (1985). Eating disorders in women athletes. In J. Puhl, C. H. Brown, & R. O. Voy (Eds.), *Sport science perspectives for women* (pp. 189-197). Champaign, IL: Human Kinetics.

Telama, R. (1991). Nature as motivation for physical activity. In P. Oja & R. Telama (Eds.), *Sport for all* (pp. 607-616). Amsterdam: Elsevier.

Tipton, C. M: (1991). Exercise, training, and hypertension: An update. *Exercise and Sport Sciences Reviews*, 19, 447-506.

Tomporowski, P. D., & Ellis, N. R. (1986). Effects of exercise on cognitive processes: A review. *Psychological Bulletin*, 99, 338-346.

Torg, J. S. (1995). Little league elbow. In J. Torg & R. J. Shephard (Eds.), *Current therapy in sports medicine* (3rd ed., pp. 104-105). Philadelphia: Mosby.

Verschuur, R. (1987). *Daily physical activity and health*. Haarlem, The Netherlands: Uitgeverij de Vrieseborch.

Vuori, I. (1995a). Exercise and physical health: Musculoskeletal health and functional capabilities. *Research Quarterly for Exercise and Sport*, 66, 276-285.

Vuori, I. (1995b). Sudden death and exercise: Effects of age and type of activity. *Sports Science Reviews*, 4, 46-84.

Webster, S., Rutt, R., & Weltman, A. (1990). Physiological effects of a weight loss regimen practiced by college wrestlers. *Medicine and Science in Sports and Exercise*, 22, 229-234.

Williams, P. T., Wood, P. D., Haskell, W. L., & Vranizan, K. (1982). The effects of running mileage and duration on plasma lipoprotein levels. *Journal of the American Medical Association*, 247, 2672-2679.

Author's Notes

The author's research is supported in part by a research grant from Canadian Tire Acceptance Limited. Correspondence concerning this article should be addressed to Roy J. Shephard, MD, PhD, DPE, School of Physical and Health Education, University of Toronto, 320 Huron Street, Toronto, Ontario, Canada M5S 1A1.

— by Roy J. Shephard

Roy J. Shephard is a professor emeritus of applied physiology in the School of Physical and Health Education at the University of Toronto and a professor in the Department of Preventive Medicine and Biostatistics in the Faculty of Medicine at the University of Toronto. He is also the Canadian Tire Acceptance Limited Resident Scholar in Health Studies at Brock University in St. Catharines, Ontario, Canada.

Chapter 15

Fitness for Kids

Contents

Section 15.1

Children's Sedentary Lifestyle a Forerunner of Unhealthy Adulthood

From *USA Today* (Magazine), May 1998, vol. 126, no. 2636, p. 58(2). © 1998
Society for the Advancement of Education; reprinted with permission.

The 1996 Surgeon General's Report on Physical Activity and Health provides considerable evidence that regular physical activity dramatically can improve health and quality of life. Among the findings are that physical activity reduces the risks of coronary heart disease, hypertension, diabetes, and premature death. In addition, it lessens feelings of anxiety and depression; helps control body weight; maintains healthy bones, muscles, and joints; and promotes psychological well-being. There also is evidence that regular physical activity significantly reduces the risk of breast cancer.

In spite of these widely recognized benefits, 75% of American adolescents and young adults do not engage in daily light to moderate activity. Of particular concern is that participation in all types of physical activity declines sharply as children get older, particularly for females. Moreover, several studies investigating health-related fitness levels of elementary school pupils have suggested that American youngsters are consistently below desirable fitness standards. Although recent evidence suggests that the "youth fitness crisis" may be exaggerated, it is clear that the fitness levels of young children have declined over the past 20 years. More specifically, research suggests that cardiovascular fitness has decreased and percentage of body fat has increased over the past two decades.

At least 25% of elementary school pupils are above desirable weight standards, and that figure is rising steadily. This finding may not be surprising in light of the fact that kids aged six through eleven watch television about 25 hours per week. Of particular concern is the fact that several researchers have demonstrated that unfit and overweight youngsters show early signs of coronary heart disease, high cholesterol levels, and elevated blood pressure. In fact, 40% of children aged five through eight have at least one heart disease risk factor.

If there is a primary target for intervention, it is during the early school years. The development of positive attitudes toward physical activity and fitness during childhood may have a positive impact on the level of physical activity during adult life. There is evidence that activities learned at a young age contribute to healthy lifestyles. For these reasons, several professional organizations have directed their attention toward early childhood intervention.

Two primary objectives identified in the U.S. Public Health Service's 1992 program, Healthy Children 2000, were to increase youngsters' physical activity and raise the number participating in daily physical education. More recently, the Surgeon General's 1996 report recommended targeting elementary school physical education to increase children's physical activity. Similarly, the President's Council on Physical Fitness and Sports suggested that same year that elementary schools provide activity opportunities before or after school in an effort to help kids develop lifetime habits. These goals, however, are not being achieved, as less than 20% of elementary school pupils participate in daily school physical education.

Until recently, researchers knew very little about proper exercise guidelines for children. For this reason, adult exercise prescriptions focusing on high-intensity and sustained physical activity were applied to youngsters. Studies clearly indicate that this is not appropriate. They found that children do raise their heart rates into the appropriate target zone, but not for the 20-minute criterion recommended for adults.

Even though kids are not continuously active, they still accumulate far more minutes of activity than teenagers or adults do. In light of these findings, experts now recommend that children be encouraged to participate in high-volume, moderate-intensity activity and accumulate 30-60 minutes of exertion each day.

These recommendations make the challenge of enhancing health-related fitness in children a bit more attainable. Using the 1990 American College of Sports Medicine guidelines in terms of duration (20 minutes of continuous activity), frequency (three times a week), and intensity (moderate to vigorous), few children could attain these goals. The revised recommendations of 30-60 minutes of moderate-intensity exercising makes it possible for parents and teachers to plan developmentally appropriate activities that promote health-related fitness.

Changing Behavior

Although increasing physical activity levels is a worthwhile goal of physical education class and after-school programs, activity without behavioral change is not enough. Children must learn about the benefits of regular physical activity and enjoy the process of attaining them. One way to achieve the goals of increasing their activity level and knowledge about health-related fitness is through quality daily physical education.

There are indications that elementary school students who take physical education classes five times a week might be more fit than those who have class the usual two times per week. Data from a recent study show that those who participate in daily physical education (150 minutes a week) receive enough moderate to vigorous activity to achieve desirable fitness levels, whereas those participating in weekly gym classes (60 minutes a week) do not.

As part of the study, a national fitness test was administered to 434 students in grades one to five. Results revealed that daily physical education participants were superior on all four of the test items (mile run, body composition, sit and reach, and sit-ups) across the five grades. Furthermore, a comparison of the results to national norms showed the daily exercise participants generally to be above the 50th or 75th percentile and the weekly participants to be below the 50th or 25th percentile. When these same students entered a middle school program that offered gym only twice weekly, their cardiovascular endurance decreased significantly after one year of participation.

These results provide strong support for a switch to daily physical education instruction. While this would help to avert the national crisis in children's health, there is stiff resistance to changing to a five-day program. Lack of funding is a key problem. Many school districts are struggling to keep enough gym teachers employed for the twice-a-week classes. Moreover, experts in other curriculum areas such as art and music are pushing for the same type of daily instruction.

A second way to achieve the goal of increasing children's activity levels is to offer after-school programs that are both enjoyable and non-competitive. Such initiatives should provide time-on-task games and activities that allow children to exercise in a target heart rate zone for the majority of the sessions. Perpetual tag games, scavenger hunts, swimming, and obstacle courses where everyone participates are far superior to more competitive games that might leave a child bored in right field or inactive on the bench.

One example is the Ball State Fit Kids Program in Muncie, Indiana. It consists of a variety of running games, water and step aerobics, and team-building activities. Muscular strength and flexibility are included as well. The heart rate intensity goal of each session is set at 150-200, and children are encouraged to stay in this target zone as much as possible. Specific goals of this after-school program are to increase youngsters' physical activity levels and develop self-management skills necessary for an active lifestyle.

One way that children learn about the benefits of activity is through the use of heart rate monitors. These consist of a chest strap with a transmitter and a wrist monitor that continuously displays the heart rate. The data can be transferred to a personal computer and printed for the wearer to review. Since each youngster receives continuous feedback about the intensity of the activity, there is the opportunity to learn a great deal about self-regulating of the workout intensity to stay within the target heart rate zone.

In addition, the heart rate monitor provides specific feedback about the principles of exercise such as resting heart rate, exercise heart rate, recovery heart rate, and target heart rate zone. These benefits are especially important for the low-fit child. Experts recommended that the 25% of kids who are at risk because of low fitness should be identified and programs to help them improve should be implemented.

Preliminary findings suggest the Ball State initiative has been successful as participants exercise in their target heart rate zone about 70% of the hour-long session each day. On program days, therefore, they meet the daily physical activity recommendations of 30-60 minutes. The monitors appear to be a motivating force since the children set individual heart rate goals on each Monday of the program and do their best to attain them by checking their watches regularly. Mile-run times tend to improve significantly over the 10-week sessions. Perhaps more importantly, feedback from parents, teachers, and the children themselves indicate that the program has been successful in educating youngsters about the important benefits of daily physical activity.

Whether or not these benefits will produce a permanent change in activity levels remains to be seen. Certainly, parents must become involved in the process of teaching their offspring about the importance of healthy lifestyles. The schools and after-school programs cannot be depended upon totally to regulate children's activity patterns. Parents, relatives, and friends can help by taking walks with kids or playing goal-oriented games that enhance self-esteem. Youngsters need to see an active lifestyle to develop one.

— by Arlene Ignico

Section 15.2

A Parent's Guide to Fitness for Kids Who Hate Sports

From KidsHealth at http://www.kidshealth.org. Copyright 2000. The Nemours Foundation. Used with permission.

Eight-year-old Bradley is a terror on the ice—he lives for hockey practice and spends much of his free time at home slapping a puck around in the driveway. But Bradley's 10-year-old brother, Michael, has no interest in hockey or in any organized sports. He would rather be in his room with a book or riding his bike around the park than playing hockey or basketball with his friends.

The boys' parents worry about Michael's lack of interest in team sports, but do they really have anything to be concerned about? Read this section to find out how you can help to promote fitness in a child who dislikes team sports.

Why Does My Child Hate Sports?

If your child isn't interested in team sports, you should attempt to get to the root of the issue rather than force her to join a team. Kids may not want to participate in sports for many reasons—some of them physical, others emotional.

Children who are physically self-conscious or who feel different from their peers may feel uncomfortable about participating in team activities. Whether this difference is real or imagined, it may lead to self-esteem and body image problems.

Fear of failure or public embarrassment—as well as fear of letting their parents down—can also make some children reluctant to play team sports. Other children may lack, or believe they lack, the grace or coordination needed to succeed at a particular sport. They may also be afraid of injury or may simply be cautious by nature.

Some children, like many adults, may just not be interested in team sports, but they can still maintain an excellent level of fitness by engaging in other activities that don't emphasize competition. As long

198

as your child does not become sedentary, there's no reason to worry if she resists joining organized sports activities.

Encourage your child to take up lifelong activities like cycling or running—activities that can promote fitness on an individual, non-competitive level, suggests Michael Stanwood, PT, ATC, coordinator of sports medicine at the Alfred I. duPont Hospital for Children in Wilmington, Delaware. He also suggests sports such as wrestling or tennis. "Wrestling takes place one on one, but the participants still earn team points."

Ruling out Any Problems

Before beginning any sports or fitness program, your child should have a physical examination by her doctor. Children with undiagnosed medical conditions, vision or hearing problems, or other disorders may have difficulty participating in certain activities. If your child shows uncharacteristic resistance to a particular activity or sudden reluctance to participate in a sport that she previously enjoyed, a visit to her doctor may be in order to rule out any health problems that may be hindering her enjoyment and performance.

Can I Help My Child Learn to Like Sports?

Although you should share your interests with your child, it's never a good idea to force your child into an activity just because you once excelled in it. In fact, many children may worry that they won't be able to measure up to the success their parents once enjoyed playing a particular sport. Your child needs to know that although you would love to share your love of softball or basketball with her, it would be equally acceptable if she would rather play golf or tennis, or take up gymnastics or karate.

You should also keep your expectations realistic: Most children never make it to the city finals or become Olympic medalists no matter how hard they try. The ultimate goal is to help and encourage your child to become fit, healthy, and happy.

Parents should try to remain open-minded about their child's chosen sport. For example, it's possible that your child may enjoy a sports activity that is not offered at her school or that is not offered for girls. If your child wants to try football or ice hockey, help her find a local league or talk to school officials about starting up a new team. Boys may prefer figure skating or ballet. Let your kids know that no matter which sport they choose, they have your support.

199

You'll also need to be patient with your child if she has difficulty choosing and sticking to an activity. It often takes several tries before a child finds an activity with which she feels comfortable.

Even if your child never belongs to a sports team, there are many other areas of her life where she can learn important skills like teamwork, competition, and cooperation. Clubs, school and volunteer activities, band or music lessons, acting or debating groups, and many other activities teach children to work and get along with others. Fortunately, there are also many alternative ways to keep fit and active other than organized sports.

What Activities Can My Child Do to Stay Fit?

Many children choose not to join teams, and prefer activities that can be done alone or with friends. Suggested fitness alternatives include:

- cycling
- horseback riding
- in-line skating
- skateboarding
- martial arts

- swimming
- dancing
- running
- hiking

These activities help children build self-esteem, strength, coordination, and general fitness.

How Can I Be a Good Fitness Role Model for My Child?

Parents who live sedentary lifestyles may have a hard time motivating their children to stay fit. Try to make exercise a part of your family life by finding fun fitness activities that the whole family can do together, such as swimming, cycling, canoeing, tennis, nature hikes, or walks with the family dog.

Maintain a positive attitude toward exercise and physical activity—be careful not to treat it as a punishment or a chore.

Encourage your child to come up with creative suggestions for family fitness activities; she will be more likely to enjoy an activity if she has a role in planning it.

Parents who attend regular fitness classes or work out at a gym may find it fairly easy to be good fitness role models. Although Stanwood recommends that children under the age of 12 or 13 not get involved in weight training, many gyms offer activities that may interest older children. Some gyms and community centers also offer "Mommy and Me" classes, which introduce fitness to toddlers and preschoolers.

Finally, emphasize the importance of having both a healthy mind and a healthy body, and make it clear to your child that physical activity is an integral part of daily life. By creating a supportive environment, acting as a positive role model, and providing your child with a wide range of fitness choices, you can help your child develop good habits that will last a lifetime.

Chapter 16

Fitness and Exercise for Teens

Contents

Section 16.1

Looking Good

From *Current Health 2*, September 1996, vol. 23, no. 1, p. 22(2). © 1996 Weekly Reader Corporation; reprinted with permission.

You look in every mirror you pass to make sure you haven't gained any weight. You're sure that if you lose 10 pounds, all your problem is will go away. You know that the actors and actresses on television and the models in magazines have what seem like "ideal bodies."

But no one has a "perfect body." Everyone, however, can look good—and feel good.

Instead of striving for the perfect body, make your goal that of being physically fit. Your image of your body will improve along with your fitness.

Forget the "thin is fit" myth. Thin is not necessarily fit nor ideal. Weight loss is not the most important factor in improving body image.

Physical fitness has more to do with how well you can perform certain physical activities than with how much you weigh. A physically fit person has good endurance, strength, and heart and lung capacity.

The body of a fit person turns fat tissue into muscle tissue. Muscles weigh more than fat because they are denser. Muscles need more calories than fat. As you start getting more muscle tissue, you'll find you can eat more without gaining weight.

How Do You Get Fit?

The American College of Sports Medicine recommends some physical activities every day, and vigorous activities for 20 to 30 minutes three or four times a week. While most teens claim they do an hour a day of physical activity, a 1994 study found that only about 50 percent of the boys and 25 percent of the girls exercise vigorously. One study showed that as teens get older, they exercise less.

You may walk to school every day, but unless you're doing four to five miles per hour for a half hour, you can't count it as the kind of vigorous exercise you get with activities such as brisk walking, jogging, basketball, racquet sports, dance, swimming laps, skating, bicycling, and strength (resistance) training. All these activities get you moving quickly and breathing hard for sustained periods of time.

One way to tell if you're exercising hard enough is to check your target heart rate. To get your target heart rate, subtract your age from 220, and multiply that number by .65 and .85 (example: 220 - 16 = 204 x .65 = 133; 204 x .85 = 173.) For a maximum workout that burns fat, your pulse rate should be between those numbers.

Do something you like. Let's face it: doing something you hate will only encourage you to avoid exercise. Catch up on the latest news while you and a friend jog together. If you're alone, doing a variety of activities will keep you from getting bored and will exercise different muscles.

Carrie Sowiak, athletic director of The Oxford Club in Denver, Colorado, recommends weight training to increase your percentage of muscle. Muscle tissue demands energy and increases your metabolism (the rate at which you burn calories).

Carrie has found that once teens start developing muscle and upper body strength, they don't worry about losing weight. The muscle definition makes them look better, and they have a new body image.

Be sure you get instruction in weight training. If you don't use the correct techniques, you can tear or strain your muscles. Carrie recommends a trainer who has a degree in a health-related field and is also certified by an accredited organization such as the American College of Sports Medicine.

Some of your exercises should be aerobic—activities that use a lot of oxygen such as jogging, bicycling, dancing, and swimming. If you haven't done the activity before, start slowly and build up to longer times and greater distance over a period of weeks. Always start your session with some stretches to give your muscles a chance to warm up, and end with a few minutes of slower exercises and stretches to cool down.

Do, Not Overdo

Avoid the "weekend athlete syndrome," saving up your daily exercise and spending it all on the weekends. If you do, you're likely to set yourself up for a sports injury. You'll want to set up a program that will strengthen you for your chosen weekend activity.

On the other hand, don't overdo exercise. Some teens decide that more is better and start exercising every spare minute. Soon they're obsessed with the idea of going longer distances and losing more weight.

Some of the signs that you are overdoing things are weighing yourself every day, or seeing yourself as fat no matter how much you weigh. You need some fat to provide insulation and store energy.

Get off to a good start this school year—get moving. Exercise is great. A regular exercise program can help you tone muscles and get in shape. You'll feel better—and look good, too.

—by Carolyn Gard

Section 16.2

Running for Brain Power

From *Current Health 2*, October 1995, vol. 22, no. 2, p. 22(2). © 1995 Weekly Reader Corporation; reprinted with permission.

Have you ever heard the phrase "jog your memory"? There's more to it than just an old cliche. Imagine yourself taking a history test. You've studied for weeks and know the textbook backward and forward. You even know which page talks about the civil war. But then, your mind draws a blank. You can't think of the answer to the next question. What do you do?

If you're like most people, you'll try different ways to "jog your memory." You might try to picture the page and the words in your mind. You might try to think of something that's associated with the same topic. You might even try to think of where you were when you studied that question. These are some ways to try to trigger a memory. But did you know that jogging (really running and working up a sweat) can actually benefit your memory as well as your intelligence?

Exercise stimulates the growth of developing brains. Dan Landers, Ph.D., looked at 13 different studies, and in each one, students under 16 years old showed the greatest link between exercise and brain power. In fact, these studies indicate that young people who exercise regularly become smarter than those who don't. And that goes for older people too. Professor Brad Hatfield found that men who did aerobic activities (exercise that really gets your heart and lungs working for at least 20 minutes) did much better in math and in concentration than men who didn't work out regularly.

More Oxygen, Higher IQ?

Now what about that history test that has you stumped? Dr. Roy J. Shephard found that young people who jog or do other aerobic activities for an hour each day did better on their school tests than those who were less active. Studies are now finding that there is a direct link between fitness and intelligence. So why is it that going out for a jog not only works your heart and lungs but your mind too? It's simple: The answer is oxygen! When you expand the heart and lungs, your body is able to take in more oxygen. The brain depends on oxygen to function properly, and a healthy heart gets more oxygen to the brain. Robert Dustman, Ph.D., acknowledges this vital link to the brain: "Improve your heart and lungs and you get smarter." Scott Hinkle and Bruce Tuckman tested students in fourth, fifth, sixth, and eighth grades. Half of each group ran for a semester and the other half didn't. The kids who ran showed greater gains on their end-of-the-semester creativity tests than those who didn't run.

So when you can't figure out the right answer for your history test, don't get too bummed out. Go for a jog! Jogging actually makes you feel better. It can help clear your mind of worries, which can free you up to think of new strategies for problem solving. In fact, more doctors are becoming aware of the benefits jogging can have on changing moods. Some even prescribe exercise programs for people who are depressed. Higher amounts of the hormone called noradrenaline are found in people who run regularly. This hormone helps to put you in a better mood. Some people who once needed drugs to feel better are now exercising instead. Regular exercise is a natural, drug-free way to better health and self-esteem. When you're feeling down, go for a jog and feel the difference!

If You Think You Can

Picture yourself winning a race, making every free throw you attempt, kicking field goal after field goal. Does this sound impossible? Thinking it is actually the first step in doing it. On May 11, 1995, the American Academy of Neurology met in Seattle, Washington. Dr. Alvaro Pascual-Leone explained his research on mental practice. He studied three groups of people: one that practiced a physical skill, one that visualized themselves doing the activity, and one that practiced both physically and mentally. The group that had the best performance improvement after five days was the group that practiced the activity both physically and mentally. He found that this was true for any skill needing rehearsal, not just sports activities. If you are going to give a speech or perform music or drama, mental practice can make dramatic improvements.

A Win-Win Situation

Working the body to help the mind perform and working the mind to help the body is a win-win situation. Exercise helps you feel better about yourself and shapes up your body. Jogging can escalate your creativity, chase the blues away, and elevate your IQ. It's a total body workout. Remember: "Practice makes perfect." Imagine yourself running and doing well on a run. But don't stop there. Imagine yourself doing other things too, and doing them well.

For More Information

Brochure: "An Introduction to Running: One Step at a Time," single copy free. Write to:

President's Council on Physical Fitness and Sports
701 Pennsylvania Avenue NW
Suite 250
Washington, DC 20004

Pamphlet: "AR&FA's Guide to Running and Racing," free with self-addressed, stamped, business-size envelope. Write to:

American Running and Fitness Association
4405 East West Highway, Suite 405
Bethesda, MD 20814
Toll-Free: 800-776-2732
Phone: 301-913-9517
Fax: 301-913-9520
Website: http://www.americanrunning.org
E-Mail: run@americanrunning.org

— by Tracy Early

Section 16.3

Promoting Lifelong Physical Activity Among Young People

From *Morbidity and Mortality Weekly Report (MMWR)*, March 7, 1997 / 46(RR-6);1-36, Centers for Disease Control and Prevention.

Summary

Regular physical activity is linked to enhanced health and to reduced risk for all-cause mortality and the development of many chronic diseases in adults. However, many U.S. adults are either sedentary or less physically active than recommended. Children and adolescents are more physically active than adults, but participation in physical activity declines in adolescence. School and community programs have the potential to help children and adolescents establish lifelong, healthy physical activity patterns.

This report summarizes recommendations for encouraging physical activity among young people so that they will continue to engage in physical activity in adulthood and obtain the benefits of physical activity throughout life. These guidelines were developed by CDC in collaboration with experts from universities and from national, federal, and voluntary agencies and organizations. They are based on an in-depth review of research, theory, and current practice in physical education, exercise science, health education, and public health.

The guidelines include recommendations about 10 aspects of school and community programs to promote lifelong physical activity among young people: policies that promote enjoyable, lifelong physical activity; physical and social environments that encourage and enable physical activity; physical education curricula and instruction; health education curricula and instruction; extracurricular physical activity programs that meet the needs and interests of students; involvement of parents and guardians in physical activity instruction and programs for young people; personnel training; health services for children and adolescents; developmentally appropriate community sports and recreation programs that are attractive to young people;

and regular evaluation of physical activity instruction, programs, and facilities.

Introduction

In recent years the public health benefits of reducing sedentary lifestyles and promoting physical activity have become increasingly apparent.[1-8] The Surgeon General's report on physical activity and health emphasizes that regular participation in moderate physical activity is an essential component of a healthy lifestyle.[1] Although regular physical activity enhances health and reduces the risk for all-cause mortality[9-18] and the development of many chronic diseases among adults,[10,12-14,17,19-45] many adults remain sedentary.[46] Although young people are more active than adults are,[1] many young people do not engage in recommended levels of physical activity.[47,48] In addition, physical activity declines precipitously with age among adolescents.[47,48] Comprehensive school health programs have the potential to slow this age-related decline in physical activity and help students establish lifelong, healthy physical activity patterns.[49,50]

This report is one in a series of CDC documents that provide guidelines for school health programs to promote healthy behavior among children and adolescents.[51-53] These physical activity guidelines address school instructional programs, school psychosocial and physical environments, and various services schools provide. Because the physical activity of children and adolescents is affected by many factors beyond the school setting, these guidelines also address parental involvement, community health services, and community sports and recreation programs for young people.

The guidelines are written for professionals who design and deliver physical activity programs for young people. At the local level, teachers and other school personnel, community sports and recreation program personnel, health service providers, community leaders, and parents may use the guidelines to promote enjoyable, lifelong physical activity among children and adolescents. Policymakers and local, state, and national health and education agencies and organizations may use them to develop initiatives that promote physical activity among young people. In addition, personnel at postsecondary institutions may use these guidelines to train professionals in education, public health, sports and recreation, and medicine.

CDC developed these guidelines by reviewing published research; considering the recommendations in national policy documents; convening experts in physical activity; and consulting with national, federal, and voluntary agencies and organizations. When possible, these guidelines are based on research; however, many are based on behavioral theory and standards for exemplary practice in physical education, exercise science, health education, and public health. More research is needed on the relationship between physical activity and health among young people, the relationship between physical activity during childhood and adolescence and that during adulthood, the determinants of physical activity among children and adolescents, and the effectiveness of school and community programs promoting physical activity among young people.

Physical Activity, Exercise and Physical Fitness

Distinctions between physical activity, exercise, and physical fitness are useful in understanding health research. Physical activity is "any bodily movement produced by skeletal muscles that results in energy expenditure.... Exercise is a subset of physical activity that is planned, structured, and repetitive" and is done to improve or maintain physical fitness. Physical fitness is "a set of attributes that are either health- or skill-related." Health-related fitness includes cardiorespiratory endurance, muscular strength and endurance, flexibility, and body composition; skill-related fitness includes balance, agility, power, reaction time, speed, and coordination.[54]

Specific forms of physical activity and exercise in which young people might participate include walking, bicycling, playing actively (i.e., unstructured physical activity), participating in organized sports, dancing, doing active household chores, and working at a job that has physical demands. The places or settings in which young people can engage in physical activity and exercise include the home, school, playgrounds, public parks and recreation centers, private clubs and sports facilities, bicycling and jogging trails, summer camps, dance centers, and religious facilities.

Health Benefits of Physical Activity and Physical Fitness

Regular moderate physical activity results in many health benefits for adults. For example, it improves cardiorespiratory endurance, flexibility, and muscular strength and endurance.[1,55] Physical activity may also reduce obesity,[56-60] alleviate depression and anxiety,[61-65] and build bone mass density.[66-71] Physically active and physically fit adults are less likely than sedentary adults to develop the chronic diseases that cause most of the morbidity and mortality in the United States: cardiovascular disease,[10,12-14,17,19-29,72-77] hypertension,[30-32,78] non-insulin-dependent diabetes mellitus,[33-37] and cancer of the colon.[38-45] All-cause mortality rates are lower among physically active than sedentary people.[9-18]

Although more research is needed on the association between physical activity and health among young people,[79-81] evidence shows that physical activity results in some health benefits for children and adolescents. For example, regular physical activity improves aerobic endurance[82-86] and muscular strength.[82,86] Among healthy young people, physical activity and physical fitness may favorably affect risk factors for cardiovascular disease (e.g., body mass index, blood lipid profiles, and resting blood pressure).[87-100] Regular physical activity among children and adolescents with chronic disease risk factors is important:[101-105] it decreases blood pressure in adolescents with borderline hypertension,[81] increases physical fitness in obese children,[106,107] and decreases the degree of overweight among obese children.[108-111] Physical activity among adolescents is consistently related to higher levels of self-esteem and self-concept and lower levels of anxiety and stress.[112] Although the relationship between physical activity during youth and the development of osteoporosis later in life is unclear,[113] evidence exists that weight-bearing exercise increases bone mass density among young people.[114,115]

Recommended Physical Activity for Young People

Increased awareness of the health benefits of physical activity has led to increased recognition of the need for initiatives to reduce sedentary lifestyles.[1-3,5-8,116-127] The International Consensus Conference on Physical Activity Guidelines for Adolescents recommends that "all adolescents...be physically active daily, or nearly every day, as part of play, games, sports, work, transportation, recreation, physical education, or planned exercise, in the context of family, school, and community activities" and that "adolescents engage in three or more sessions per week of activities that last 20 minutes or more at a time and that require moderate to vigorous levels of exertion."[128]

Prevalence of Physical Activity among Young People

Although children and adolescents are more physically active than adults, many young people do not engage in moderate or vigorous physical activity at least 3 days a week.[47,48,129-131] For example, among high school students, only 52% of girls and 74% of boys reported that they exercised vigorously on at least 3 of the previous 7 days.[48] Physical activity among both girls and boys tends to decline steadily during adolescence. For example, 69% of young people 12-13 years of age but only 38% of those 18-21 years of age exercised vigorously on at least 3 of the preceding 7 days,[47] and 72% of 9th-grade students but only 55% of 12th-grade students engaged in this level of physical activity.[48]

Factors Influencing Physical Activity

Demographic, individual, interpersonal, and environmental factors are associated with physical activity among children and adolescents. Demographic factors include sex, age, and race or ethnicity. Girls are less active than boys, older children and adolescents are less active than younger children and adolescents, and among girls, blacks are less active than whites.[47,48,132-134]

Individual factors positively associated with physical activity among young people include confidence in one's ability to engage in exercise (i.e., self-efficacy),[133,135, 136] perceptions of physical or sport competence,[137-141] having positive attitudes toward physical education,[133,138] and enjoying physical activity.[142,143] Perceiving benefits from engaging in physical activity or being involved in sports is positively associated with increased physical activity among young people.[133,137, 138] These perceived benefits include excitement and having fun; learning and improving skills; staying in shape; improving appearance; and increasing strength, endurance, and flexibility.[132,137,144-147] Conversely, perceiving barriers to physical activity, particularly lack of time, is negatively associated with physical activity among adolescents.[133,137,148] In addition, a person's stage of change (i.e., readiness to begin being physically active)[149-153] influences physical activity among adults and may also influence physical activity among young people.

Interpersonal and environmental factors positively associated with physical activity among young people include peers' or friends' support for and participation in physical activity.[133,142,154] Among older children and adolescents, physical activity is positively associated with that of siblings,[155,156] and research generally reveals a positive relationship between the physical activity level of parents and that of their children, particularly adolescents.[133,135,141,142,154,156-163] Parental support for physical activity is correlated with active lifestyles among adolescents.[133,141, 154,157] Physical activity among young people is also positively correlated with having access to convenient play

213

spaces,[133,160] sports equipment,[142,157] and transportation to sports or fitness programs.[158]

Objectives for Physical Activity among Young People

The following national health promotion and disease prevention objectives for the year 2000 are related to physical activity and fitness among children and adolescents.[164]

1.2   Reduce overweight to a prevalence of less than or equal to 20% among people aged greater than or equal to 20 years and less than or equal to 15% among adolescents aged 12-19 years.

1.3   Increase to greater than or equal to 30% the proportion of people aged greater than or equal to 6 years who engage regularly, preferably daily, in light to moderate physical activity for greater than or equal to 30 minutes per day.

1.4   Increase to greater than or equal to 20% the proportion of people aged greater than or equal to 18 years and to greater than or equal to 75% the proportion of children and adolescents aged 6-17 years who engage in vigorous physical activity that promotes the development and maintenance of cardiorespiratory fitness greater than or equal to 3 days per week for greater than or equal to 20 minutes per occasion.

1.5   Reduce to less than or equal to 15% the proportion of people aged greater than or equal to 6 years who engage in no leisure-time physical activity.

1.6   Increase to greater than or equal to 40% the proportion of people aged greater than or equal to 6 years who regularly perform physical activities that enhance and maintain muscular strength, muscular endurance, and flexibility.

1.7   Increase to greater than or equal to 50% the proportion of overweight people aged greater than or equal to 12 years who have adopted sound dietary practices combined with regular physical activity to attain an appropriate body weight.

1.8   Increase to greater than or equal to 50% the proportion of children and adolescents in 1st through 12th grade who participate in daily school physical education.

1.9   Increase to greater than or equal to 50% the proportion of school physical education class time that students spend being physically active, preferably engaged in lifetime physical activities.

1.11 Increase community availability and accessibility of physical activity and fitness facilities.

1.12 Increase to greater than or equal to 50% the proportion of primary care providers who routinely assess and counsel their patients regarding the frequency, duration, type, and intensity of each patient's physical activity practices.

Rationale for School and Community Efforts to Promote Physical Activity among Young People

Schools and communities should promote physical activity among children and adolescents because many young people already have risk factors for chronic diseases associated with adult morbidity and mortality.[165] For example, the prevalence of overweight is at an all-time high among children and adolescents.[166] In addition, physical activity has a beneficial effect on the physical and mental health of young people.[81-100,106-112,114,115]

People begin to acquire and establish patterns of health-related behaviors during childhood and adolescence;[167] thus, young people should be encouraged to engage in physical activity. However, many children are less physically active than recommended.[47,48,129-131] Physical activity declines during adolescence,[47,48] and enrollment in daily physical education has decreased.[48,168]

Schools and communities have the potential to improve the health of young people by providing instruction, programs, and services that promote enjoyable, lifelong physical activity.[116-121,124,125] Schools are an efficient vehicle for providing physical activity instruction and programs because they reach most children and adolescents.[49,125,169] Communities are essential because most physical activity among young people occurs outside the school setting.[129,170]

Schools and communities should coordinate their efforts to make the best use of their resources in promoting physical activity among young people.[49,50] School personnel, students, families, community organizations, and businesses should collaborate to develop, implement, and evaluate physical activity instruction and programs for young people. One way to achieve this collaboration is to form a coalition.[171] National, state, and local resources that might be useful in promoting physical activity among young people are available to schools and community groups.

Within the school, efforts to promote physical activity among students should be part of a coordinated, comprehensive school health program, which is "an integrated set of planned, sequential, and school-affiliated strategies, activities, and services designed to promote the optimal physical, emotional, social, and educational development of students. The program involves and is supportive of families and is determined by the local community based on community needs, resources, standards, and requirements. It is coordinated by a multidisciplinary team and accountable to the community for program quality and effectiveness."[172] This coordinated program should include health education; physical education; health services; school counseling and social services; nutrition services; the psychosocial and biophysical environment; faculty and staff health promotion; and integrated efforts of schools, families, and communities.[173] These programs have the potential to improve both the health and the educational prospects of students.[49,50]

Some school health programs have implemented educational and environmental interventions to promote physical activity among students.[132,174-187] These programs have been effective in enhancing students' physical activity-related knowledge,[174,175,183] attitudes,[187] and behavior[132,186] and their physical fitness.[183] Programs that seem to be most effective focus on social factors that influence physical activity (e.g., peers' support for physical activity.[188])

Recommendations for School and Community Programs Promoting Physical Activity among Young People

Listed below are 10 broad recommendations for school and community programs to promote physical activity among young people. Following this list, each recommendation is described in detail.

1. **Policy:** Establish policies that promote enjoyable, lifelong physical activity among young people.

2. **Environment:** Provide physical and social environments that encourage and enable safe and enjoyable physical activity.

3. **Physical education:** Implement physical education curricula and instruction that emphasize enjoyable participation in physical activity and that help students develop the knowledge,

attitudes, motor skills, behavioral skills, and confidence needed to adopt and maintain physically active lifestyles.

4. **Health education:** Implement health education curricula and instruction that help students develop the knowledge, attitudes, behavioral skills, and confidence needed to adopt and maintain physically active lifestyles.

5. **Extracurricular activities:** Provide extracurricular physical activity programs that meet the needs and interests of all students.

6. **Parental involvement:** Include parents and guardians in physical activity instruction and in extracurricular and community physical activity programs, and encourage them to support their children's participation in enjoyable physical activities.

7. **Personnel training:** Provide training for education, coaching, recreation, health-care, and other school and community personnel that imparts the knowledge and skills needed to effectively promote enjoyable, lifelong physical activity among young people.

8. **Health services:** Assess physical activity patterns among young people, counsel them about physical activity, refer them to appropriate programs, and advocate for physical activity instruction and programs for young people.

9. **Community programs:** Provide a range of developmentally appropriate community sports and recreation programs that are attractive to all young people.

10. **Evaluation:** Regularly evaluate school and community physical activity instruction, programs, and facilities.

Recommendation 1. Policy: Establish policies that promote enjoyable, lifelong physical activity among young people.

Policies provide formal and informal rules that guide schools and communities in planning, implementing, and evaluating physical activity programs for young people. School and community policies related to physical activity should comply with state and local laws and with recommendations and standards provided by national, state, and local agencies and organizations. These policies should be included in a written document that incorporates input from administrators, teachers, coaches, athletic trainers, parents, students, health-care providers, public health professionals, and other school and community personnel and should address the following requirements.

- **Require comprehensive, daily physical education for students in kindergarten through grade 12.** Physical education instruction can increase students' knowledge,[183] physical activity in physical education class,[177,179,189] and physical fitness.[183,190-195] Daily physical education from kindergarten through 12th grade is recommended by the American Heart Association[118] and the National Association for Sport and Physical Education[196] and is also a national health objective for the year 2000.[164] The minimum amount of physical education required for students is usually set by state law. Although most states (94%) and school districts (95%) require some physical education,[173,197] only one state requires it daily from kindergarten through 12th grade. Less than two thirds (60%) of high school students are enrolled in physical education classes, and only 25% take physical education daily.[48] Enrollment in both physical education (9th grade, 81%; 12th grade, 42%) and daily physical education (9th grade, 41%; 12th grade, 13%) declines at higher grades, and enrollment in daily physical education and active time in physical education classes decreased from 1991 to 1995 among high school students[48]. Further, 30% of schools exempt students from physical education if the students participate in band, chorus, cheerleading, or interscholastic sports.[197] Substitution of these programs for physical education reduces students' opportunities to develop knowledge, attitudes, motor skills, behavioral skills, and confidence related to physical activity.[196,198]

- **Require comprehensive health education for students in kindergarten through grade 12.** Comprehensive health education, which includes instruction on physical activity topics, can complement the instruction students receive in comprehensive physical education.[179] Health education may improve students' health knowledge, attitudes, and behaviors.[199] Many educational organizations recommend that students receive planned and sequential health education from kindergarten through 12th grade,[200-203] and such education is a national health objective for the year 2000.[164] Although many states (90%) and school districts (91%) require that schools offer health education, fewer school districts require that a separate course be devoted to health topics (elementary school, 19%; middle school, 44%; senior high school, 66%).[204] Administrators of public schools and parents of adolescents in public schools believe that these students should be taught more health information and skills.[205]

- **Require that adequate resources, including budget and facilities, be committed for physical activity instruction and programs.** The National Association for Sport and Physical Education and the Joint Committee for National Health Education Standards note that adequate budget and facilities are necessary for physical education, health education, extracurricular physical activities, and community sports and recreation programs to be successful.[198,206-208] However, these programs rarely have sufficient resources.[168,209] Schools and communities should be vigilant in ensuring that physical education, health education, and physical activity programs have sufficient financial and facility resources to ensure safe participation by young people.[198,206-208] Schools should have policies that ensure that teacher-to-student ratios in physical education are comparable to those in other subjects[198,206,207,210] and that physical education spaces and facilities are not usurped for other events. Schools should have policies requiring that physical education classes be scheduled so that students in each class are of similar physical maturity and grade level.[198,206,207]

- **Require the hiring of physical education specialists to teach physical education in kindergarten through grade 12, elementary school teachers trained to teach health education, health education specialists to teach health education in middle and senior high schools, and qualified people to direct school and community physical activity programs and to coach young people in sports and recreation programs.** Planning, implementing, and evaluating physical activity instruction and programs require specially trained personnel.[125,198,206-208,211] Physical education specialists teach longer lessons, spend more time on developing skills, impart more knowledge, and provide more moderate and vigorous physical activity than do classroom teachers.[189,212] Schools should have policies requiring that physical education specialists teach physical education in kindergarten through grade 12, elementary school teachers trained to teach health education do so in elementary schools, health education specialists teach health education in middle and senior high schools, and qualified people direct school and community physical activity programs and coach young people in sports and recreation programs.[198,206-208,211]

Some states have established minimum standards for teachers. Eighty-four percent of states require physical education certification for secondary school physical education teachers, and 16% require such certification for elementary school physical education teachers.[197] Only 69% of states require health education certification for secondary school health education teachers.[204] These data indicate the need for a greater commitment to hiring professionally trained physical education specialists and health education specialists for our nation's schools.

Some states have established minimum standards for athletic coaches. Both schools and communities should have policies that require employing people who have the coaching competency appropriate to participants' developmental and skill levels.[213] Coaches who work with beginning athletes should meet at least the Level I, if not Level II, coaching competencies identified by the National Association for Sport and Physical Education.[213] Entry-level interscholastic coaches and master coaches should achieve at least Level III and Level IV coaching competencies, respectively.[213]

- **Require that physical activity instruction and programs meet the needs and interests of all students.** All students, irrespective of their sex, race/ethnicity, health status, or physical and cognitive ability or disability should have access to physical education, health education, extracurricular physical activity programs, and community sports and recreation programs that meet their needs and interests.[214,215] In addition, physical activity programs that overemphasize a limited set of team sports and underemphasize noncompetitive, lifetime fitness and recreational activities (e.g., walking or bicycling) could exclude or be unattractive to potential participants.[131,216]

Adolescents' interests and participation in physical activity differ by sex.[47, 48,217] For example, compared with boys, girls engage in less physical activity,[47,48] are less likely to participate in team sports,[47,48,218] and are more likely to participate in aerobics or dance.[47] Girls and boys also perceive different benefits of physical activity;[132,137,145,147] for example, boys more often cite competition and girls more often cite weight management as a reason for engaging in physical activity.[132,137] Because boys are more likely than girls to have higher perceptions of self-efficacy[136] and physical competence,[137,219] physical activity programs serving girls should provide instruction and experiences that increase girls' confidence in participating in physical activity, opportunities for them to participate in physical activities, and social environments that support their involvement in a range of physical activities. Adolescents' participation in physical activity also differs by race and ethnicity.[47,48]

Children and adolescents who are obese or who have physical or cognitive disabilities, chronic health conditions (e.g., diabetes, heart disease, or asthma), or low levels of fitness need instruction and programs in which they can develop motor skills, improve fitness, and experience enjoyment and success.[3,124,143,164,220] Young people who have these disabilities or health concerns are often overtly or unintentionally discouraged from engaging in regular physical activity even though they may be in particular need of it.[220,221] For example, 59% of high schools allow students who have physical disabilities to be exempt from physical education courses.[197] Schools should be required to provide modified physical education and health education for these students.[221,222] By modifying physical education, health education, extracurricular physical activities, and community sports and recreation programs, schools and communities can help these young people acquire the physical, mental, and social benefits of physical activity.

Physical education, health education, extracurricular physical activity programs, and community sports and recreation programs can also provide opportunities for multicultural experiences (e.g., American Indian and African dance). These experiences can meet children's and adolescents' interests and foster their awareness and appreciation of different physical activities enjoyed by different cultural groups.[223]

Recommendation 2. Environment: Provide physical and social environments that encourage and enable safe and enjoyable physical activity.

The physical and social environments of children and adolescents should encourage and enable their participation in safe and enjoyable physical activities. These environments are described by the following guidelines.

- **Provide access to safe spaces and facilities for physical activity in the school and the community.** School spaces and facilities should be available to young people before, during, and after the school day, on weekends, and during summer and other vacations. These spaces and facilities should also be readily available to community agencies and organizations offering physical activity programs.[3,118,119,124,127,198,200, 206,207,224]

  National health objective 1.11 calls for increased availability of facilities for physical activity (e.g., hiking, bicycling, and fitness trails; public swimming pools; and parks and open spaces for recreation).[164] Community coalitions should coordinate the availability of these open spaces and facilities. Some communities may need to build new facilities, whereas others may need only to coordinate existing community spaces and facilities. The needs of all children and adolescents, particularly those who have disabilities, should be incorporated into the building of new facilities and the coordination of existing ones.

  Schools and communities should ensure that spaces and facilities meet or exceed recommended safety standards for design, installation, and maintenance.[206,207, 225,226] For example, playgrounds should have cool water and adequate shade for play and rest.[227] Young people also need places that are free from violence and free from exposure to environmental hazards (e.g., fumes from incinerators or motor vehicles). Spaces and facilities for physical activity should be regularly inspected, and hazardous conditions should be immediately corrected.[206,207,228]

- **Establish and enforce measures to prevent physical activity-related injuries and illnesses.** Minimizing physical activity-related injuries and illnesses among young people is the joint responsibility of teachers, administrators, coaches, athletic trainers, other school and community personnel, parents, and young people.[226] Preventing injuries and illness includes having appropriate adult supervision, ensuring compliance with safety rules and the use of protective clothing and equipment, and avoiding the effects of extreme weather conditions. Explicit safety rules should be taught to, and followed by, young people in physical education, health education, extracurricular physical activity programs, and community sports and recreation programs.[164,206,229-231] Adult supervisors should consistently reinforce safety rules.[231]

Adult supervisors should be aware of the potential for physical activity-related injuries and illnesses among young people so that the risks for and consequences of these injuries and illnesses can be minimized.[228,229] These adults should receive medical information relevant to each student's participation in physical activity (e.g., whether the child has asthma), be able to provide first aid and cardiopulmonary resuscitation, and practice precautions to prevent the spread of bloodborne pathogens (e.g., the human immunodeficiency virus).[198,207] Written policies on providing first aid and reporting injuries and illnesses to parents and to appropriate school and community authorities should be established and followed.[198,207] Adult supervisors can take the following steps to avoid injuries and illnesses during structured physical activity for young people: require physical assessment before participation, provide developmentally appropriate activities, ensure proper conditioning, provide instruction on the biomechanics of specific motor skills, appropriately match participants according to size and ability, adapt rules to the skill level of young people and the protective equipment available, avoid excesses in training, modify rules to eliminate unsafe practices, and ensure that injuries are healed before further participation.[198,207,227,228]

Children and adolescents should be provided with, and required to use, protective clothing and equipment appropriate to the type of physical activity and the environment.[164,198,206,207,227-229,231] Protective clothing and equipment includes footwear appropriate for the specific activity; helmets for bicycling; helmets, face masks, mouth guards, and protective pads for football and ice hockey; and reflective clothing for walking and running. Protective gear and athletic equipment should be frequently inspected, and they should be replaced if worn, damaged, or outdated.

Exposure to the sun can be minimized by use of protective hats, clothing, and sunscreen; avoidance of midday sun exposure; and use of shaded spaces or indoor facilities.[164,227,232] Heat-related illnesses can be prevented by ensuring that children and adolescents frequently drink cool water, have adequate rest and shade, play during cool times of the day, and are supervised by people trained to recognize the early signs of heat exhaustion and heat stroke.[227] Cold-related injuries can be avoided by ensuring that young people wear multilayered clothing for outside play and exercise, increasing the intensity of outdoor activities, using indoor facilities during extremely cold weather, ensuring proper water temperature for aquatic activities, and providing supervision by persons trained to recognize the early signs of frostbite and hypothermia.[227] Measures should be taken to avoid health problems associated with poor air quality (e.g., reduce the intensity of physical activity or hold physical education classes or programs indoors).

Teachers, parents, coaches, athletic trainers, and health-care providers should promote a range of healthy behaviors. These adults should encourage young people to abstain from tobacco, alcohol, and other drugs; to maintain a healthy diet; and to practice healthy weight management techniques.[227] Adult supervisors should be aware of the signs and symptoms of eating disorders and take steps to prevent eating disorders among young people.[227]

- **Provide time within the school day for unstructured physical activity.** During the school day, opportunities for physical activity exist within physical education classes, during recess, and immediately before and after school. For example, students in grades one through four have an average recess period of 30 minutes.[233] School personnel should encourage students to be physically active during these times. The use of time during the school day for unstructured physical activity should complement rather than substitute for the physical activity and instruction children receive in physical education classes.

- **Discourage the use or withholding of physical activity as punishment.** Teachers, coaches, and other school and community personnel should not force participation in or withhold opportunities for physical activity as punishment. Using physical activity as a punishment risks creating negative associations with physical activity in the minds of young people. Withholding physical activity deprives students of health benefits important to their well-being.

- **Provide health promotion programs for school faculty and staff.** Enabling school personnel to participate in physical activity and other healthy behaviors should help them serve as role models for students. School-based health promotion programs have been effective in improving teachers' participation in vigorous exercise, which in turn has improved their physical fitness, body composition, blood pressure, general well-being, and ability to handle job stress.[234,235] In addition, participants in school-based health promotion programs may be less likely than non-participants to be absent from work.[235]

Recommendation 3. Physical education: Implement physical education curricula and instruction that emphasize enjoyable participation in physical activity and that help students develop the knowledge, attitudes, motor skills, behavioral skills, and confidence needed to adopt and maintain physically active lifestyles.

Physical education curricula and instruction are vital parts of a comprehensive school health program. One of the main goals of these curricula should be to help students develop an active lifestyle that will persist into and throughout adulthood.[3,174,180,236,237]

- **Provide planned and sequential physical education curricula from kindergarten through grade 12 that promote enjoyable, lifelong physical activity.** School physical education curricula are often mandated by state laws or regulations. Many states (76%) and school districts (89%) have written goals, objectives, or outcomes for physical education (CDC, unpublished data), and only 26% of states require a senior high school physical education course promoting physical activities that can be enjoyed throughout life.[197] Planned and sequential physical education curricula should emphasize knowledge about the benefits of physical activity and the recommended amounts and types of physical activity needed to promote health.[3,116-118,124,164] Physical education should help students develop the attitudes, motor skills, behavioral skills, and confidence they need to engage in lifelong physical activity.[116-118,122,125,164,237] Physical education should emphasize skills for lifetime physical activities (e.g., dance, strength training, jogging, swimming, bicycling, cross-country skiing, walking, and hiking) rather than those for competitive sports.[116-118,164,197,237-239]

If physical fitness testing is used, it should be integrated into the curriculum and emphasize health-related components of physical fitness (e.g., cardiorespiratory endurance, muscular strength and endurance, flexibility, and body composition). The tests should be administered only after students are well oriented to the testing procedures. Testing should be a mechanism for teaching students how to apply behavioral skills (e.g., self-assessment, goal setting, and self-monitoring) to physical fitness development and for providing feedback to students and parents about students' physical fitness. The results of physical fitness testing should not be used to assign report card grades.[193,240,241] Also, test results should not be used to assess program effectiveness; the validity of these measurements may be unreliable, and physical fitness and improvements in physical fitness are influenced by factors (e.g., physical maturation, body size, and body composition) beyond the control of teachers and students.[193,240,241]

- **Use physical education curricula consistent with the national standards for physical education.** The national standards for physical education[211] describe what students should know and be able to do as a result of physical education. A student educated about physical activity "has learned skills necessary to perform a variety of physical activities, is physically fit, does participate regularly in physical activity, knows the implications of and the benefits from involvement in physical activities, (and) values physical activity and its contribution to a healthful lifestyle."[196] The national standards emphasize the development of movement competency and proficiency, use of cognitive information to enhance motor skill acquisition and performance, establishment of regular participation in physical activity, achievement of health-enhancing physical fitness, development of responsible personal and social behavior, understanding of and respect for individual differences, and awareness of values and benefits of physical activity participation.[211] These standards provide a framework that should be used to design, implement, and evaluate physical education curricula that promote enjoyable, lifelong physical activity.

- **Use active learning strategies and emphasize enjoyable participation in physical education class.** Enjoyable physical education experiences are believed to be essential in promoting physical activity among children and adolescents.[3,124,125] Physical education experiences that are enjoyable and actively involve students in learning may help foster positive attitudes toward and encourage participation in physical education and physical activity.[133,138] Active learning strategies that involve the student in learning physical activity concepts, motor skills, and behavioral skills include brainstorming, cooperative groups, simulation, and situation analysis.

- **Develop students' knowledge of and positive attitudes toward physical activity.** Knowledge of physical activity is viewed as an essential component of physical education curricula.[117,118,124,125,164] Related concepts include the physical, social, and mental health benefits of physical activity; the components of health-related fitness; principles of exercise; injury prevention; precautions for preventing the spread of bloodborne pathogens; nutrition and weight management; social influences on physical activity; and the development of safe and effective individualized physical activity programs. For both young people and adults, knowledge about how to be physically active may be a more important influence on physical activity than is knowledge about why to be active.[237,242]

  Positive attitudes toward physical activity may affect young people's involvement in physical activity.[116-118,124,125,164] Positive attitudes include perceptions that physical activity is important and that it is fun. Ways to generate positive attitudes include providing students with enjoyable physical education experiences that meet their needs and interests, emphasizing the many benefits of physical activity, supporting students who are physically active, and using active learning strategies.

- **Develop students' mastery of and confidence in motor and behavioral skills for participating in physical activity.** Physical education should help students master[243-245] and gain confidence in[3,125,219,242] motor and behavioral skills used in physical activity. Students should become competent in many motor skills and proficient in a few to use in lifelong physical activities.[117,118,122,124,164,211] Elementary school students should develop basic motor skills that allow participation in a variety of physical activities, and older students should become competent in a select number of lifetime physical activities they enjoy and succeed in. Students' mastery of and confidence in motor skills occurs when these skills are broken down into components and the tasks are ordered from easy to hard.[246] In addition, students need opportunities to observe others performing the skills and to receive encouragement, feedback, and repeated opportunities for practice during physical education class.[246]

Behavioral skills (e.g., self-assessment, self-monitoring, decision making, goal setting, and communication) may help students establish and maintain regular involvement in physical activity. Active student involvement and social learning experiences that focus on building confidence may increase the likelihood that children and adolescents will enjoy and succeed in physical education and physical activity.[246]

- **Provide a substantial percentage of each student's recommended weekly amount of physical activity in physical education classes.** For physical education to make a meaningful and consistent contribution to the recommended amount of young people's physical activity, students at every grade level should take physical education classes that meet daily and should be physically active for a large percentage of class time.[3,125,164,247] National health objective 1.9 calls for students to be physically active for at least 50% of physical education class time,[164] but many schools do not meet this objective,[212,248-251] and the percentage of time students spend in moderate or vigorous physical activity during physical education classes has decreased over the past few years.[48]

- **Promote participation in enjoyable physical activity in the school, community, and home.** Physical education teachers should encourage students to be active before, during, and after the school day. Physical education teachers can also refer students to community physical sports and recreation programs available in their community[3] and promote participation in physical activity at home by assigning homework that students can do on their own or with family members.[122]

Recommendation 4. Health education: Implement health education curricula and instruction that help students develop the knowledge, attitudes, behavioral skills, and confidence needed to adopt and maintain physically active lifestyles.

Health education can effectively promote students' health-related knowledge, attitudes, and behaviors.[199,252,253] The major contribution of health education in promoting physical activity among students should be to help them develop the knowledge, attitudes, and behavioral skills they need to establish and maintain a physically active lifestyle.[208,209,254]

- **Provide planned and sequential health education curricula from kindergarten through grade 12 that promote lifelong participation in physical activity.** Many states (65%) and school districts (82%) require that physical activity and physical fitness topics be part of a required course in health education.[204] Planned and sequential health education curricula, like physical education curricula, should draw on social cognitive theory[188] and emphasize physical activity as a component of a healthy lifestyle.

- **Use health education curricula consistent with the national standards for health education.** The national standards for health education developed by the Joint Committee for National Health Education Standards[208] describe what health-literate students should know and be able to do as a result of school health education. Health literacy is "the capacity of individuals to obtain, interpret, and understand basic health information and services and the competence to use such information and services in ways which enhance health."[208] The standards specify that, as a result of health education, students should be able to comprehend basic health concepts; access valid health information and health-promoting products and services; practice health-enhancing behaviors; analyze the influence of culture and other factors on health; use interpersonal communication skills to enhance health; use goal-setting and decision-making skills to enhance health; and advocate for personal, family, and community health. These standards emphasize the development of students' skills and can be used as the basis for health education curricula.

- **Promote collaboration among physical education, health education, and classroom teachers as well as teachers in related disciplines who plan and implement physical activity instruction.** Physical education and health education teachers in about one third of middle and senior high schools collaborate on activities or projects.[197,204] Collaboration allows coordinated physical activity instruction and should enable teachers to provide range and depth of physical activity-related content and skills. For example, health education and physical education teachers can collaborate to reinforce the link between sound dietary practices and regular physical activity for weight management. Collaboration also allows teachers to highlight the influence of other behaviors on the capacity to engage in physical activity (e.g., using alcohol or other drugs) or behaviors that interact with physical activity to reduce the risk of developing chronic diseases (e.g., not using tobacco).

- **Use active learning strategies to emphasize enjoyable participation in physical activity in the school, community, and home.** Health education instruction should include the use of active learning strategies. Such strategies may encourage students' active involvement in learning and help them develop the concepts, attitudes, and behavioral skills they need to engage in physical activity.[209,254] Additionally, health education teachers should encourage students to adopt healthy behaviors (e.g., physical activity) in the school, community, and home.

- **Develop students' knowledge of and positive attitudes toward healthy behaviors, particularly physical activity.** Health education curricula should provide information about physical activity concepts.[3] These concepts should include the physical, social, and mental health benefits of physical activity; the components of health-related fitness; principles of exercise; injury prevention and first aid; precautions for preventing the spread of bloodborne pathogens; nutrition, physical activity, and weight management; social influences on physical activity; and the development of safe and effective individualized physical activity programs.

  Health instruction should also generate positive attitudes toward healthy behaviors. These positive attitudes include perceptions that it is important and fun to participate in physical activity. Ways to foster positive attitudes include emphasizing the multiple benefits of physical activity, supporting children and adolescents who are physically active, and using active learning strategies.

- **Develop students' mastery of and confidence in the behavioral skills needed to adopt and maintain a healthy lifestyle that includes regular physical activity.** Children and adolescents should develop behavioral skills that may enable them to adopt healthy behaviors.[116,164] Certain skills (e.g., self-assessment, self-monitoring, decision making, goal setting, identifying and managing barriers, self-regulation, reinforcement, communication, and advocacy) may help students adopt and maintain a healthy lifestyle that includes regular physical activity. Active learning strategies give students opportunities to practice, master, and develop confidence in these skills.[209,254]

Recommendation 5. Extracurricular activities: Provide extracurricular physical activity programs that meet the needs and interests of all students.

Extracurricular activities are any activities offered by schools outside of formal classes. Interscholastic athletics, intramural sports, and sports and recreation clubs are believed to contribute to the physical and social development of young people,[196] and schools should extend these benefits to the greatest possible number of students. These activities can help meet the goals of comprehensive school health programs by providing students with opportunities to engage in physical activity and to further develop the knowledge, attitudes, motor skills, behavioral skills, and confidence needed to adopt and maintain physically active lifestyles.

- **Provide a diversity of developmentally appropriate competitive and noncompetitive physical activity programs for all students.** Interscholastic athletic programs are typically limited to the secondary school level and usually consist of a few highly competitive team sports. Intramural sports programs are not common but, where they are offered, usually emphasize competitive team sports. Such programs usually underserve students who are less skilled, less physically fit, or not attracted to competitive sports.[145,255,256] One reason that participation in sports declines steadily during late childhood and adolescence is that undue emphasis is placed on competition.[145]

  After the needs and interests of all students are assessed, interscholastic, intramural, and club programs should be modified and expanded to offer a range of competitive and noncompetitive activities. For example, noncompetitive lifetime physical activities include walking, running, swimming, and bicycling.[118]

- **Link students to community physical activity programs, and use community resources to support extracurricular physical activity programs.** Schools should work with community organizations to enhance the appropriate use of out-of-school time among children and adolescents[224] and to develop effective systems for referring young people from schools to community agencies and organizations that can provide needed services. To help students learn about community resources, schools can sponsor information fairs that represent community groups, physical education and health education teachers can provide information about community resources as part of the curricula,[3] and community-based program personnel can be speakers or demonstration lecturers in school classes.

Frequently schools have the facilities but lack the personnel to deliver extracurricular physical activity programs. Community resources can expand existing school programs by providing intramural and club activities on school grounds. For example, community agencies and organizations can use school facilities for after-school physical fitness programs for children and adolescents, weight management programs for overweight or obese young people, and sports and recreation programs for young people with disabilities or chronic health conditions.

Recommendation 6. Parental involvement: Include parents and guardians in physical activity instruction and in extracurricular and community physical activity programs, and encourage them to support their children's participation in enjoyable physical activities.

Parental involvement in children's physical activity instruction and programs is key to the development of a psychosocial environment that promotes physical activity among young people.[116,117,208,231,257,258] Involvement in these programs provides parents opportunities to be partners in developing their children's physical activity-related knowledge, attitudes, motor skills, behavioral skills, confidence, and behavior. Thus, teachers, coaches, and other school and community personnel should encourage and enable parental involvement. For example, teachers can assign homework to students that must be done with their parents and can provide flyers designed for parents that contain information and strategies for promoting physical activity within the family.[259] Parents can also join school health advisory councils, booster clubs, and parent-teacher organizations.[209,259] Parents who have been trained by professionals can also serve as volunteer coaches for or leaders of extracurricular physical activity programs and community sports and recreation programs.

- **Encourage parents to advocate for quality physical activity instruction and programs for their children.** Parents may be able to influence the quality and quantity of physical activity available to their children by advocating for comprehensive, daily physical education in schools and for school and community physical activity programs that promote lifelong physical activity among young people.[164] Parents should also advocate for safe spaces and facilities that provide their children opportunities to engage in a range of physical activities.[164,257]

- **Encourage parents to support their children's participation in appropriate, enjoyable physical activities.** Parents should ensure that their children participate in physical education classes, extracurricular physical activity programs, and community sports and recreation programs in which the children will experience enjoyment and success.[145] Parents should learn what their children want from extracurricular and community physical activity programs and then help select appropriate activities.[145] Fun and skill development, rather than winning, are the primary reasons most young people participate in physical activity and sports programs.[145,255] Parents should help their children gain access to toys and equipment for physical activity and transportation to activity sites.[145]

- **Encourage parents to be physically active role models and to plan and participate in family activities that include physical activity.** Parental support is a determinant of physical activity among children and adolescents,[133,141,154,157] and parents' attitudes toward physical activity may influence children's involvement in physical activity.[260] Parents and guardians should try to be role models for physical activity behavior and should plan and participate in family activities (e.g., going to the community swimming pool or using the community trails for bicycling or walking).[3,116,117,164,231,239,257,258]

Because peers and friends influence children's physical activity behavior,[133, 142,154] parents can encourage their children to be active with their friends. Children's participation in sedentary activities (e.g., watching television or playing video games) should be monitored and replaced with physical activity,[164,242] and parents should encourage their children to play outside in safe places and in supervised playgrounds and parks.[231,261]

Recommendation 7. Personnel training: Provide training for education, coaching, recreation, health-care, and other school and community personnel that imparts the knowledge and skills needed to effectively promote enjoyable, lifelong physical activity among young people.

The lack of trained personnel is a barrier to implementing safe, organized, and effective physical activity instruction and programs for young people. National, state, and local education and health agencies; institutions of higher education; and national and state professional organizations should collaborate to provide teachers, coaches, administrators, and other school personnel pre-service and in-service training in promoting enjoyable, lifelong physical activity among young people.[116,121,124,164,247,262] Instructor training has proven to be efficacious; for example, physical education specialists teach longer and higher quality lessons,[189,212] and teacher training is important in successful implementation of innovative health education curricula.[263,264] Institutions of higher education should use national guidelines such as those for athletic coaches,[213] entry-level physical education teachers,[265] entry-level health education teachers,[266] and elementary school classroom teachers[267] to plan, implement, and evaluate professional preparation programs for school personnel. In addition, physicians, school nurses, and others who provide health services to young people need pre-service training in promoting physical activity and providing physical activity assessment, counseling, and referral.[116, 121,124,164]

Although many states and school districts provide in-service training on physical education topics (72% and 50%, respectively),[197] all states and school districts need to do so. School personnel often want more training than they receive. For example, more than one third of lead physical education teachers want additional training in developing individualized fitness programs, increasing students' physical activity inside and outside of class, and involving families in physical activity.[197]

- **Train teachers to deliver physical education that provides a substantial percentage of each student's recommended weekly amount of physical activity.** The proportion of physical education class time spent on moderate or vigorous physical activity is insufficient to meet national health objective 1.9.[212,248-251] In-service teacher training that focuses on increasing the amount of class time spent on moderate or vigorous physical activity is effective in increasing students' physical activity during physical education classes.[176,177,179,189] Although 52% of states have offered training to physical education teachers on increasing students' physical activity during class, only 15% of school districts have provided this training.[197] National, state, and local education and health agencies; institutions of higher education; and national and state professional organizations should augment efforts to provide this training to teachers.

- **Train teachers to use active learning strategies needed to develop students' knowledge about, attitudes toward, skills in, and confidence in engaging in physical activity.** Physical education and health education teachers should observe experienced teachers using active learning strategies, have hands-on practice in using these strategies, and receive feedback.[268] Such training should increase teachers' use of these strategies.

- **Train school and community personnel how to create psychosocial environments that enable young people to enjoy physical activity instruction and programs.** Pre-service and in-service training should help teachers, coaches, and other school and community personnel plan and implement physical education as well as extracurricular and community physical activity programs that meet a range of students' needs and interests. Training should also encourage these school and community personnel to place less emphasis on competition and more emphasis on students' having fun and developing skills.

- **Train school and community personnel how to involve parents and the community in physical activity instruction and programs.** Few teachers, coaches, and other school personnel have been trained to involve families and the community in physical activity instruction and programs.[197] Instruction on communication skills for interacting with parents and the community as well as strategies for obtaining adults' support for physical activity instruction and programs is beneficial.[124,259] Teachers should have the knowledge, skills, and materials for creating fact sheets for parents and assigning physical education and health education homework for students to complete with their families.[259]

- **Train volunteers who coach sports and recreation programs for young people.** Volunteer coaches who work with beginning athletes in schools and communities should have the Level I coaching competency delineated by the National Association for Sport and Physical Education.[213] Like professional coaches, volunteer coaches should receive professional training on how to provide experiences for young people that emphasize fun, skill development, confidence-building, and self-knowledge[145] and injury prevention, first aid, cardiopulmonary resuscitation, precautions against contamination by bloodborne pathogens, and promotion of other healthy behaviors (e.g., dietary behavior).

Recommendation 8. Health services: Assess physical activity patterns among young people, counsel them about physical activity, refer them to appropriate programs, and advocate for physical activity instruction and programs for young people.

Physicians, school nurses, and other people who provide health services to young people have a key role in promoting healthy behaviors. Health-care providers are important in promoting physical activity, especially among children and adolescents who have physical and cognitive disabilities or chronic health conditions.

- **Regularly assess the physical activity patterns of young people, reinforce physical activity among active young people, counsel inactive young people about physical activity, and refer young people to appropriate physical activity programs.** As a routine part of care, health-care providers should assess the physical activity of their young patients.[117,164,230,231,258,269] Young people and their families should be counseled about the importance of physical activity and be provided information that enable young people to initiate and maintain regular, safe, and enjoyable participation in physical activity.[3,164,230,231,239,258] Children and adolescents who are already active should be encouraged to continue their physical activity. Health-care providers should work with inactive young people and their families to develop exercise prescriptions and should refer these young people to school and community physical activity programs appropriate to the youths' needs and interests.[117,258] Children with chronic diseases, risk factors for chronic diseases, and physical and cognitive disabilities have special physical activity needs.[257,269] Obese children and adolescents, for example, should be referred to a physical activity and nutrition program for overweight young people.

- **Advocate for school and community physical activity instruction and programs that meet the needs of young people.** To help create physical and social environments that encourage physical activity, health-care providers should advocate for physical education curricula, extracurricular activities, and community sports and recreation programs that emphasize lifetime physical activities and that enable participation in safe, enjoyable physical activities.[116,239,257,258] Physicians, school nurses, and other health-care professionals can support physical activity among children and adolescents by becoming involved in school and community physical activity initiatives. Within schools, many nurses are already involved in joint activities or projects with physical education teachers and health education teachers.[270] Physicians can volunteer to serve as advisors to schools and other community organizations that provide physical activity instruction and programs to young people.[269] Health-care providers should advocate that coaches be trained to ensure that young people compete safely and thrive physically, emotionally, and socially.[271] Health-care providers also should encourage parents to be role models for their children, plan physical activities that involve the whole family, and discuss with their children the value of healthy behaviors such as physical activity.[117,231,239,258,269]

Recommendation 9. Community programs: Provide a range of developmentally appropriate community sports and recreation programs that are attractive to all young people.

Most physical activity among children and adolescents occurs outside the school setting.[129] Thus, community sports and recreation programs are integral to promoting physical activity among young people.[3] These community programs can complement the efforts of schools by providing children and adolescents opportunities to engage in the types and levels of physical activity that may not be offered in school. Community sports and recreation programs also provide an avenue for reaching out-of-school young people.

- **Provide a diversity of developmentally appropriate community sports and recreation programs for all young people.** Young people become involved in structured physical activity programs for various reasons: to develop competence, to build social relationships, to enhance fitness, and to have fun.[145,272] However, adolescents' participation in community sports and recreation programs declines with age.[48,145] Many young people drop out of these programs because the activities are not fun, are too competitive, or demand too much time.[145,256] Because definitions of fun and success vary with each person's age, sex, and skill level, community sports and recreation programs should assess and try to meet the needs and interests of all young people. These programs should also try to match the skill level of the participants with challenges that encourage skill development and fun and to develop programs that are not based exclusively on winning.[145,255]

- **Provide access to community sports and recreation programs for young people.** In most communities, physical activity programs for young people exist, but these opportunities often require transportation, fees, or special equipment. These limitations often discourage children and adolescents from low-income families from participating. Communities should ensure that all young people, irrespective of their family's income, have access to these programs. For example, community sports and recreation programs can collaborate with schools and other community organizations (e.g., places of worship) to provide transportation to these programs. Communities can also ask businesses to sponsor youth physical activity programs and to provide children and adolescents from low-income families appropriate equipment, clothing, and footwear for participation in physical activity.

Recommendation 10. Evaluation: Regularly evaluate school and community physical activity instruction, programs, and facilities.

Evaluation can be used to assess and improve physical activity policies, spaces and facilities, instruction, programs, personnel training, health services, and student achievement. All groups involved in and affected by school and community programs to promote lifelong physical activity among young people should have the opportunity to contribute to evaluation. Valid evaluations may increase support for and involvement in these programs by students, parents, teachers, and other school and community personnel.

- **Evaluate the implementation and quality of physical activity policies, curricula, instruction, programs, and personnel training.** Evaluation is useful for gaining insight about the implementation and quality of physical activity policies, physical activity spaces and facilities, physical education and health education curricula and instruction, extracurricular and community sports and recreation programs, and pre-service and in-service training programs for personnel. The Child and Adolescent Trial for Cardiovascular Health (CATCH)[180] has developed a model that can be used to assess the quantity and quality of physical education instruction, lesson content, fidelity of curriculum implementation, and opportunities for other physical activity.[273,274] National competency frameworks, including Quality Sports, Quality Coaches: National Standards for Athletic Coaches,[213] National Standards for Beginning Physical Education Teachers,[265] A Guide for the Development of Competency-Based Curricula for Entry Level Health Educators,[266] and Health Instruction Responsibilities and Competencies for Elementary (K-6) Classroom Teachers[267] can be used to assess the competencies of coaches, entry-level physical education and health education teachers, and elementary school teachers and the quality of professional training programs for these people. Parents and guardians can use the checklist developed by the National Association for Sport and Physical Education to evaluate the quality of sports and physical activity programs for their children.[275] Other guidelines exist to assess the provision of health services for children and adolescents[231,258] and the safety of playgrounds.[225,226]

- **Measure students' attainment of physical activity knowledge, achievement of motor skills and behavioral skills, and adoption of healthy behaviors.** Measuring students' achievement in physical education requires a comprehensive assessment of their knowledge, motor and behavioral skills, and behavior related to physical activity. Measuring students' achievement in health education requires an assessment of their knowledge, behavioral skills, and behaviors. *Moving into the Future: National Standards for Physical Education*[211] and *National Health Education Standards: Achieving Health Literacy*[208] describe what students should know and be able to do as a result of comprehensive physical education and health education programs. Student's achievement may be measured using paper-and-pencil tests that assess knowledge and performance tests that assess motor and behavioral skills. Portfolios of students' work that reflect their knowledge, motor and behavioral skills, and progress toward personal physical activity goals are appropriate for assessing students' achievement.[276] Although fitness testing is a common component of many school physical education programs, the test results should not be used to assign report card grades or assess program effectiveness.[193,240,241]

Conclusion

School and community programs that promote regular physical activity among young people could be among the most effective strategies for reducing the public health burden of chronic diseases associated with sedentary lifestyles. Programs that provide students with the knowledge, attitudes, motor skills, behavioral skills, and confidence to participate in physical activity may establish active lifestyles among young people that continue into and throughout their adult lives. These programs can promote physical activity by establishing physical activity policies; providing physical and social environments that enable safe and enjoyable participation in physical activity; implementing planned and sequential physical education and health education curricula and instruction from kindergarten through 12th grade; providing extracurricular physical activity programs; including parents and guardians in physical activity instruction and programs; providing personnel training in methods to effectively promote physical activity; providing health services that encourage and support physical activity; providing community-based sports and recreation programs; and evaluating school and community physical activity instruction, programs, and facilities.

References

1. U.S. Department of Health and Human Services. *Physical activity and health: a report of the Surgeon General*. Atlanta: U.S. Department of Health and Human Services, Centers for Disease Control and Prevention, National Center for Chronic Disease Prevention and Health Promotion, 1996.

2. McGinnis JM. The public health burden of a sedentary lifestyle. *Med Sci Sports Exercise* 1992;24(6 suppl):S196-S200.

3. Pate RR, Pratt M, Blair SN, et al. Physical activity and public health: a recommendation from the Centers for Disease Control and Prevention and the American College of Sports Medicine. *JAMA* 1995;273(5):402-7.

4. Powell KE, Blair SN. The public health burdens of sedentary living habits: theoretical but realistic estimates. *Med Sci Sports Exercise* 1994;26(7):851-6.

5. Morris JN. Exercise in the prevention of coronary heart disease: today's best buy in public health. *Med Sci Sports Exercise* 1994;26(7):807-14.

6. McGinnis JM, Foege WH. Actual causes of death in the United States. *JAMA* 1993; 270(18):2207-12.

7. Hahn RA, Teutsch SM, Rothenberg RB, Marks JS. Excess deaths from nine chronic diseases in the United States, 1986. *JAMA* 1990;264(20):2654-9.

8. Powell KE, Kreuter MW, Stephens T, Marti B, Heinemann L. The dimensions of health promotion applied to physical activity. *J Public Health Policy* 1991;12(4):492-509.

9. Kaplan GA, Seeman TE, Cohen RD, Knudsen LP, Guralnik J. Mortality among the elderly in the Alameda County Study: behavioral and demographic risk factors. *Am J Public Health* 1987;77(3):307-12.

10. Slattery ML, Jacobs DR Jr, Nichaman MZ. Leisure time physical activity and coronary heart disease death: the US Railroad Study. *Circulation* 1989;79:304-11.

11. Leon AS, Connett J. Physical activity and 10.5 year mortality in the Multiple Risk Factor Intervention Trial (MRFIT). *Int J Epidemiol* 1991;20(3):690-7.

12. Linsted KD, Tonstad S, Kuzma JW. Self-report of physical activity and patterns of mortality in Seventh-Day Adventist men. *J Clin Epidemiol* 1991;44(4/5):355-64.

13. Chang-Claude J, Frentzel-Beyme R. Dietary and lifestyle determinants of mortality among German vegetarians. *Int J Epidemiol* 1993;22(2):228-36.

14. Paffenbarger RS Jr, Hyde RT, Wing AL, Lee I-M, Jung DL, Kampert JB. The association of changes in physical-activity level and other lifestyle characteristics with mortality among men. *N Engl J Med* 1993;328:538-45.

15. Paffenbarger RS Jr, Hyde RT, Wing AL, Lee I-M, Kampert JB. Some interrelations of physical activity, physiological fitness,

health, and longevity. In: Bouchard C, Shephard RJ, Stephens T, eds. *Physical activity, fitness, and health: international proceedings and consensus statement*. Champaign, IL: Human Kinetics, 1994:119-33.

16. Paffenbarger RS Jr, Kampert JB, Lee I-M, Hyde RT, Leung RW, Wing AL. Changes in physical activity and other lifeway patterns influencing longevity. *Med Sci Sports Exercise* 1994; 26(7):857-65.

17. Lee I-M, Hsieh C-C, Paffenbarger RS Jr. Exercise intensity and longevity in men: the Harvard Alumni Health Study. *JAMA* 1995;273(15):1179-84.

18. Haapanen N, Miilunpalo S, Vuori I, Oja P, Pasanen M. Characteristics of leisure time physical activity associated with decreased risk of premature all-cause and cardiovascular disease mortality in middle-aged men. *Am J Epidemiol* 1996;143(9):870-80.

19. Lapidus L, Bengtsson C. Socioeconomic factors and physical activity in relation to cardiovascular disease and death: a 12 year follow up of participants in a population study of women in Gothenburg, Sweden. *Br Heart J* 1986;55:295-301.

20. Kannel WB, Belanger A, D'Agostino R, Israel I. Physical activity and physical demand on the job and risk of cardiovascular disease and death: the Framingham Study. *Am Heart J* 1986; 112(4):820-5.

21. Leon AS, Connett J, Jacobs DR Jr, Rauramaa R. Leisure-time physical activity levels and risk of coronary heart disease and death: the Multiple Risk Factor Intervention Trial. *JAMA* 1987; 258(17):2388-95.

22. Donahue RP, Abbott RD, Reed DM, Yano K. Physical activity and coronary heart disease in middle-aged and elderly men: the Honolulu Heart Program. *Am J Public Health* 1988;78(6):683-5.

23. Pekkanen J, Nissinen A, Marti B, Tuomilehto J, Punsar S, Karvonen MJ. Reduction of premature mortality by high physical activity: a 20-year follow-up of middle-aged Finnish men. *Lancet* 1987;1(8548):1473-7.

24. Salonen JT, Slater JS, Tuomilehto J, Rauramaa R. Leisure time and occupational physical activity: risk of death from ischemic heart disease. *Am J Epidemiol* 1988;127(1):87-94.

25. Arraiz GA, Wigle DT, Mao Y. Risk assessment of physical activity and physical fitness in the Canada health survey mortality follow-up study. *J Clin Epidemiol* 1992;45(4):419-28.

26. Hein HO, Suadicani P, Gyntelberg F. Physical fitness or physical activity as a predictor of ischaemic heart disease? A 17 year follow-up in the Copenhagen Male Study. *J Intern Med* 1992;232:471-9.

27. Rodriguez BL, Curb JD, Burchfiel CM, et al. Physical activity and 23-year incidence of coronary heart disease morbidity and mortality among middle-aged men: the Honolulu Heart Program. *Circulation* 1994;89:2540-4.

28. Gartside PS, Glueck CJ. The important role of modifiable dietary and behavioral characteristics in the causation and prevention of coronary heart disease hospitalization and mortality: the prospective NHANES I follow-up study. *J Am Coll Nutr* 1995;14(1):71-9.

29. Yeager KK, Anda RF, Macera CA, Donehoo RS, Eaker ED. Sedentary lifestyle and state variation in coronary heart disease mortality. *Public Health Rep* 1995;110(1):100-2.

30. Paffenbarger RS Jr, Wing AL, Hyde RT, Jung DL. Physical activity and incidence of hypertension in college alumni. *Am J Epidemiol* 1983;117(3):245-57.

31. Stamler R, Stamler J, Gosch FC, et al. Primary prevention of hypertension by nutritional-hygienic means: final report of a randomized, controlled trial. *JAMA* 1989;262(13):1801-7.

32. Folsom AR, Prineas RJ, Kaye SA, Munger RG. Incidence of hypertension and stroke in relation to body fat distribution and other risk factors in older women. *Stroke* 1990;21:701-6.

33. Helmrich SP, Ragland DR, Leung RW, Paffenbarger RS Jr. Physical activity and reduced occurrence of non-insulin-dependent diabetes mellitus. *N Engl J Med* 1991;325(3):147-52.

34. Manson JE, Rimm EB, Stampfer MJ, et al. Physical activity and incidence of non-insulin-dependent diabetes mellitus in women. *Lancet* 1991;338:774-8.

35. Manson JE, Nathan DM, Krolewski AS, Stampfer MJ, Willett WC, Hennekens CH. A prospective study of exercise and incidence of diabetes among US male physicians. *JAMA* 1992;268(1):63-7.

36. Helmrich SP, Ragland DR, Paffenbarger RS Jr. Prevention of non-insulin-dependent diabetes mellitus with physical activity. *Med Sci Sports Exercise* 1994;26(7):824-30.

37. Burchfiel CM, Sharp DS, Curb JD, et al. Physical activity and incidence of diabetes: the Honolulu Heart Program. *Am J Epidemiol* 1995;141(4):360-8.

38. Gerhardsson M, Floderus B, Norell SE. Physical activity and colon cancer risk. *Int J Epidemiol* 1988;17(4):743-6.

39. Slattery ML, Schumacher MC, Smith KR, West DW, Abd-Elghany N. Physical activity, diet, and risk of colon cancer in Utah. *Am J Epidemiol* 1988;128(5):989-99.

40. Gerhardsson de Verdier M, Steineck G, Hagman U, Rieger, Norell SE. Physical activity and colon cancer: a case-referent study in Stockholm. *Int J Cancer* 1990;46:985-9.

41. Whittemore AS, Wu-Williams AH, Lee M, et al. Diet, physical activity, and colorectal cancer among Chinese in North American and China. *J Natl Cancer Inst* 1990;82(11):915-26.

42. Lee I-M, Paffenbarger RS Jr, Hsieh C-C. Physical activity and risk of developing colorectal cancer among college alumni. *J Natl Cancer Inst* 1991;83:1324-9.

43. Markowitz S, Morabia A, Garibaldi K, Wynder E. Effect of occupational and recreational activity on the risk of colorectal cancer among males: a case-control study. *Int J Epidemiol* 1992; 21(6):1057-62.

44. Giovannucci E, Ascherio A, Rimm EB, Colditz GA, Stampfer MJ, Willet WC. Physical activity, obesity, and risk for colon cancer and adenoma in men. *Ann Intern Med* 1995;122:327-34.

45. Longnecker MP, Gerhardsson de Verdier M, Frumkin H, Carpenter C. A case-control study of physical activity in relation to risk of cancer of the right colon and rectum in men. *Int J Epidemiol* 1995;24(1):42-50.

46. Siegel PZ, Brackbill RM, Frazier EL, et al. Behavioral risk factor surveillance, 1986-1990. *MMWR* 1991;40(SS-4):1-22.

47. Adams PF, Schoenborn CA, Moss AJ, Warren CW, Kann L. *Health-risk behaviors among our nation's youth: United States, 1992.* Hyattsville, MD: U.S. Department of Health and Human Services, Public Health Service, CDC, 1995. DHHS publication no. (PHS) 95-1520. (Vital and health statistics; series 10, no. 192.)

48. CDC. Youth Risk Behavior Surveillance—United States, 1995. *MMWR* 1996;45(SS-4).

49. Kolbe LJ. An essential strategy to improve the health and education of Americans. *Prev Med* 1993;22:544-60.

50. McGinnis JM. The year 2000 initiative: implications for comprehensive school health. *Prev Med* 1993;22:493-8.

51. CDC. Guidelines for school health programs to promote lifelong healthy eating. *MMWR* 1996; 45(RR-9):1-41.

52. CDC. Guidelines for effective school health education to prevent the spread of AIDS. *MMWR* 1988;37(S-2):1-14.

53. CDC. Guidelines for school health programs to prevent tobacco use and addiction. *MMWR* 1994;43(RR-2):1-18.

54. Caspersen CJ, Powell KE, Christenson GM. Physical activity, exercise, and physical fitness: definitions and distinctions for health-related research. *Public Health Rep* 1985;100(2):126-31.

55. Bouchard C, Shephard RJ. Physical activity, fitness, and health: the model and key concepts. In: Bouchard C, Shephard RJ, Stephens T, eds. *Physical activity, fitness, and health: international proceedings and consensus statement.* Champaign, IL: Human Kinetics, 1994:77-88.

56. Dannenberg AL, Keller JB, Wilson PWF, Castelli WP. Leisure time physical activity in the Framingham Offspring Study. *Am J Epidemiol* 1989;129(1):76-88.

57. Slattery ML, McDonald A, Bild DE, et al. Associations of body fat and its distribution with dietary intake, physical activity, alcohol, and smoking in blacks and whites. *Am J Clin Nutr* 1992;55:943-9.

58. Williamson DF, Madans J, Anda RF, Kleinman JC, Kahn HS, Byers T. Recreational physical activity and ten-year weight change in a US national cohort. *Int J Obes* 1993; 17:279-86.

59. French SA, Jeffery RW, Forster JL, McGovern PG, Kelder SH, Baxter JE. Predictors of weight change over two years among a population of working adults: the Healthy Worker Project. *Int J Obes* 1994;18:145-54.

60. Ching PLYH, Willett WC, Rimm EB, Colditz GA, Gortmaker SL, Stampfer MJ. Activity level and risk of overweight in male health professionals. *Am J Public Health* 1996;86(1):25-30.

61. Farmer ME, Locke BZ, Mocicki EK, Dannenberg AL, Larson DB, Radloff LS. Physical activity and depressive symptoms: the NHANES I Epidemiologic Follow-up Study. *Am J Epidemiol* 1988;128(6):1340-51.

62. Ross CE, Hayes D. Exercise and psychologic well-being in the community. *Am J Epidemiol* 1988;127(4):762-71.

63. Stephens T. Physical activity and mental health in the United States and Canada: evidence from four population surveys. *Prev Med* 1988;17:35-47.

64. Camacho TC, Roberts RE, Lazarus NB, Kaplan GA, Cohen RD. Physical activity and depression: evidence from the Alameda County Study. *Am J Epidemiol* 1991;134(2):220-31.

65. Weyerer S. Physical inactivity and depression in the community. *Int J Sports Med* 1992:13(6):492-6.

66. Lane NE, Bloch DA, Jones HH, Marshall WH, Wood PD, Fries JF. Long-distance running, bone density, and osteoarthritis. *JAMA* 1986;255(9):1147-51.

67. Aloia JF, Vaswani AN, Yeh JK, Cohn SH. Premenopausal bone mass is related to physical activity. *Arch Intern Med* 1988;148:121-3.

68. Dalsky GP, Stocke KS, Ehsani AA, Slatopolsky E, Lee WC, Birge SJ Jr. Weight-bearing exercise training and lumbar bone mineral content in postmenopausal women. *Ann Intern Med* 1988;108:824-8.

69. Michel BA, Bloch DA, Fries JF. Weight-bearing exercise, over-exercise, and lumbar bone density over age 50 years. *Arch Intern Med* 1989;149:2325-9.

70. Pruitt LA, Jackson RD, Bartels RL, Lehnhard HJ. Weight-training effects on bone mineral density in early postmeno-pausal women. *J Bone Miner Res* 1992;7(2):179-85.

71. Greendale GA, Barrett-Connor E, Edelstein S, Ingles S, Haile R. Lifetime leisure exercise and osteoporosis: the Rancho Bernardo Study. *Am J Epidemiol* 1995;141(10):951-9.

72. Sobolski J, Kornitzer M, De Backer G, et al. Protection against ischemic heart disease in the Belgian Fitness Study: physical fitness rather than physical activity? *Am J Epidemiol* 1987; 125(4):601-10.

73. Ekelund L-G, Haskell WL, Johnson JL, Whaley FS, Criqui MH, Sheps DS. Physical fitness as a predictor of cardiovascu-lar mortality in asymptomatic North American men. *N Engl J Med* 1988;319(21):1379-84.

74. Slattery ML, Jacobs DR Jr. Physical fitness and cardiovascu-lar disease mortality: the US Railroad Study. *Am J Epidemiol* 1988;127(3):571-80.

75. Blair SN, Kohl HW III, Paffenbarger RS Jr, Clark DG, Cooper KH, Gibbons LW. Physical fitness and all-cause mortality. *JAMA* 1989;262(17):2395-401.

76. Sandvik L, Erikssen J, Thaulow E, Erikssen G, Mundal R, Rodahl K. Physical fitness as a predictor of mortality among healthy, middle-aged Norwegian men. *N Engl J Med* 1993; 328(8):533-7.

77. Blair SN, Kohl HW III, Barlow CE, Paffenbarger RS Jr, Gib-bons LW, Macera CA. Changes in physical fitness and all-cause mortality: a prospective study of healthy and unhealthy men. *JAMA* 1995;273(14):1093-8.

78. Blair SN, Goodyear NN, Gibbons LW, Cooper KH. Physical fitness and incidence of hypertension in healthy normotensive men and women. *JAMA* 1984;252(4):487-90.

79. Bar-Or O, Baranowski T. Physical activity, adiposity, and obesity among adolescents. *Pediatr Exercise Sci* 1994;6:348-60.

80. Armstrong N, Simons-Morton B. Physical activity and blood lipids in adolescents. *Pediatr Exercise Sci* 1994;6:381-405.

81. Alpert BS, Wilmore JH. Physical activity and blood pressure in adolescents. *Pediatr Exercise Sci* 1994;6:361-80.

82. Dotson CO, Ross JG. Relationships between activity patterns and fitness. *J Physical Educ Recreation Dance* 1985;56(1):86-90.

83. Pate RR, Ross JG. Factors associated with health-related fitness. *J Physical Educ Recreation Dance* 1987;58(9):93-5.

84. Tell GS, Vellar OD. Physical fitness, physical activity, and cardiovascular disease risk factors in adolescents: the Oslo Youth Study. *Prev Med* 1988;17:12-24.

85. Aaron DJ, Kriska AM, Dearwater SR, et al. The epidemiology of leisure physical activity in an adolescent population. *Med Sci Sports Exercise* 1993;25(7):847-53.

86. Sallis JF, McKenzie TL, Alcaraz JE. Habitual physical activity and health-related physical fitness in fourth-grade children. *Am J Dis Child* 1993;147:890-6.

87. Berkowitz RI, Agras WS, Korner AF, Kraemer HC, Zeanah CH. Physical activity and adiposity: a longitudinal study from birth to childhood. *J Pediatr* 1985;106:734-8.

88. Fripp RR, Hodgson JL, Kwiterovich PO, Werner JC, Schuler HG, Whitman V. Aerobic capacity, obesity, and atherosclerotic risk factors in male adolescents. *Pediatrics* 1985;75(5):813-8.

89. Sallis JF, Patterson TL, Buono MJ, Nader PR. Relation of cardiovascular fitness and physical activity to cardiovascular disease risk factors in children and adults. *Am J Epidemiol* 1988; 127(5):933-41.

90. Treiber FA, Strong WB, Arensman RW, Gruber M. Relationship between habitual physical activity and cardiovascular responses to exercise in young children. In: Oseid S, Carlsen

K-H, eds. *Children and exercise XIII*. Champaign, IL: Human Kinetics, 1989:285-93.

91. Gutin B, Basch C, Shea S, et al. Blood pressure, fitness, and fatness in 5- and 6-year-old children. *JAMA* 1990; 264(9):1123-7.

92. Suter E, Howes MR. Relationship of physical activity, body fat, diet, and blood lipid profile in youths 10-15 yr. *Med Sci Sports Exercise* 1993;25(6):748-54.

93. Blessing DL, Keith RE, Williford HN, Blessing ME, Barksdale JA. Blood lipid and physiological responses to endurance training in adolescents. *Pediatr Exercise Sci* 1995;7:192-202.

94. Zonderland ML, Erich WBM, Kortlandt W, Erkelens DW. Additional physical education and plasma lipids and apoproteins: a 3-year intervention study. *Pediatr Exercise Sci* 1994;6:128-39.

95. Panico S, Celentano E, Krogh V, et al. Physical activity and its relationship to blood pressure in school children. *J Chron Dis* 1987;40(10):925-30.

96. Strazzullo P, Cappuccio FP, Trevisan M, et al. Leisure time physical activity and blood pressure in schoolchildren. *Am J Epidemiol* 1988;127:726-33.

97. Brandon LJ, Fillingim J. Health fitness training responses of normotensive and elevated normotensive children. *Am J Health Promot* 1990;5(1):30-5.

98. Hansen HS, Froberg K, Hyldebrandt N, Nielsen JR. A controlled study of eight months of physical training and reduction of blood pressure in children: the Odense schoolchild study. *Br Med J* 1991;303:682-5.

99. Bazzano C, Cunningham LN, Varrassi G, Falconio T. Health related fitness and blood pressure in boys and girls ages 10 to 17 years. *Pediatr Exercise Sci* 1992;4:128-35.

100. Shea S, Basch CE, Gutin B, et al. The rate of increase in blood pressure in children 5 years of age is related to changes in aerobic fitness and body mass index. *Pediatrics* 1994;94(4):465-70.

101. Tomassoni TL. Introduction: the role of exercise in the diagnosis and management of chronic disease in children and youth. *Med Sci Sports Exercise* 1996;28(4):403-5.

102. Nixon PA. Role of exercise in the evaluation and management of pulmonary disease in children and youth. *Med Sci Sports Exercise* 1996;28(4):414-20.

103. Tomassoni TL. Role of exercise in the management of cardiovascular disease in children and youth. *Med Sci Sports Exercise* 1996;28(4):406-13.

104. Bar-Or O. Role of exercise in the assessment and management of neuromuscular disease in children. *Med Sci Sports Exercise* 1996;28(4):421-7.

105. Epstein LH, Coleman KJ, Myers MD. Exercise in treating obesity in children and adolescents. *Med Sci Sports Exercise* 1996;28(4):428-35.

106. Ignico AA, Mahon AD. The effects of a physical fitness program on low-fit children. *Res Q Exercise Sport* 1995;66(1):85-90.

107. Gutin B, Cucuzzo N, Islam S, Smith C, Stachura ME. Physical training, lifestyle education, and coronary risk factors in obese girls. *Med Sci Sports Exercise* 1996;28(1):19-23.

108. Brownell KD, Kaye FS. A school-based behavior modification, nutrition education, and physical activity program for obese children. *Am J Clin Nutr* 1982;35:277-83.

109. Sasaski J, Shindo M, Tanaka H, Ando M, Arakawa K. A long-term aerobic exercise program decreases the obesity index and increases the high density lipoprotein cholesterol concentration in obese children. *Int J Obesity* 1987;11:339-45.

110. Epstein LH, Valoski A, Wing RR, McCurley J. Ten-year follow-up of behavioral, family-based treatment for obese children. *JAMA* 1990;264(19):2519-23.

111. Epstein LH, Valoski AM, Vara LS, et al. Effects of decreasing sedentary behavior and increasing activity on weight change in obese children. *Health Psychol* 1995;14(2):109-15.

112. Calfas KJ, Taylor WC. Effects of physical activity on psychological variables in adolescents. *Pediatr Exercise Sci* 1994;6:406-23.

113. Bailey DA, Martin AD. Physical activity and skeletal health in adolescents. *Pediatr Exercise Sci* 1994;6:330-47.

114. McCulloch RG, Bailey DA, Whalen RL, Houston CS, Faulkner RA, Craven BR. Bone density and bone mineral content of adolescent soccer athletes and competitive swimmers. *Pediatr Exercise Sci* 1992;4:319-30.

115. Rubin K, Schirduan V, Gendreau P, Sarfarazi M, Mendola R, Dalsky G. Predictors of axial and peripheral bone mineral density in healthy children and adolescents, with special attention to the role of puberty. *J Pediatr* 1993;123:863-70.

116. American College of Sports Medicine. Opinion statement on physical fitness in children and youth. *Med Sci Sports Exercise* 1988;20(4):422-3.

117. Fletcher GF, Blair SN, Blumenthal J, et al. Statement on exercise. Benefits and recommendations for physical activity programs for all Americans. *Circulation* 1992;86(1):340-4.

118. American Heart Association. Strategic plan for promoting physical activity. Dallas, TX: American Heart Association, 1995.

119. Ibrahim MA, Yankauer A. The promotion of exercise. *Am J Public Health* 1988;78(11):1413-4.

120. Iverson DC, Fielding JE, Crow RS, Christenson GM. The promotion of physical activity in the United States population: the status of programs in medical, worksite, community, and school settings. *Public Health Rep* 1985;100(2):212-23.

121. King AC. Community and public health approaches to the promotion of physical activity. *Med Sci Sports Exercise* 1994;26(11):1405-12.

122. King AC, Jeffery RW, Fridinger FW, et al. Environmental and policy approaches to cardiovascular disease prevention through physical activity: issues and opportunities. *Health Educ Q* 1995;22(44):499-511.

123. Schmid TL, Pratt M, Howze E. Policy as intervention: environmental and policy approaches to the prevention of cardiovascular disease. *Am J Public Health* 1995;85(9):1207-11.

124. Owen N, Lee C. Development of behaviorally-based policy guidelines for the promotion of exercise. *J Public Health Policy* 1989;10(1):43-61.

125. McGinnis JM, Kanner L, DeGraw C. Physical education's role in achieving national health objectives. *Res Q Exercise Sport* 1991;62(2):138-42.

126. Winkleby MA. The future of community-based cardiovascular disease intervention studies. *Am J Public Health* 1994;84(9):1369-72.

127. Blair SN, Booth M, Gyarfas I, et al. Development of public policy and physical activity initiatives internationally. *Sports Med* 1996;21(3):157-63.

128. Sallis JF, Patrick K. Physical activity guidelines for adolescents: consensus statement. *Pediatr Exercise Sci* 1994;6:302-14.

129. Simons-Morton BG, O'Hara NM, Parcel GS, Huang IW, Baranowski T, Wilson B. Children's frequency of participation in moderate to vigorous physical activities. *Res Q Exercise Sport* 1990;61(4):307-14.

130. Pate RR, Long BJ, Heath G. Descriptive epidemiology of physical activity in adolescents. *Pediatr Exercise Sci* 1994;6:434-47.

131. Sallis JF. Epidemiology of physical activity and fitness in children and adolescents. *Crit Rev Food Sci Nutr* 1993;33(4/5):403-8.

132. Kelder SH, Perry CL, Peters RJ Jr, Lytle LL, Klepp K-I. Gender differences in the Class of 1989 Study: the school component of the Minnesota Heart Health Program. *J Health Educ* 1995;26 (2 suppl):S36-S44.

133. Zakarian JM, Hovell MF, Hofstetter CR, Sallis JF, Keating KJ. Correlates of vigorous exercise in a predominantly low SES and minority high school population. *Prev Med* 1994;23:314-21.

134. Robinson TN, Killen JD. Ethnic and gender differences in the relationships between television viewing and obesity, physical activity, and dietary fat intake. *J Health Educ* 1995;26(2 suppl):S91-S98.

135. Reynolds KD, Killen JD, Bryson SW, et al. Psychosocial predictors of physical activity in adolescents. *Prev Med* 1990;19:541-51.

136. Trost SG, Pate RR, Dowda M, Saunders R, Ward DS, Felton G. Gender differences in physical activity and determinants of physical activity in rural fifth grade children. *J Sch Health* 1996; 66(4):145-50.

137. Tappe MK, Duda JL, Menges-Ehrnwald P. Personal investment predictors of adolescent motivational orientation toward exercise. *Can J Sport Sci* 1990;15(3):185-92.

138. Ferguson KJ, Yesalis CE, Pomrehn PR, Kirkpatrick MB. Attitudes, knowledge, and beliefs as predictors of exercise intent and behavior in schoolchildren. *J Sch Health* 1989;59(3):112-5.

139. Dempsey JM, Kimiecik JC, Horn TS. Parental influence on children's moderate to vigorous physical activity participation: an expectancy-value approach. *Pediatr Exercise Sci* 1993;5:151-67.

140. Biddle S, Armstrong N. Children's physical activity: an exploratory study of psychological correlates. *Soc Sci Med* 1992;34(3):325-31.

141. Biddle S, Goudas M. Analysis of children's physical activity and its association with adult encouragement and social cognitive variables. *J Sch Health* 1996;66(2):75-8.

142. Stucky-Ropp RC, DiLorenzo TM. Determinants of exercise in children. *Prev Med* 1993;22:880-9.

143. Tinsley BJ, Holtgrave DR, Reise SP, Erdley C, Cupp RG. Developmental status, gender, age, and self-reported decision-making influences on students' risky and preventive health behaviors. *Health Educ Q* 1995;22(2):244-59.

144. McCullagh P, Matzkanin KT, Shaw SD, Maldonado M. Motivation for participation in physical activity: a comparison of parent-child perceived competencies and participation motives. *Pediatr Exercise Sci* 1993;5:224-33.

145. Athletic Footwear Association. *American youth and sports participation*. North Palm Beach, FL: Athletic Footwear Association, 1990.

146. Borra ST, Schwartz NE, Spain CG, Natchipolsky MM. Food, physical activity, and fun: inspiring America's kids to more healthful lifestyles. *J Am Diet Assoc* 1995;95(7):816-8.

147. Godin G, Shephard RJ. Psychosocial factors influencing intentions to exercise of young students from grades 7 to 9. *Res Q Exercise Sport* 1986;57(1):41-52.

148. Tappe MK, Duda JL, Ehrnwald PM. Perceived barriers to exercise among adolescents. *J Sch Health* 1989;59(4):153-5.

149. Marcus BH, Eaton CA, Ross JS, Harlow LL. Self-efficacy, decision-making, and stages of change: an integrative model of physical exercise. *J Appl Soc Psychol* 1994;24(6):489-508.

150. Calfas KJ, Sallis JF, Lovato CY, Campbell J. Physical activity and its determinants before and after college graduation. *Med Exercise Nutr Health* 1994;3:323-34.

151. Cardinal BJ. The stages of exercise scale and stages of exercise behavior in female adults. *J Sports Med Physical Fitness* 1995;35(2):87-92.

152. Marcus BH, Simkin LR. The transtheoretical model: applications to exercise behavior. *Med Sci Sports Exercise* 1994;26(11):1400-4.

153. Armstrong CA, Sallis JF, Hovell MF, Hofstetter CR. Stages of change, self-efficacy, and the adoption of vigorous exercise: a prospective analysis. *J Sport Exercise Psychol* 1993;15:390-402.

154. Anderssen N, Wold B. Parental and peer influences on leisure-time physical activity in young adolescents. *Res Q Exercise Sport* 1992;63(4):341-8.

155. Perusse L, Tremblay A, LeBlanc C, Bouchard C. Genetic and environmental influences on level of habitual physical activity and exercise participation. *Am J Epidemiol* 1989;129(5):1012-22.

156. Sallis JF, Patterson TL, Buono MJ, Atkins CJ, Nader PR. Aggregation of physical activity habits in Mexican-American and Anglo families. *J Behav Med* 1988;11(1):31-41.

157. Butcher J. Longitudinal analysis of adolescent girls' participation in physical activity. *Sociol Sport J* 1985;2:130-43.

158. Sallis JF, Alcaraz JE, McKenzie TL, Hovell MF, Kolody B, Nader PR. Parental behavior in relation to physical activity and fitness in 9-year-old children. *Am J Dis Child* 1992;146:1383-8.

159. McMurray RG, Bradley CB, Harrell JS, Bernthal PR, Frauman AC, Bangdiwala SI. Parental influences on childhood fitness and activity patterns. *Res Q Exercise Sport* 1993;64(3):249-55.

160. Garcia AW, Norton Broda MA, Frenn M, Coviak C, Pender NJ, Ronis DL. Gender and developmental differences in exercise beliefs among youth and prediction of their exercise behavior. *J Sch Health* 1995;65(6):213-9.

161. Freedson PS, Evenson S. Familial aggregation in physical activity. *Res Q Exercise Sport* 1991; 62(4):384-9.

162. Gottlieb NH, Chen M-S. Sociocultural correlates of childhood sporting activities: their implications for heart health. *Soc Sci Med* 1985;21(5):533-9.

163. Poest CA, Williams JR, Witt DD, Atwood ME. Physical activity patterns of preschool children. *Early Childhood Res Q* 1989;4:367-76.

164. Public Health Service. *Healthy People 2000: national health promotion and disease prevention objectives*. Full report, with commentary. Washington, DC: U.S. Department of Health and Human Services, Public Health Service, 1991. DHHS publication no. (PHS) 91-50212.

165. Nicklas TA, Webber LS, Johnson CC, Srinivasan SR, Berenson GS. Foundations for health promotion with youth: a review of observations from the Bogalusa Heart Study. *J Health Educ* 1995;26(2 suppl):S18-S26.

166. Troiano RP, Flegal KM, Kuczmarksi RJ, Campbell SM, Johnson CL. Overweight prevalence and trends for children and adolescents. *Arch Pediatr Adolesc Med* 1995;149:1085-91.

167. Kelder SH, Perry CL, Klepp K-I, Lytle LL. Longitudinal tracking of adolescent smoking, physical activity, and food choice behaviors. *Am J Public Health* 1994;84(7):1121-6.

168. Public Health Service. *Healthy People 2000: midcourse review and 1995 revisions*. Washington, DC: U.S. Department of Health and Human Services, Public Health Service, 1995.

169. Kann L, Collins JL, Pateman BC, Small ML, Ross JG, Kolbe LJ. The School Health Policies and Programs Study (SHPPS): rationale for a nationwide status report on school health programs. *J Sch Health* 1995;65(8):291-4.

170. Ross JG, Dotson CO, Gilbert GG, Katz SJ. After physical education.... Physical activity outside of school physical education programs. *J Physical Educ Recreation Dance* 1985;56(1):77-81.

171. CDC. *Promoting physical activity: a guide for community action*. Atlanta: U.S. Department of Health and Human Services, Public Health Service, CDC (in press).

172. Allensworth D, Wyche J, Lawson E, Nicholson L, eds. *Defining a comprehensive school health program: an interim statement*. Washington, DC: National Academy Press, 1995.

173. Kolbe LJ, Kann L, Collins JL, Small ML, Pateman BC, Warren CW. The School Health Policies and Programs Study (SHPPS): context, methods, general findings, and future efforts. *J Sch Health* 1995;65(8):339-43.

174. Bush PJ, Zuckerman AE, Theiss PK, et al. Cardiovascular risk factor prevention in black schoolchildren: two-year results of the "Know Your Body" program. *Am J Epidemiol* 1989; 129(3):466-82.

175. Bush PJ, Zuckerman AE, Taggart VS, Theiss PK, Peleg EO, Smith SA. Cardiovascular risk factor prevention in black school children: the "Know Your Body" evaluation project. *Health Educ Q* 1989;16(2):215-27.

176. Simons-Morton BG, Parcel GS, O'Hara NM. Implementing organizational changes to promote healthful diet and physical activity at school. *Health Educ Q* 1988;15(1):115-30.

177. Simons-Morton BG, Parcel GS, Baranowski T, Forthofer R, O'Hara NM. Promoting physical activity and a healthful diet among children: results of a school-based intervention study. *Am J Public Health* 1991;81(8):986-91.

178. Parcel GS, Simons-Morton BG, O'Hara NM, Baranowski T, Kolbe LJ, Bee DE. School promotion of healthful diet and exercise behavior: an integration of organizational change and social learning theory interventions. *J Sch Health* 1987;57(4):150-6.

179. Luepker RV, Perry CL, McKinlay SM, et al. Outcomes of a field trial to improve children's dietary patterns and physical activity: the Child and Adolescent Trial for Cardiovascular Health (CATCH). *JAMA* 1996;275(10):768-76.

180. Perry CL, Stone EJ, Parcel GS, et al. School-based cardiovascular health promotion: the Child and Adolescent Trial for Cardiovascular Health (CATCH). *J Sch Health* 1990;60(8):406-13.

181. Perry CL, Parcel GS, Stone E, et al. The Child and Adolescent Trial for Cardiovascular Health (CATCH): overview of the intervention program and evaluation methods. *Cardiovasc Risk Factors* 1992;2(1):36-44.

182. Stone EJ. Foreword. *Health Educ Q* 1994;suppl 2:S3-S4.

183. Arbeit ML, Johnson CC, Mott DS, et al. The Heart Smart cardiovascular school health promotion: behavior correlates of risk factor change. *Prev Med* 1992;21:18-32.

184. Butcher AH, Frank GC, Harsha DW, et al. Heart Smart: a school health program meeting the 1990 objectives for the nation. *Health Educ Q* 1988;5(1):17-34.

185. Downey AM, Frank GC, Webber LS, et al. Implementation of "Heart Smart:" a cardiovascular school health promotion program. *J Sch Health* 1987;57(3):98-104.

186. Kelder SH, Perry CL, Klepp K-I. Community-wide youth exercise promotion: long-term outcomes of the Minnesota Heart Health Program and the Class of 1989 Study. *J Sch Health* 1993;63(5):218-23.

187. Prokhorov AV, Perry CL, Kelder SH, Klepp K-I. Lifestyle values of adolescents: results from Minnesota heart health youth program. *Adolescence* 1993;28(111):637-47.

188. Bandura A. Social foundations of thought and action: a social cognitive theory. Englewood Cliffs, NJ: Prentice-Hall, 1986.

189. McKenzie TL, Sallis JF, Faucette N, Roby JJ, Kolody B. Effects of a curriculum and inservice program on the quantity and quality of elementary physical education classes. *Res Q Exercise Sport* 1993;64(2):178-87.

190. Duncan B, Boyce WT, Itami R, Puffenbarger N. A controlled trial of a physical fitness program for fifth grade students. *J Sch Health* 1983;53(8):467-71.

191. Dwyer T, Coonan WE, Worsley A, Leitch DR. An assessment of the effects of two physical activity programmes on coronary heart disease risk factors in primary school children. *Community Health Stud* 1979;3(3):196-202.

192. Dwyer T, Coonan WE, Leitch DR, Hetzel BS, Baghurst RA. An investigation of the effects of daily physical activity on the health of primary school students in South Australia. *Int J Epidemiol* 1983;12:308-13.

193. Shephard RJ, Lavallee H. Changes of physical performance as indicators of the response to enhanced physical education. *J Sports Med Physical Fitness* 1994;34(4):323-35.

194. Shephard RJ, Lavallee H. Impact of enhanced physical education on muscle strength of the prepubescent child. *Pediatr Exercise Sci* 1994;6:75-87.

195. Vandongen R, Jenner DA, Thompson C, et al. A controlled evaluation of a fitness and nutrition intervention program on cardiovascular health in 10- to 12-year-old children. *Prev Med* 1995;24:9-22.

196. National Association for Sport and Physical Education. *Sport and physical education advocacy kit*. Reston, VA: National Association for Sport and Physical Education, 1994.

197. Pate RR, Small ML, Ross JG, Young JC, Flint KH, Warren CW. School physical education. *J Sch Health* 1995;65(8):312-8.

198. National Association for Sport and Physical Education. *Guidelines for secondary school physical education*. Reston, VA: National Association for Sport and Physical Education, 1992.

199. Connell DB, Turner RR, Mason EF. Summary of findings of the School Health Education Evaluation: health promotion

effectiveness, implementation, and costs. *J Sch Health* 1985; 55(8):316-21.

200. The National Commission on the Role of the School and the Community in Improving Adolescent Health. *Code blue: uniting for healthier youth*. Alexandria, VA: National Association of State Boards of Education, 1990.

201. National School Boards Association. *School health: helping children learn*. Alexandria, VA: National School Boards Association, 1991.

202. Council of Chief State School Officers. *Beyond the health room*. Washington, DC: Council of Chief State School Officers, 1993.

203. Comprehensive School Health Education Workshop. National action plan for comprehensive school health education. *J Sch Health* 1993;63(1):46-53.

204. Collins JL, Small ML, Kann L, Pateman BC, Gold RS, Kolbe LJ. School health education. *J Sch Health* 1995;65(8):302-11.

205. Gallup Organization. *Values and opinions of comprehensive school health education in US public schools: adolescents, parents, and school district administrators*. Atlanta: American Cancer Society, 1994.

206. National Association for Sport and Physical Education. *Guidelines for elementary school physical education*. Reston, VA: National Association for Sport and Physical Education, 1994.

207. National Association for Sport and Physical Education. *Guidelines for middle school physical education*. Reston, VA: National Association for Sport and Physical Education, 1992.

208. Joint Committee on National Health Education Standards. *National health education stan-dards: achieving health literacy. An investment in the future*. Atlanta: American Cancer Society, 1995.

209. Lavin AT. Comprehensive school health education: barriers and opportunities. *J Sch Health* 1993;63(1):24-7.

210. National Association for Sport and Physical Education. *Appropriate practices for middle school physical education*. Reston,

VA: National Association for Sport and Physical Education, 1995.

211. National Association for Sport and Physical Education. *Moving into the future: national stan-dards for physical education. A guide to content and assessment*. Reston, VA: Mosby, 1995.

212. McKenzie TL, Feldman H, Woods SE, et al. Children's activity levels and lesson context during third-grade physical education. *Res Q Exercise Sport* 1995;66(3):184-93.

213. National Association for Sport and Physical Education. *Quality sports, quality coaches: national standards for athletic coaches*. Reston, VA: Kendall/Hunt Publishing Company, 1995.

214. Millstein SG, Nightingale EO, Petersen AC, Mortimer AM, Hamburg DA. Promoting the healthy development of adolescents. *JAMA* 1993;269(11):1413-5.

215. Grahm G. Physical education through students' eyes and in students' voices: implications for teachers and researchers. *J Teaching Physical Educ* 1995;14:478-82.

216. Portman PA. Who is having fun in physical education classes? Experiences of sixth-grade students in elementary and middle schools. *J Teaching Physical Educ* 1995;14:445-53.

217. Stone EJ, Baranowski T, Sallis JF, Cutler JA. Review of behavioral research for cardiopulmonary health: emphasis on youth, gender, and ethnicity. *J Health Educ* 1995;26(2 suppl):S9-S17.

218. Faucette N, Sallis JF, McKenzie T, Alcaraz J, Kolody B, Nugent P. Comparison of fourth grade students' out-of-school physical activity levels and choices by gender: Project SPARK. *J Health Educ* 1995;26(2 suppl):S82-S90.

219. Lirgg CD. Gender differences in self-confidence in physical activity: a meta-analysis of recent studies. *J Sport Exercise Psychol* 1991;8:294-310.

220. Pate RR, Hohn RC. Health-related physical education—A direction for the 21st century. In: Pate RR, Hohn RC, eds. *Health and fitness through physical education*. Champaign, IL: Human Kinetics, 1994:215-7.

221. Ward DS. Exercise for children with special needs. In: Pate RR, Hohn RC, eds. *Health and fitness through physical education*. Champaign, IL: Human Kinetics, 1994:99-111.

222. American Association for Active Lifestyles and Fitness and the National Association for Sport and Physical Education. *Including students with disabilities in physical education*. Reston, VA: National Association for Sport and Physical Education, 1995.

223. DeSensi JT. Understanding multiculturalism and valuing di versity: a theoretical perspective. *Quest* 1995;47:34-43.

224. Carnegie Council on Adolescent Development. A matter of time: risk and opportunity in the out-of-school hours. Recommendations for strengthening community programs for youth. New York, NY: Carnegie Corporation of New York, 1994.

225. U.S. Consumer Product Safety Commission. *Handbook for public playground safety*. Washington, DC: U.S. Government Printing Office, 1991. Publication no. 305-724.

226. Jambor T, Palmer SD. Playground safety manual. Birmingham, AL: Alabama Chapter of the American Academy of *Pediatrics*, 1991.

227. Dyment PG, ed. Sports medicine: health care for young athletes. 2nd ed. Elk Grove Village, IL: American Academy of *Pediatrics*, 1991.

228. Wilson MH, Baker SP, Teret SP, Shock S, Garbarino J. *Saving children: a guide to injury prevention*. New York, NY: Oxford University Press, 1991.

229. Macera CA, Wooten W. Epidemiology of sports and recreation injuries among adolescents. *Pediatr Exercise Sci* 1994;6:424-33.

230. Budetti PP, Feinson C. Ensuring adequate health care benefits for children and adolescents. In: Solloway MR, Budetti PP, eds. *Child health supervision: analytical studies in the financing, delivery, and cost-effectiveness of preventive and health promotion services for infants, children, and adolescents*. Arlington, VA: National Center for Education in Maternal and Child Health, 1995:77-100.

231. Green M, ed. *Bright futures: guidelines for health supervision of infants, children, and adolescents.* Arlington, VA: National Center for Education in Maternal and Child Health, 1994.

232. Buller DB, Callister MA, Reichert T. Skin cancer prevention by parents of young children: health information sources, skin cancer knowledge, and sun-protection practices. *Oncol Nurs Forum* 1995;22(10):1559-66.

233. Ross JG, Pate RR, Corbin CB, Delpy LA, Gold RS. What is going on in the elementary physical education program? *J Physical Educ Recreation Dance* 1987;58(9):78-84.

234. Blair SN, Collingwood TR, Reynolds R, Smith M, Hagan RD, Sterling CL. Health promotion for educators: impact on health behaviors, satisfaction, and general well-being. *Am J Public Health* 1984;74(2):147-9.

235. Blair SN, Smith M, Collingwood TR, Reynolds R, Prentice MC, Sterling CL. Health promotion for educators: impact on absenteeism. *Prev Med* 1986;15:166-75.

236. Ross JG, Gilbert GG. A summary of findings. *J Physical Educ Recreation Dance* 1985;56(1):45-50.

237. Sallis JF, McKenzie TL. Physical education's role in public health. *Res Q Exercise Sport* 1991;62(2):124-37.

238. Pate RR, Hohn RC. A contemporary mission for physical education. In: Pate RR, Hohn RC, eds. *Health and fitness through physical education.* Champaign, IL: Human Kinetics, 1994:1-8.

239. American Academy of Pediatrics. Physical fitness and the schools. *Pediatrics* 1987;80(3):449-50.

240. Corbin CB, Pangrazi RP. Are American children and youth fit? *Res Q Exercise Sport* 1992;63(2):96-106.

241. Freedson PS, Rowland TW. Youth activity level versus youth fitness: let's redirect our efforts. *Res Q Exercise Sport* 1992;63(2):133-6.

242. Sallis JF. Determinants of physical activity behavior in children. In: Pate RR, Hohn RC, eds. *Health and fitness through physical education.* Champaign, IL: Human Kinetics, 1994:31-43.

243. Silverman S. Relationship of engagement and practice trials to student achievement. *J Teaching Physical Educ* 1985;5:13-21.

244. Graham KC. A description of academic work and student performance in a middle school volleyball unit. *J Teaching Physical Educ* 1987;7:22-37.

245. Buck M, Harrison JM, Bryce GR. An analysis of learning trials and their relationship to achievement in volleyball. *J Teaching Physical Educ* 1990;10:134-52.

246. Perry CL, Baranowski T, Parcel GS. How individuals, environments, and health behavior interact: social learning theory. In: Glanz K, Lewis FM, Rimer RK, eds. *Health behavior and health education: theory, research, and practice.* San Francisco, CA: Jossey-Bass, 1990:161-86.

247. Nelson MA. The role of physical education and children's activity in public health. *Res Q Exercise Sport* 1991;62(2):148-50.

248. Quinn PB, Strand B. A comparison of two instructional formats on heart rate intensity and skill development. *Physical Educator* 1995;52(2):62-9.

249. Li XJ, Dunham P Jr. Fitness load and exercise time in secondary physical education classes. J Teaching Physical Educ 1993;12:180-7.

250. Simons-Morton BG, Taylor WC, Snider SA, Huang IW. The physical activity of fifth-grade students during physical education classes. *Am J Public Health* 1993;83(2):262-4.

251. Simons-Morton BG, Taylor WC, Snider SA, Huang IW, Fulton JE. Observed levels of elementary and middle school children's physical activity during physical education classes. *Prev Med* 1994;23:437-41.

252. Tolsma DD, Koplan JP. Health behaviors and health promotion. In: Last JM, Wallace RB, eds. *Public health and preventive medicine. 13th ed.* Norwalk, CT: Appleton & Lange, 1992:701-14.

253. Mullen PD, Evans D, Forster J, et al. Settings as an important dimension in health education/promotion policy, programs, and research. *Health Educ Q* 1995;22(3):329-45.

254. Allensworth DD. The research base for innovative practices in school health education at the secondary level. *J Sch Health* 1994;64(5):180-7.

255. Petlichkoff LM. Youth sport participation and withdrawal: is it simply a matter of fun? *Pediatr Exercise Sci* 1992;4:105-10.

256. Seefeldt V, Ewing M, Walk S. *Overview of youth sports programs in the United States.* Washington, DC: Carnegie Council on Adolescent Development, 1993.

257. Strong WB. Physical activity and children. *Circulation* 1990;81(5):1697-701.

258. Elster AB, Kuznets NJ. *AMA Guidelines for Adolescent Preventive Services (GAPS): recommendations and rationale.* Baltimore, MD: Williams & Wilkins, 1994.

259. Birch DA. Involving families in school health education: implications for professional preparation. *J Sch Health* 1994;64(7):296-9.

260. Brustad RJ. Who will go out and play? Parental and psychological influences on children's attraction to physical activity. *Pediatr Exercise Sci* 1993;5:210-23.

261. Nader PR, Sallis JF, Broyles SL, et al. Ethnic and gender trends for cardiovascular risk behaviors in Anglo and Mexican American children ages four to seven. *J Health Educ* 1995;26(2 suppl):S27-S35.

262. Haywood KM. The role of physical education in the development of active lifestyles. *Res Q Exercise Sport* 1991;62(2):151-6.

263. Gold RS. The science base for comprehensive school health education. In: Cortese P, Middleton K, eds. *The comprehensive school health challenge. Volume 2: promoting health through education.* Santa Cruz, CA: ETR Associates, 1994:545-73.

264. Burks A, Fox E. Why is inservice training essential? In: Cortese P, Middleton K, eds. The comprehensive school health challenge. Volume 2: promoting health through education. Santa Cruz, CA: ETR Associates, 1994:783-99.

265. National Association for Sport and Physical Education. *National standards for beginning physical education teachers.*

Reston, VA: National Association for Sport and Physical Education, 1995.

266. National Task Force on the Preparation and Practice of Health Educators. *A guide for the development of competency-based curricula for entry level health educators.* New York, NY: National Task Force for the Preparation and Practice of Health Educators, 1983.

267. Joint Committee of the Association for the Advancement of Health Education and the American School Health Association. Health instruction responsibilities and competencies for elementary (K-6) classroom teachers. *J Health Educ* 1992;23(6):352-4.

268. Tappe MK, Galer-Unti RA, Bailey KC. Long-term implementation of the Teenage Health Teaching Modules by trained teachers: a case study. *J Sch Health* 1995;65(10):411-5.

269. DuRant RH, Hergenroeder AC. Promotion of physical activity among adolescents by primary health care providers. *Pediatr Exercise Sci* 1994;6:448-63.

270. Small ML, Majer LS, Allensworth DD, Farquhar BK, Kann L, Pateman BC. School health services. *J Sch Health* 1995;65(8):319-26.

271. Brown BR Jr, Butterfield SA. Coaches: a missing link in the health care system. *Am J Dis Child* 1992;146:211-7.

272. Scanlan TK, Carpenter PJ, Lobel M, Simons JP. Sources of enjoyment for youth sport athletes. *Pediatr Exercise Sci* 1993;5:275-85.

273. McKenzie TL, Strikmiller PK, Stone EJ, et al. CATCH: physical activity process evaluation in a multicenter trial. *Health Educ Q* 1994;suppl 2:S73-S89.

274. Edmundson EW, Luton SC, McGraw SA, et al. CATCH: classroom process evaluation in a multicenter trial. *Health Educ Q* 1994;suppl 2:S27-S50.

275. National Association for Sport and Physical Education. *Parent/guardian's checklist for quality sport and physical activity programs for children and youth.* Reston, VA: National Association for Sport and Physical Education, n.d.

276. Nugent P, Faucette N. Marginalized voices: constructions of and responses to physical education and grading practices by students categorized as gifted or learning disabled. *J Teaching Physical Educ* 1995;14:418-30.

Technical Advisors

Tom Baranowski, Ph.D. M.D. Anderson Cancer Center University of Texas Houston, TX; Oded Bar-Or, M.D. McMaster University Hamilton, Canada; Steven Blair, P.E.D. Cooper Institute for Aerobics Research Dallas, TX; Charles Corbin, Ph.D. Arizona State University Tempe, AZ; Marsha Dowda, M.S.P.H.* University of South Carolina Columbia, SC; Patty Freedson, Ph.D. University of Massachusetts Amherst, MA; Russell Pate, Ph.D.* University of South Carolina Columbia, SC; Sharon Plowman, Ph.D. Northern Illinois University De Kalb, IL; James Sallis, Ph.D. San Diego State University San Diego, CA; Ruth Saunders, Ph.D.* University of South Carolina Columbia, SC; Vernon Seefeldt, Ph.D. Michigan State University East Lansing, MI; Daryl Siedentop, P.E.D. Ohio State University Columbus, OH; Bruce Simons-Morton, Ed.D., M.P.H. National Institute for Child Health and Human Development Bethesda, MD; Christine Spain, M.A. President's Council on Physical Fitness and Sports Washington, DC; Marlene Tappe, Ph.D.* Centers for Disease Control and Prevention Atlanta, GA; Dianne Ward, Ed.D.* University of South Carolina Columbia, SC;

*Assisted in the preparation of this report.

Chapter 17

99 Tips for Family Fitness Fun

Introduction

A Message from Dr. Koop on Healthy Weight and Physical Fitness

"A survey conducted by Shape Up America! has revealed that child care responsibilities are interfering with the efforts of many families to get more exercise and at the same time we know many children are now overweight or obese. The solution is a commitment on the part of the entire family to spend more time together. I encourage you to choose activities you can do together and support and reward each other's efforts to be more active at home, at school, at work, and in your communities. I urge you to replace the use of food as a reward for good behavior and offer to take a walk with your child instead. The pleasure of your company is the best reward your child can receive and the best gift you can give."

— *Dr. C. Everett Koop*

Getting Started

1. Schedule a regular time throughout the week for physical activity.

From "99 Tips for Family Fitness Fun," a cooperative effort of the National Association for Sport and Physical Education, Shape Up America!, and MET-RX Foundation for Health Management; reprinted with permission. Available at http://www.shapeup.org/publications/99.tips.for.family.fitness.fun/index.html.

2. Take turns selecting an activity for the family to do as a group each week.

3. Start a log of daily fitness activities for each family member.

4. Adapt all activities to suit those with special needs and preferences.

5. Help everyone to find something active that makes them feel successful.

Remember: It does not have to cost a lot of money to activate the family!

Tips for the Home

6. Designate indoor and outdoor play areas where rolling, climbing, jumping, and tumbling are allowed.

7. Buy toys or equipment that promote physical activity.

8. Select fitness-oriented gifts with the recipient's skills and interests in mind.

9. Limit time spent watching television programs, videotapes, and playing computer games.

10. Use physical activity rather than food as a reward (e.g., family goes in-line skating).

11. Include grandparents, other relatives, and friends whenever possible.

12. Emphasize the importance of having fun and learning; avoid a push "to win."

13. Get off the couch and change the channel manually—or better yet, turn it off!

14. Spend as much time outdoors as possible.

Tips for the Kitchen

15. Pack your own nutritious snacks and meals for family outings.

16. Keep fresh fruit and vegetables washed, cut-up, chilled and readily available for post-exercise snacking.

17. Have attractive containers of water available during and after workouts.

18. Take the family grocery shopping so everyone can learn to read the nutrition labels (find the cereal that offers the most fiber per serving; find the tastiest non-fat cheese).

Tips for School

19. Talk to the physical education teacher about your child's physical education program and how you can provide support.

20. Encourage your school board to make physical education a priority.

21. Volunteer to help with physical activity events at your child's school.

22. Join a marching band for excellent exercise.

23. Encourage your school physical education teacher to coordinate family evening and weekend activities in the gymnasium or in the schoolyard.

Tips for Work

24. Stop every hour or two to walk and stretch.

25. Devote a portion of your lunch break to physical activity (e.g., walking).

26. Collect data on dollars spent and days of work lost due to illness related to overweight and/or sedentary lifestyles and encourage your employer to install facilities and provide incentives to support physical activity in order to avoid such disorders as:

    - diabetes
    - cardiovascular disease
    - breast cancer
    - hypertension
    - stroke
    - and others

27. Walk to a co-worker's desk rather than using the intercom.

28. Make plans with a co-worker to go to a gym or participate in a sport on a weekly basis.

Tips for Anywhere

29. Pack a lunch for work if it's hard to find restaurants and delis that offer whole grains, fruits and vegetables.

30. Always use the stairs.

31. Carry items such as book bags, groceries, and picnic baskets to build strength.

32. Walk, jog, or skip instead of driving (to and from school, grocery store, library, park, etc.).

33. Make chores YOUR chance to be active.

34. Get off the bus a few stops early and walk.

35. Park the car AS FAR AWAY from the entrance as possible.

The Great Outdoors

36. Discover what free and low-cost physical activity areas are near your home (park, bike trail, hiking trail, tennis court, swimming pool, etc.).

37. Rake leaves ... then jump in them!

38. Shovel snow; build a snow sculpture; make snow angels; build a snow house.

39. Dig and plant in the garden; help everyone plant their own vegetables, fruits and flowers.

40. Chop and stack wood; end with a campfire and sing-a-long.

41. Take a long walk or jog on the beach.

42. Cross country ski around town and into the woods.

43. Use a compass to map out a course—then set out on a walk, jog, or bike hike.

44. Canoe or raft for an entire afternoon.

45. Ice skate for a great winter workout.

46. Skiing always gives the family a lift.

47. Jump into water sports—enjoy water walking and aerobics.

48. Play mixed-age water volleyball.

49. Visit outdoor education centers.

50. Take a nature hike.

51. Go up, up and away with a kite-flying day.

52. Go to a driving range or enjoy a game of miniature golf.

53. Go camping where you can pitch a tent, gather firewood, fish, bike, and walk.

54. Visit farms throughout the year where you can pick your own strawberries, peaches, and apples.

55. Plan cycling trips on safe trails by calling your local bike shop or bike club.

In Your Own Backyard

56. Run, jog, and walk in a family treasure hunt.

57. Toss around as many different-shaped balls/objects as you can find.

58. Juggle with the entire family.

59. Play "Hit and Go" croquet—hit the ball and run to it—across the whole yard.

60. Count hula hoop rotations.

61. Jump rope—practice rhythms, rhymes and tricks.

62. Play a "hot potato" game of Frisbee.

63. Play an action-packed game of badminton. Serve from where the birdie drops.

64. Jump on Pogo stick and count bounces.

65. Build stilts and walk on them to create laughter and exercise.

66. Ride on a skateboard (with knee, wrist and elbow pads and helmets).

67. Play hopscotch and organize a family tournament.

68. Run and dodge in a "Tag and You're It" game.

69. Play traditional and modified backyard sports: basketball, softball, volleyball, and tetherball.

70. Practice on in-line skates (with knee and elbow pads and helmets)—go further and get faster each day.

71. Take the family pet for a walk or jog.

72. Wash the car...enjoy an active game with the hose.

Tips for the Neighborhood, Community, and Beyond

73. Create your own Olympic events at a family reunion or neighborhood block party.

74. Organize a family swim outing—be sure to swim with a buddy in supervised areas.

75. Enjoy a weekend afternoon of physical activities at a local community center.

76. Enter and walk in holiday parades, ethnic festivals, and charity fundraisers.

77. Walk or bike to a nearby playground—challenge family members to try their skills swinging, crossing a horizontal ladder.

78. Take a historical (or architectural) walk or cycling tour.

79. Plan a "block fitness festival," including relay races.

80. Adopt a highway, park, or beach, and keep it clean.

81. Participate in a "volksmarch." It's German for a "people's walk," is social in nature, and usually 10 kilometers (6.2 miles).

82. Help organize mall walks—especially in bad weather.

83. Help organize your building, development, or community to exercise on preset routes at preset times so you can keep each other company.

84. Enter a "Fun Run" or a "Bike-a-Thon."

85. Encourage local religious and civic organizations to allow halls to be used for indoor family activities.

Take Advantage of Facilities in Your Neighborhood

86. Join the Y or a health club.

87. Organize a party at an indoor ice or roller skating rink.

88. Bowl to your heart's content.

89. Participate in a mixed-age martial arts class.

Don't Be Stuck—Liven Up!

On rainy days or when stormy weather keeps you indoors, don't let your fitness fun fail. Music makes it easy!

90. Create a family video of exercise routines.

91. Invite friends and neighbors over for some country western line dancing.

92. Invent a new dance and name it after your family.

93. Host a dance fever contest.

94. Share dances from each generation in your family.

95. Throw an ethnic/multi-cultural dance party.

Take Advantage of What You've Got around the House

96. Use a bench or steps for step-aerobic workout.

97. Play "Twister" or other indoor active games.

98. Encourage everyone to "act out" a story as you read it.

99. Build an obstacle course in the basement or garage on a rainy day.

And there are at least 99,000 more! Make up your own—and be on your way to becoming a fit family.

Keeping Track

Now that you have made good physical activity choices, keep a record in a log. A sample is shown in Table 17.1.

Table 17.1. Sample physical activity log.

Date	Activity	How Long	How Many	Who With	Reactions
6/10	rode bike	1 hour		Mom	fun
6/11	chin-ups		10	self	difficult today
6/12	walked	1 hour		spouse	enjoyable!

273

Chapter 18

Exercise for Older Adults

Introduction

A Word about Words

Terms used to discuss exercise can be confusing. We want to explain a few key words that will prepare you to read this chapter.

- You probably have heard the term "aerobics" or "aerobic exercises." We call them "endurance exercises" or "endurance activities." They are activities that increase your heart rate and breathing for an extended period of time.

- The term "cardiovascular" refers to your heart and circulatory systems.

- The word "frailty" has more than one meaning. In this chapter, we use it to mean the physical condition that results, in part, from severe muscle loss—the kind of muscle loss seen in people who have been inactive for many years. Frail people have severe loss of strength, and an inability to perform everyday tasks is often the outcome.

- One of the biggest concerns older adults have is that they will become dependent on other people and won't be able to live in

"Exercise: A Guide from the National Institute on Aging," National Institute on Aging, National Institutes of Health Publication No. NIH 99-4258, 1999.

their own homes. We frequently use the word "independence"; in this chapter, it means older adults' ability to live and do things on their own. Being independent doesn't necessarily mean doing things alone; it means being able to do for yourself, in your tasks of everyday living and your leisure activities, to the greatest extent possible.

- Exercises that build muscle have a variety of names, including "strength-training," "resistance-training," "weight-training," or "weight-lifting." In this chapter, we call them "muscle-building" or "strength" exercises.

- What is considered a physical activity and what is considered an exercise? A physical activity is any voluntary body movement that burns calories. Exercise is physical activity that follows a planned format. It's done with repeated movements, with the goal of improving or keeping up one or more specific areas of physical fitness.

What Can Exercise Do for Me?

The notion that exercise is good for you is something everyone just always seems to have known. Somehow, though, older adults have been left out of the picture—until recently. A clear new picture is emerging from research: Older people of all ages and physical conditions have very much to gain from exercise and from staying physically active. They also have very much to lose if they become physically inactive—some degree of health and ability, for example.

Exercise isn't just for older adults in the younger age range, who live independently and are able to go on brisk jogs, although this chapter is very much for them, too. Researchers studied the question of whether exercise and physical activity also can improve the health of people who are 90 or older, who are frail, or who have the diseases that seem to accompany aging. We now know from reliable scientific studies that it can help. Staying physically active and exercising regularly can help prevent or delay some diseases and disabilities as people grow older. In some cases, it can improve health for older people who already have diseases and disabilities, if it's done on a long-term, regular basis.

What Kinds of Activities Improve Health and Ability?

Endurance exercises are activities that increase your breathing and heart rate. They improve the health of your heart, lungs, and circulatory system. Having more endurance not only helps keep you healthier; it can also improve your stamina for the tasks you need to do to live and do things on your own—climbing stairs and grocery shopping, for example. Endurance exercises also may delay or prevent many diseases associated with aging, such as diabetes, colon cancer, heart disease, stroke, and others, and have been shown to reduce the overall death and hospitalization rates.

Strength exercises build your muscles, but they do more than just make you stronger. They may improve your independence by giving you more strength to do things on your own. Even very small increases in muscle can make a big difference in ability, especially for frail people. Strength exercises also increase your metabolism, helping to keep your weight and blood sugar in check. That's important, because obesity and diabetes are major health problems for older adults. Studies suggest that strength exercises also may help prevent osteoporosis.

Balance exercises help prevent a common problem in older adults: falls. In older people, falling is a major cause of broken hips and other injuries that often lead to disability and loss of independence. Some balance exercises build up your leg muscles; others improve your balance by requiring you to do simple activities like briefly standing on one leg.

Flexibility exercises are stretching exercises. They are thought to help keep your body limber by stretching your muscles and the tissues that hold your body's structures in place. Although research hasn't proven, yet, that stretching exercises can improve your ability to live on your own and do things independently, studies are under way. Already, physical therapists and other health professionals recommend certain stretching exercises to help their patients recover from injuries and to prevent injuries from happening in the first place. Flexibility also may play a part in preventing falls.

Which Ones Should I Do, and How Much Should I Do?

As you read this chapter, you will learn more about which of these types of exercises will help you meet your health goals and about how you should do them. Some types of exercise improve just one area of health or ability. More often, though, an exercise has many different benefits.

In other words, as much as you can, it's best to increase both the types and amounts of exercises and physical activities you do. Gradually build up to include all four areas: endurance, strength, balance, and flexibility.

You might be enthusiastic about getting started, now that you have read about all the benefits exercise can bring. Throughout this chapter, we emphasize the importance of starting out at a level you can manage and working your way up gradually. That's good advice to follow.

For one thing, if you do too much too quickly, you can damage your muscles and tissues, and that can keep you on the sidelines. For another, your enthusiasm needs to be with you for a lifetime. The benefits of exercise and physical activity come from making them a permanent habit. Starting out with one or two types of exercises that you really can manage and that you really can fit into your schedule, then adding more as you adjust, is one way of ensuring that you will stick with it.

One physician who specializes in exercise for older people puts it this way: "It's like starting out on a journey. You start with a single step."

How much you do depends on you and on your unique situation. For some of you, muscle-building exercise might mean pushing more than a hundred pounds of weight at the local gym to keep your legs in shape for hiking or jogging. For others, it might mean lifting one pound of weight to strengthen your arm muscles enough to use a washcloth. That might mean the dignity that comes from being able to wash yourself, instead of having someone else do it for you. That's a good place to start, for some older adults. The goal is to improve from wherever you are right now.

Some people are reluctant to start exercising because they are afraid it will be too strenuous. Researchers have found that you don't have to do strenuous exercises to gain health benefits; moderate exercises are effective, too. (You will read more about the difference between vigorous and moderate exercises later in this chapter.)

How Much Physical Activity Is Enough?

Everyday physical activities can accomplish some of the same goals as exercise. But if you decide to do everyday physical activities instead of exercise, just how much should you do to get health benefits?

We can't always give you answers, yet, but we can point you in the right direction by giving examples of what researchers have found out. For instance, bus and taxi drivers, who are physically inactive on the job, were found to have a higher rate of heart disease than were men in other occupations. And studies show that people who remain physically active have a lower death rate than people who don't.

In another study, researchers measured muscle strength in 75-year-olds who regularly did tasks like housework and gardening and in 75-year-olds who were inactive. The researchers measured muscle strength in the same people five years later and found that the active people, who had been using their muscles in everyday tasks, kept more of their strength than did the inactive people.

While we can't yet tell you exactly how much everyday physical activity you should get to gain specific health benefits in areas like strength, the message these types of studies are sending is clear: Whatever your age, stay physically active.

Doing the exercises we show later in this chapter may be helpful to you for several reasons. For one, we give you specific amounts of exercises to do. These exercises are intended to help you not only maintain your current levels of strength and fitness, but also to build them up. For another, our examples might encourage you to exercise muscles and joints that you have stopped using during everyday activities or that you use less without even realizing it.

Is It Safe for Me to Exercise?

"Too old" and "too frail" are not, in and of themselves, reasons to prohibit physical activity. In fact, there aren't very many health reasons to keep older adults from becoming more active.

Most older people think in terms of getting their doctor's approval to start exercising. As you will see in this chapter, that's a good idea for some people. But given what we now know about the importance of exercise for older adults and about the health risks of not exercising, we feel that there should be another side to the discussion. Your doctor can talk to you not only about whether it's all right for you to exercise; he or she also can talk to you about how important exercise is for older adults.

Chronic Diseases: Not Necessarily a Barrier

Chronic diseases are illnesses that can't be cured, but usually can be controlled with medications and other treatments throughout a person's life. They are common among older adults, and include diabetes, cardiovascular disease (such as high blood pressure), and arthritis, among many others.

Traditionally, exercise has been discouraged in people with certain chronic conditions. But researchers have found that exercise can actually improve some chronic conditions in most older people, as long as it's done during periods when the condition is under control.

Congestive heart failure (CHF) is an example of a serious chronic condition common in older adults. In people with CHF, the heart can't empty its load of blood with each beat, resulting in a backup of fluid throughout the body, including the lungs. Disturbances in heart rhythm also are common in CHF. Older adults are hospitalized more often for this disease than for any other.

No one is sure why, but muscles throughout the body tend to waste away badly in people with CHF, leaving them weak, sometimes to the point that a person can't perform everyday tasks. No medicine has been shown to have a direct muscle-strengthening effect in people with CHF, but muscle-building exercises (lifting weights, for example) have, indeed, been shown to improve muscle strength in these people.

Having a chronic disease like CHF probably doesn't mean you can't exercise. But it does mean that keeping in touch with your doctor is important if you do exercise. For example, some studies suggest that endurance exercises, like brisk walking, may improve how well the heart and lungs work in people with CHF, but only in people who are in a stable phase of the disease. CHF, like most chronic diseases, has periods when the disease gets better, then worse, then better again, off and on. The same endurance exercises that might help people in a stable phase of CHF could be very harmful to people who are in an unstable phase; that is, when their lungs are experiencing a fluid build-up or their heart's rhythm has become irregular.

If you have a chronic condition, you are probably asking yourself how you can tell whether your disease is stable; that is, how to know when exercise wouldn't be bad for you and when it would.

Chances are good that, if you have a chronic disease, you are being seen regularly by a physician (if you aren't, you should be, for many reasons). Your doctor should have discussed with you symptoms that mean trouble—a flare-up, or what doctors call an acute phase or exacerbation of your disease. If you have CHF, you know by now that the acute phase of this disease should be taken very, very seriously. You should not exercise when warning symptoms of the acute phase of CHF, or any other chronic disease, appear. It could be dangerous.

But you and your doctor also should have discussed, by now, how you feel when you are free of those symptoms—in other words, stable; under control. This is the time to exercise.

If you have a chronic disease, your doctor should be keeping up to date on your condition. Before you start exercising, let your doctor know. He or she might agree that it's fine to start, as long as you are free of symptoms, or might ask you to come in for a visit.

By listening to your lungs, your doctor can hear signs of fluid build-up that could signal the unstable phase of CHF. He or she can see changes in heart rhythm that warn of an acute phase of CHF, or clues about the status of other chronic conditions. Your doctor also can put your mind at ease by letting you know when it's fine to exercise because your chronic condition is stable. He or she may refer you to a qualified professional who can start you on an exercise plan.

Diabetes is another chronic condition common among older people. Too much sugar in the blood is a hallmark of diabetes. It can cause damage throughout the body. Exercise can help your body "use up" some of the damaging sugar.

The most common form of diabetes is linked to physical inactivity. In other words, you are less likely to get it, in the first place, if you stay physically active.

If you do have diabetes and it has caused changes in your body—cardiovascular disease, eye disease, or changes in your nervous system, for example—check with your doctor to find out what exercises will help you and whether you should avoid certain types of activity. If you take insulin or a pill that helps lower your blood sugar, your doctor might need to adjust your dose so that your blood sugar doesn't get too low.

Your doctor might find that you don't have to modify your exercises at all, if you are in the earlier stages of diabetes or if your condition is stable.

If you are at high risk for any chronic disease—for example, if you have a family history of heart disease or diabetes, or if you smoke or are obese—you should check with your doctor before increasing your physical activity. You should also see your doctor first if you just suspect that you have some risk factors and you haven't had a checkup lately.

Checkpoints

You have already read about precautions you should take if you have a chronic condition. Other circumstances require caution, too. You shouldn't exercise until checking with a doctor if you have:

- any new, undiagnosed symptom
- chest pain

- irregular, rapid, or fluttery heart beat

- severe shortness of breath

- significant, ongoing weight loss that hasn't been diagnosed

- infections, such as pneumonia, accompanied by fever

- fever itself, which can cause dehydration and a rapid heart beat

- acute deep-vein thrombosis (blood clot)

- a hernia that is causing symptoms

- foot or ankle sores that won't heal

- joint swelling

- persistent pain or a disturbance in walking after you have fallen. You might have a fracture and not know it, and exercise could cause further injury.

- certain eye conditions, such as bleeding in the retina or detached retina. Before you exercise after a cataract or lens implant, or after laser treatment or other eye surgery, check with your physician.

If you are a man over 40 or a woman over 50, you should check with your doctor first if you plan to start doing vigorous, as opposed to moderate, physical activities. Vigorous activity could be a problem for people who have "hidden" heart disease—that is, people who have heart disease, but don't know it because they don't have any symptoms.

How can you tell if the activity you plan to do is vigorous? There are a couple of ways. If the activity makes you breathe hard and sweat hard (if you tend to sweat, that is), you can consider it vigorous. Charts later in this chapter explain more about how to tell if your exercise is moderate or vigorous.

For some people, running is a vigorous activity, but for others, walking could be considered just as vigorous. It depends on you—on the shape you are in and on your medical conditions.

If you have had a heart attack recently, your doctor or cardiac rehabilitation therapist should have given you specific exercises to do when you were discharged from the hospital or your cardiac rehabilitation program. Research has shown that exercises done as part of a cardiac rehabilitation program can improve fitness and even reduce your risk of dying. If you didn't get instructions before leaving the hospital, call your doctor to discuss exercise before you begin increasing your physical activity.

For some conditions, vigorous exercise is dangerous and should not be done, even in the absence of symptoms. It's especially important to check with a physician before beginning any kind of exercise program if you have either of the following conditions:

- abdominal aortic aneurysm, a weakness in the wall of the heart's major outgoing artery (unless it has been surgically repaired or is so small that your doctor tells you that you can exercise vigorously)

- critical aortic stenosis, a narrowing of one of the valves of the heart.

Most older adults, regardless of age or condition, will do just fine in increasing their physical activity. You might want to show your doctor this chapter, to open the door to discussions about exercise.

How to Keep Going

"Definitely NOT!" That's what 75-year-old Emma King told us when we asked her if she ever intended to stop exercising. Ms. King lives in Durham, North Carolina, and has taken long walks at least 4 or 5 days a week, for years. Last year, she took part in a study of exercise for older adults and added stretching to her weekly routine. "I can really tell the difference if I miss 2 or 3 days. I don't know what it would be like not to exercise," she said.

For many older adults, motivation to keep exercising and doing physical activities isn't a problem. They say that regular physical activity makes them feel so much better that it would be hard to stop.

Others say that, while physical activity makes them feel better, a little extra motivation helps them get going.

For example, Georgia Burnette, 68, of Amherst, New York, told us that she used to put on headphones and listen to recorded s borrowed from the library to make her 40-minute walks more interesting. Now, she mall-walks for an hour, 5 days a week, with a friend. Having that companionship is a good motivator, Ms. Burnette said.

We have included this section on motivation because physical activity needs to be a regular, permanent habit to produce benefits like those listed earlier. So does staying motivated!

Recording your scores and watching them improve can be an excellent motivator to exercise, and we have included charts at the end of this chapter so you can do that. On the other hand, if you see that your scores have improved by only a few seconds or just one or two lifts of a weight, you might get discouraged.

Putting it in perspective might help. While your test scores might rise by what looks like only a tiny amount, in terms of real-life benefits, those slight improvements are multiplied many times over as you include them in your everyday activities, probably without even realizing it. You incorporate that extra little bit of endurance and extra little bit of strength into everything you do, and it adds up to a lot.

But no matter how enthusiastic you are about exercise, there may be times when you need extra motivation. It's common for beginning exercisers, especially those who are frail, to make fast progress at first. You might get discouraged when the improvements you were making taper off at times.

These leveling-off periods are normal. You are probably doing your activities correctly, and you are probably still benefiting from them. Often, these leveling-off periods mean that it's time to gradually make your activities more challenging. If you have any doubts about whether you are doing the right things to progress, check the guidelines listed under each type of exercise later in this chapter or check with a qualified fitness professional or doctor.

For times that you need extra motivation, try the following:

- Ask someone to be your exercise buddy. Many of the older adults we talked to agreed that having someone to exercise with helps keep them going.

- Follow Georgia Burnette's advice: Listen to recorded music while you do endurance activities.

- Set a goal, and decide on a reward you will get when you reach it.

- Give yourself physical activity homework assignments for the next day or the next week

- Think of your exercise sessions as appointments, and mark them on your calendar.

- Keep a record of what you do and of your progress. Understand that there will be times that you don't show rapid progress and that you are still benefiting from your activities during those times.

- Plan ahead for vacations, bad weather, and house guests. For example, you might want to have an exercise video so you can exercise indoors when the weather is bad.

Sticking with It: What Works

According to the U.S. Surgeon General's report, you are more likely to keep doing physical activities if you:

- think that, overall, you will benefit from them
- include activities you enjoy
- feel you can do the activities correctly and safely
- have access to the activities on a regular basis
- can fit the activities into your daily schedule
- feel that the activities don't impose financial or social costs you aren't willing to take on
- have few negative consequences from doing your activities (such consequences might include injury, lost time, and negative peer pressure)

In other words, you are more likely to stick with your exercises if you set yourself up to succeed from the start. You can help do that by choosing realistic goals, learning to do the exercises correctly and safely, and charting your progress to see your improvement. Take a minute to think carefully about the points in this list before you start planning your exercises and activities.

Finding a Qualified Fitness Professional

Most older people will exercise just fine on their own, without advice from a fitness instructor. Some have special needs and may want to consult a professional. If you decide to seek advice, how can you tell whom to trust? Anyone can call himself or herself a fitness professional, and many people do—but that doesn't always mean they have the training to help older people exercise safely and effectively.

Instructors who aren't trained to work with older adults, specifically, might not be aware of their needs. For example, they might not know that certain conditions or medications can change older people's heart rates or that people with osteoporosis risk spine fractures if they do some types of forward-bending exercises incorrectly.

Doctors who specialize in sports medicine are highly qualified to help you exercise the right way. So are professionals who have a college degree in physical therapy or exercise physiology, particularly when it comes to helping you start an exercise program tailored to your needs, building it up to your best possible level, then showing you how to continue safely on your own.

Physical therapists are legally licensed health professionals. Their training makes them well-qualified to design exercise plans for older people, especially those who have conditions affecting their muscles and skeletal systems, or nervous system conditions that affect their muscles. Some physical therapists take special training for a certification in geriatrics from their national licensing board. Although physical therapists can work with anyone, doctors often refer patients with special needs to them.

An excellent resource that trains and certifies people to work with older adults and others is the American College of Sports Medicine (ACSM). The ACSM is made up of health professionals and scientists with an interest in fitness. Some of its members are among the nation's leading experts on the topic of exercise and physical activity. If the professional you consult is ACSM-certified to work with older people, he or she is likely to be well qualified to help you design a safe, effective exercise plan. ACSM-certified fitness instructors work in a variety of settings; for example, you might find them leading hospital-based exercise programs for older adults, working with older people in exercise studies, or working as personal trainers.

Cardiologists can advise you on how to improve your cardiovascular system through endurance exercise. Orthopedic doctors can help you understand how to prevent injuries to your muscles, bones, and other structures.

Many hospitals and health maintenance organizations now include wellness centers that offer exercise programs. Some colleges and universities hold special exercise classes for older adults or conduct studies on exercise for older people. It's likely that the fitness instructors hired by these types of organizations are carefully screened and are qualified to teach you how to exercise correctly. Try calling them to find a fitness professional in your area.

Most older adults won't need to consult a fitness instructor. If you have special needs, your doctor probably will refer you to a specific, qualified professional. But if you look for an instructor independently, ask for his or her credentials. Any instructor who is qualified to work with older people is likely to be proud of his or her credentials and will be happy to share them with you. Also ask about expense. Costs vary, and insurance plans differ as to what kinds of services they will cover.

Examples of Exercises to Do at Home

A lot of different physical activities can improve your health and independence. Whether you choose to do the at-home exercises listed in this chapter or other activities that accomplish the same goals, gradually work your way up to include all four areas of fitness listed here: endurance, strength, balance, and stretching. Here are some points to keep in mind as you begin increasing your activity:

- If you stop exercising for several weeks and then return, start out at about half the effort you were putting into it when you stopped, then gradually build back up. Some of the effects of endurance and muscle-building exercises deteriorate within 2 weeks if these activities are cut back substantially, and benefits may disappear altogether if they aren't done for 2 to 8 months.

- When an exercise calls for you to bend forward, bend from the hips, not the waist. If you keep your entire back and shoulders straight as you bend forward, that will help ensure that you are bending the right way, from the hips. If you find your back or shoulders humping in any spot as you bend forward, that's a sign that you are bending incorrectly, from the waist. Bending from the waist may cause spine fractures in some people with osteoporosis.

- It's possible to combine exercises. For example, regular stair-climbing sessions improve endurance and strengthen leg muscles at the same time.

How Hard Should I Exercise?

We can't tell you exactly how many pounds to lift or how steep a hill you should climb to reach a moderate or vigorous level of exercise, because what is easy for one person might be strenuous for another. It's different for different people.

We can, however, provide some advice based on scientific research: Listen to your body. The level of effort you feel you are putting into an activity is likely to agree with what actual physical measurements would show, researchers have found. In other words, if your body tells you that the exercise you are doing is moderate, measurements of things like how hard your heart is working would probably show that it really is working at a moderate level. During moderate activity, for instance, you can sense that you are challenging yourself but that you aren't near your limit.

One way you can estimate how hard to work is by using something called the Borg scale. It was named after Gunnar Borg, the scientist who developed it. The numbers on the left of the scale don't indicate how many times or how many minutes you should do an activity; they are just a way of helping you describe how hard you feel you are working.

For endurance activities, you should gradually work your way up to level 13—the feeling that you are working at a somewhat hard level. Some people might feet that way when they are walking on flat ground; others might feel that way when they are jogging up a hill. Both are right. Only you know how hard your exercise feels to you.

Strength exercises are higher on the Borg scale. Gradually work your way up to level 15 to 17—hard to very hard—to build muscle effectively. You can tell how hard an effort you are making by comparing it to your maximum effort. How hard does your current effort feel compared to when you are lifting the heaviest weight you can lift? Once you start exerting more than a moderate amount of effort in your muscle-building exercises, your strength is likely to increase quickly.

As your body adapts and you become more fit, you can gradually keep making your activities more challenging. You might find, for

Table 18.1. The Borg Category Rating Scale

Least effort		
6		
7	very, very light	
8		
9	very light	
10		
11	fairly light	ENDURANCE
12		TRAINING
13	somewhat hard	ZONE
14		
15	hard	STRENGTH
16		TRAINING
17	very hard	ZONE
18		
19	very, very hard	
20		
Maximum effort		

example, that walking on a flat surface used to make you feel like you were working at level 13 on the Borg scale, but that now you have to walk up a mild hill to feel like you are working at level 13. Later, you might find that you need to walk up an even steeper slope to feel that you are working at level 13.

The Borg scale is simple to use. But if you feel that your level of effort doesn't match the numbers you see on the Borg scale—for example, if you feel you are doing the exercise correctly, but you aren't progressing or you feel exhausted by your effort—check with the kinds of exercise professionals described under "Finding a Qualified Fitness Professional." These experts are likely to understand the science that went into developing the Borg scale, and they can teach you how to match your level of effort with the right number on the scale.

How to Improve Your Endurance

Endurance exercises are any activity—walking, jogging, swimming, raking—that increases your heart rate and breathing for an extended period of time.

- Build up your endurance gradually, starting out with as little as 5 minutes of endurance activities at a time, if you need to.

- Starting out at a lower level of effort and working your way up gradually is especially important if you have been inactive for a long time. It may take months to go from a very longstanding sedentary lifestyle to doing some of the activities suggested in this section.

- Your goal is to work your way up, eventually, to a moderate-to-vigorous level that increases your breathing and heart rate. It should feel somewhat hard to you (level 13 on the Borg scale).

- Once you reach your goal, you can divide your exercise into sessions of no less than 10 minutes at a time, if you want to, as long as they add up to a total of at least 30 minutes at the end of the day. Doing less than 10 minutes at a time won't give you the desired cardiovascular and respiratory system benefits. (The exception to this guideline is when you have first made the decision to begin doing endurance activities, and you are just starting out).

- Your goal is to build up to a total of at least 30 minutes of endurance exercise on most or all days of the week. More often is better, and every day is best.

Tips on How to Gauge Your Effort

Here are some informal guidelines you can use to estimate how much effort you are putting into your endurance activities.

- Talking doesn't take much effort during moderate activity. During vigorous activity, talking is difficult.

- If you tend to perspire, you probably won't sweat during light activity (except on hot days). You will sweat during vigorous or sustained moderate activity.

- Your muscles may get a rubbery feeling after vigorous activity, but not after moderate activity.

- One doctor who specializes in exercise for older adults tells her patients this about how hard they should work during endurance activities: "If you can't talk while you're exercising, it's too difficult. If you can sing a song from an opera, it's too easy!"

Safety

- Endurance activities should not make you breathe so hard that you can't talk. They should not cause dizziness or chest pain.

- Do a little light activity before and after your endurance exercise session, to warm up and cool down (example: easy walking).

- Stretch after your endurance activities, when your muscles are warm.

- As you get older, your body may become less likely to trigger the urge to drink when you need water. In other words, you may need water, but you won't feel thirsty. Be sure to drink fluids when you are doing any activity that makes you lose fluid through sweat. The rule-of-thumb is that, by the time you notice you are thirsty, you are already somewhat dehydrated (low on fluid). This guideline is important year-round, but is especially important in hot weather, when dehydration is more likely.

- If your doctor has asked you to limit your fluids, be sure to check with him or her before increasing the amount of fluid you drink while exercising. Congestive heart failure and kidney disease are examples of chronic diseases that often require fluid restriction. Older adults can be affected by heat and cold more than other adults. In extreme cases, exposure to too much heat can cause heat stroke, and exposure to very cold temperatures can lead to hypothermia (a dangerous drop in body temperature). If you are exercising outdoors, dress in layers so you can add or remove clothes as needed.

- Use safety equipment to prevent injuries. For example, wear a helmet for bicycling, and wear protective equipment for activities like skiing and skating. If you walk or jog, wear stable shoes made for that purpose.

Progressing

- When you are ready to progress, build up the amount of time you spend doing endurance activities first; then build up the difficulty of your activities later. Example: First, gradually increase your time to 30 minutes over several days to weeks (or even months, depending on your condition) by walking longer distances, then start walking up steeper hills or walking more briskly.

Examples of Endurance Activities/Exercises

Examples of activities that are moderate for the average older adult are listed below. Some older adults, especially those who have been inactive for a long time, will need to work up to these activities gradually.

Moderate

- Swimming
- Bicycling
- Cycling on a stationary bicycle
- Gardening (mowing, raking)
- Walking briskly on a level surface
- Mopping or scrubbing floor
- Golf, without a cart
- Tennis (doubles)
- Volleyball
- Rowing
- Dancing

The following are examples of activities that are vigorous. People who have been inactive for a long time or who have some of the health risks listed previously should not start out with these activities.

Vigorous

- Climbing stairs or hills
- Shoveling snow
- Brisk bicycling up hills
- Digging holes
- Tennis (singles)
- Swimming laps
- Cross-country skiing
- Downhill skiing
- Hiking
- jogging

Even very small changes in muscle size can make a big difference in strength, especially in people who already have lost a lot of muscle. An increase in muscle that's not even visible to the eye can be all it takes to improve your ability to do things like get up from a chair or climb stairs.

Your muscles are active even when you are sleeping. Their cells are still doing the routine activities they need to do to stay alive. This work is called metabolism, and it uses up calories. That can help keep your weight in check, even when you are asleep!

How Muscles Work

What makes your muscles look bigger when you flex them—when you "make a muscle" with your biceps, for example?

Muscle cells contain long strands of protein lying next to each other. When you want your muscles to move, your brain signals your nerves to stimulate them. A chemical reaction in your muscles follows, causing the long strands of protein to slide toward and over each other, shortening the length of your muscle cells. When you "make a muscle" and you see your muscle bunch up and bulge, you are actually watching it shorten as the protein strands slide over each other.

When you do challenging muscle-building exercises on a regular basis, the bundles of protein strands inside your muscle cells grow bigger.

About Strength Exercises

To do most of the following strength exercises, you need to lift or push weights, and you need to keep gradually increasing the amount of weight you use. You can use the hand and ankle weights sold in sporting-goods stores, or you can use things like emptied milk jugs filled with sand or water, or socks filled with beans and tied shut at the ends.

There are many alternatives to the exercises shown here. For example, you can buy a resistance band (it looks like a giant rubber band, and stretching it helps build muscle) at a sporting-good store for under $10 to do other types of strength exercises. Or you can use the special strength-training equipment at a fitness center.

How Much, How Often

- Do strength exercises for all of your major muscle groups at least twice a week. Don't do strength exercises of the same muscle group on any 2 days in a row.

- Depending on your condition, you might need to start out using as little as 1 or 2 pounds of weight, or no weight at all. The tissues that bind the structures of your body together need to adapt to strength exercises.

- Use a minimum of weight the first week, then gradually build up the weight. Starting out with weights that are too heavy can cause injuries.

- At the same time, remember that you have to gradually add a challenging amount of weight in order to benefit from strength exercises. If you don't challenge your muscles, you won't benefit from strength exercises.

- When doing a strength exercise, do 8 to 15 repetitions in a row. Wait a minute, then do another set of 8 to 15 repetitions in a row of the same exercise. (Tip: While you are waiting, you might want to stretch the muscle you just worked or do a different strength exercise that uses a different set of muscles).

- Take 3 seconds to lift or push a weight into place; hold the position for 1 second, and take another 3 seconds to lower the weight. Don't let the weight drop; lowering it slowly is very important.

- It should feel somewhere between hard and very hard (15 to 17 on the Borg scale) for you to lift or push the weight. It should not feel very, very hard. If you can't lift or push a weight 8 times in a row, it's too heavy for you. Reduce the amount of weight. If you can lift a weight more than 15 times in a row, it's too light for you. Increase the amount of weight.

293

- Stretch after strength exercises, when your muscles are warmed up. If you stretch before strength exercises, be sure to warm up your muscles first (through light walking and arm pumping, for example).

Safety

- Don't hold your breath during strength exercises. Breathe normally. Holding your breath while straining can cause changes in blood pressure. This is especially true for people with cardiovascular disease.

- If you have had a hip repair or replacement, check with the doctor who did your surgery before doing lower-body exercises.

- If you have had a hip replacement, don't cross your legs, and don't bend your hips farther than a 90-degree angle.

- Avoid jerking or thrusting weights into position. That can cause injuries. Use smooth, steady movements. Avoid "locking" the joints in your arms and legs in a tightly straightened position. (A tip on how to straighten your knees: Tighten your thigh muscles. This will lift your kneecaps and protect them.)

- Breathe out as you lift or push, and breathe in as you relax. For example, if you are doing leg lifts, breathe out as you lift your leg, and breathe in as you lower it. This may not feel natural at first, and you probably will have to think about it as you are doing it for awhile.

- Muscle soreness lasting up to a few days and slight fatigue are normal after muscle-building exercises, but exhaustion, sore joints, and unpleasant muscle pulling aren't. The latter symptoms mean you are overdoing it.

- None of the exercises you do should cause pain. The range within which you move your arms and legs should never hurt.

Progressing

- Gradually increasing the amount of weight you use is crucial for building strength.

- When you are able to lift a weight between 8 to 15 times, you can increase the amount of weight you use at your next session.

- Here is an example of how to progress gradually: Start out with a weight that you can lift only 8 times. Keep using that weight until you become strong enough to lift it 12 to 15 times. Add more weight so that, again, you can lift it only 8 times. Use this weight until you can lift it 12 to 15 times, then add more weight. Keep repeating.

Sarcopenia: A Word You Are Likely to Hear More About

We know that muscle-building exercises can improve strength in most older adults, but many questions remain about muscle loss and aging. Researchers want to know, for example, if factors other than a sedentary lifestyle contribute to muscle loss. Does age itself cause changes in the muscles of older people? Is muscle loss related to changes in hormones or nutrition? These are the kinds of questions scientists are examining now. The answers may lead to ways of helping us keep our strength as we age.

In this chapter, we use the word "frailty" to describe the loss of muscle and strength often seen in older people, because it's a word that most people are familiar with. The problem is that "frailty" has more than one meaning. A better word to use, but one that most people haven't heard of, is "sarcopenia" (pronounced sar-ko-PEEN-ya). It's the word researchers use to mean not only the loss of muscle and strength but also the decreased quality of muscle tissue often seen in older adults. It's a word you are likely to hear more about in the future, since sarcopenia is a very active area of research.

Examples of Strength Exercises

Arm Raise

Strengthens shoulder muscles. Sit in a chair, with your back straight. Your feet should be flat on the floor, spaced apart so that they are even with your shoulders. Hold hand weights straight down at your sides, with your palms facing inward. Take 3 seconds to lift your arms straight out, sideways, until they are parallel to the ground. Hold the position for 1 second. Take 3 seconds to lower your arms so that they are straight down by your sides again. Pause. Repeat 8 to 15 times. Rest; do another set of 8 to 15 repetitions.

Summary

1. Sit in chair.

2. Feet flat on floor; keep feet even with shoulders.

3. Arms straight down at sides, palms inward.

4. Raise both arms to side, shoulder height.

5. Hold position.

6. Slowly lower arms to sides.

Chair Stand

Strengthens muscles in abdomen and thighs. Sit toward the middle or front of a chair and lean back so that you are in a half-reclining position, with back and shoulders straight, knees bent, and feet flat on the floor. Be sure to place pillows against the lower back of the chair first, to support your back and keep it straight. Using your hands as little as possible (or not at all, if you can), bring your back forward so that you are sitting upright. Your back should no longer be leaning against the pillows. Keep your back straight as you come up, so that you feel your abdominal muscles do the work; don't lean forward with your shoulders as you rise. Next, with feet flat on the floor, take at least 3 seconds to stand up, using your hands as little as possible. As you bend slightly forward to stand up, keep your back and shoulders straight. Take at least 3 seconds to sit back down. Your goal is to do this exercise without using your hands as you become stronger. Repeat 8 to 15 times. Rest; then repeat 8 to 15 times more.

Summary

1. Place pillows against back of chair.

2. Sit in middle or toward front of chair, knees bent, feet flat on floor.

3. Lean back on pillows, in half-reclining position, back and shoulders straight.

4. Raise upper body forward until sitting upright, using hands as little as possible.

5. Slowly stand up, using hands as little as possible.

6. Slowly sit back down.

7. Keep back and shoulders straight throughout exercise.

Biceps Curl

Strengthens upper-arm muscles. Sit in an armless chair, with your back supported by the back of the chair. Your feet should be flat on the floor, spaced apart so that they are even with your shoulders. Hold hand weights, with your arms straight down at your side, palms facing in toward your body. Take 3 seconds to lift your left hand weight toward your chest by bending your elbow. As you lift, turn your left hand so that your palm is facing your shoulder. Hold the position for 1 second. Take 3 seconds to lower your hand to the starting position. Pause, then repeat with right arm. Alternate until you have repeated the exercise 8 to 15 times on each side. Rest, then do another set of 8 to 15 alternating repetitions.

Summary

1. Sit in armless chair, with your back supported by back of chair.

2. Feet flat on floor, keep feet even with shoulders.

3. Hold hand weights at sides, arms straight, palms in.

4. Slowly bend one elbow, lifting weight toward chest. (Rotate palm to face shoulder while lifting weight.)

S. Hold position.

6. Slowly lower arm to starting position.

7. Repeat with other arm.

Plantar Flexion

Strengthens ankle and calf muscles. Use ankle weights, if you are ready to. Stand straight, feet flat on the floor, holding onto the edge of a table or chair for balance. Take 3 seconds to stand as high up on tiptoe as you can; hold for 1 second, then take 3 seconds to slowly lower yourself back down. Do this exercise 8 to 15 times; rest a minute, then do another set of 8 to 15 repetitions. As you become stronger, do this exercise first on your right leg only, then on your left leg only, for a total of 8 to 15 times on each leg. Rest a minute, then do another set of 8 to 15 alternating repetitions.

Summary

1. Stand straight, holding table or chair for balance.

2. Slowly stand on tiptoe, as high as possible.

3. Hold position.

4. Slowly lower heels all the way back down.

Variation, as strength increases: Do the exercise standing on one leg only, alternating legs.

Triceps Extension

Note: If your shoulders aren't flexible enough to do this exercise, see alternative "Dip" exercise.

Strengthens muscles in back of upper arm. Sit in a chair, toward the front. Your feet should be flat on the floor, spaced apart so that they are even with your shoulders. Hold a weight in your left hand, and raise your left arm all the way up, so that it's pointing toward the ceiling, palm facing in. Support your left arm by holding it just below the elbow with your right hand. Slowly bend your left arm so that the weight in your left hand now rests behind your left shoulder. Take 3 seconds to straighten your left arm so that it's pointing toward the ceiling again. Hold the position for 1 second. Take 3 seconds to lower the weight back to your shoulder by bending your elbow. Keep supporting your left arm with your right hand throughout the exercise. Pause, then repeat the bending and straightening until you have done the exercise 8 to 15 times with your left arm. Reverse positions and repeat 8 to 15 times with your right arm. Rest, then repeat another set of 8 to 15 repetitions on each side.

Summary

1. Sit in chair, near front edge.

2. Feet flat on floor; keep feet even with shoulders.

3. Raise one arm straight toward ceiling.

4. Support this arm, below elbow, with other hand.

5. Bend raised arm at elbow, bringing hand weight toward same shoulder.

6. Slowly re-straighten arm toward ceiling.

7. Hold position.

8. Slowly bend arm toward shoulder again.

Alternative "Dip" Exercise for Back of Upper Arm

Sit in a chair with armrests. Lean slightly forward, keeping your back and shoulders straight. Hold onto the arms of the chair. Your hands should be level with the trunk of your body, or slightly farther forward. Place your feet slightly under the chair, with your heels off the ground and the weight of your feet and legs resting on your toes and the balls of your feet. Slowly lift yourself up, using your arms, as high as you can. This pushing motion will strengthen your arm muscles even if you aren't yet able to lift yourself up off of the chair. Don't use your legs or feet for assistance, or use them as little as possible. Slowly lower yourself back down. Repeat 8 to 15 times. Rest; repeat another 8 to 15 times.

Summary

1. Sit in chair with armrests.

2. Lean slightly forward, back and shoulders straight.

3. Grasp arms of chair.

4. Tuck feet slightly under chair, weight on toes.

5. Slowly push body off of chair using arms, not legs.

6. Slowly lower down to starting position.

Knee Flexion

Strengthens muscles in back of thigh. Use ankle weights, if you are ready to. Stand straight, very close to a table or chair, holding it for balance. Take 3 seconds to bend your left knee so that your calf comes as far up toward the back of your thigh as possible. Don't move your upper leg at all; bend your knee only. Take 3 seconds to lower your left leg all the way back down. Repeat with right leg. Alternate legs until you have done 8 to 15 repetitions with each leg. Rest; then do another set of 8 to 15 alternating repetitions.

Summary

1. Stand straight; hold onto table for balance.

2. Slowly bend knee as far as possible.

3. Hold position.

4. Slowly lower foot all the way back down.

5. Repeat with other leg.

Hip Flexion

Strengthens thigh and hip muscles. Use ankle weights, if you are ready to. Stand to the side or behind a chair or table, holding it with one hand for balance. Take 3 seconds to bend your left knee and bring it as far toward your chest as possible. Stand straight throughout, without bending at the waist or hips. Hold position for 1 second, then take 3 seconds to lower your left leg all the way down. Repeat with right leg; alternate legs until you have done 8 to 15 repetitions on each side. Rest; then do another set of 8 to 15 alternating repetitions.

Summary

1. Stand straight, holding tall, stable object for balance.

2. Slowly bend one knee toward chest, without bending waist or hips.

3. Hold position.

4. Slowly lower leg all the way down.

5. Repeat with other leg.

Shoulder Flexion

Strengthens shoulder muscles. Sit in a chair, with your back straight. Your feet should be flat on the floor, spaced apart so that they are even with your shoulders. Hold hand weights straight down at your sides, with your palms facing inward. Take 3 seconds to lift your arms in front of you, keeping them straight and rotating them so that your palms are facing upward, until your arms are parallel to the ground. Hold the position for 1 second. Take 3 seconds to lower your arms so that they are straight down by your sides again. Pause. Repeat 8 to 15 times. Rest; do another set of 8 to 15 repetitions.

Summary

1. Sit in chair.

2. Feet flat on floor; keep feet even with shoulders.

3. Arms straight down at sides, palms inward.

4. Raise both arms in front of you (keep them straight and rotate so palms face upward) to shoulder height.

5. Hold position.

6. Slowly lower arms to sides.

Knee Extension

Strengthens muscles in front of thigh and shin. Use ankle weights, if you are ready to. Sit in a chair, with your back resting against the back of the chair. If your feet are flat on the floor in this position, you should place a rolled-up towel under your knees to lift them up. Only the balls of your foot and your toes should be resting on the floor. Rest your hands on your thighs or on the sides of the chair. Take 3 seconds to extend your right leg in front of you, parallel to the floor, until your knee is straight. With your right leg in this position, flex your foot so that your toes are pointing toward your head; hold your foot in this position for 1 to 2 seconds. Take 3 seconds to lower your right leg back to the starting position, so that the ball of your foot rests on the floor again. Repeat with left leg. Alternate legs, until you have done the exercise 8 to 15 times with each leg. Rest; then do another set of 8 to 15 alternating repetitions.

Summary

1. Sit in chair. Put rolled towel under knees, if needed.

2. Slowly extend one leg as straight as possible.

3. Hold position and flex foot to point toes toward head.

4. Slowly lower leg back down.

5. Repeat with other leg.

Hip Extension

Strengthens buttock and lower-back muscles. Use ankle weights, if you are ready to. Stand 12 to 18 inches away from a table or chair, feet slightly apart. Bend forward from the hips, at about a 45-degree angle, holding onto the table or chair for balance. In this position, take 3 seconds to lift your left leg straight behind you without bending your knee, pointing your toes, or bending your upper body any farther forward. Hold the position for 1 second. Take 3 seconds to lower your left leg back to the starting position. Repeat with right leg. Alternate legs, until you have repeated the exercise 8 to 15 times with each leg. Rest; then do another set of 8 to 15 alternating repetitions with each leg.

301

Summary

1. Stand 12 to 18 inches from table.
2. Bend at hips; hold onto a table.
3. Slowly lift one leg straight backwards.
4. Hold position.
S. Slowly lower leg.
6. Repeat with other leg.

Side Leg Raise

Strengthens muscles at sides of hips and thighs. Use ankle weights, if you are ready to. Stand up straight, directly behind a table or chair, feet slightly apart. Hold onto the table to help keep your balance. Take 3 seconds to lift your right leg 6 to 12 inches out to the side. Keep your back and both legs straight. Don't point your toes outward; keep them facing forward. Hold the position for 1 second. Take 3 seconds to lower your leg back to the starting position. Repeat with left leg. Alternate legs, until you have repeated the exercise 8 to 15 times with each leg. Rest; do another set of 8 to 15 alternating repetitions.

Summary

1. Stand straight, directly behind table, feet slightly apart.
2. Hold table for balance.
3. Slowly lift one leg to side, 6-12 inches.
4. Hold position.
5. Slowly lower leg.
6. Repeat with other leg.
7. Back and both knees are straight throughout exercise.

How to Improve Your Balance

Each year, U.S. hospitals have 300,000 admissions for broken hips, and falling is often the cause of those fractures. Balance exercises can help you stay independent by helping you avoid the disability—often permanent—that may result from falling.

As you will see, there is a lot of overlap between strength and balance exercises; very often, one exercise serves both purposes.

About Strength / Balance Exercises

Any of the lower-body exercises for strength shown in the strength section also are balance exercises. They include plantar flexion, hip flexion, hip extension, knee flexion, and side leg raise. Just do your regularly scheduled strength exercises, and they will improve your balance at the same time. They can improve your balance even more if you add the following modifications: Note that these exercises instruct you to hold onto a table or chair for balance. Hold onto the table with only one hand. As you progress, try holding on with only one fingertip. Next, try these exercises without holding on at all. If you are very steady on your feet, move on to doing the exercises using no hands, with your eyes closed. Have someone stand close by if you are unsteady.

Don't do more than your regularly scheduled strength-exercise sessions to incorporate these balance modifications; remember that doing strength exercises too often can do more harm than good. Simply do your strength exercises, and incorporate these balance techniques as you progress. Also do the knee-extension exercise shown in the strength section. It helps you keep your balance by increasing muscle strength in your upper thighs.

Examples of Strength/Balance Exercises

Plantar Flexion

Plantar flexion is already included in your strength exercises (described in previous section). When you do your strength exercises, add these modifications to plantar flexion as you progress: Hold table with one hand, then one fingertip, then no hands; then do exercise with eyes closed, if steady.

Summary

1. Stand straight, holding onto a table or chair for balance.

2. Slowly stand on tip toe, as high as possible.

3. Hold position.

4. Slowly lower heels all the way back down.

5. Repeat 8 to 15 times.

6. Rest a minute, then do another 8 to 15 repetitions.

7. Add modifications as you progress.

Knee Flexion

Do knee flexion as part of your regularly scheduled strength exercises, and add these modifications as you progress: Hold table with one hand, then one fingertip, then no hands; then do exercise with eyes closed, if steady.

Summary

1. Stand straight; hold onto table or chair for balance.
2. Slowly bend one knee as far as possible, so foot lifts up behind you.
3. Hold position.
4. Slowly lower foot all the way back down.
5. Repeat with other leg.
6. Add modifications as you progress.

Hip Flexion

Do hip flexion as part of your regularly scheduled strength exercises, and add these modifications as you progress: Hold table with one hand, then one fingertip, then no hands; then do exercise with eyes closed, if steady.

Summary

1. Stand straight; holding onto a table or chair for balance.
2. Slowly bend one knee toward chest, without bending waist or hips.
3. Hold position.
4. Slowly lower leg all the way down.
5. Repeat with other leg.
6. Add modifications as you progress.

Hip Extension

Do hip extension as part of your regularly scheduled strength exercises, and add these modifications as you progress: Hold table with one hand, then one fingertip, then no hands; then do exercise with eyes closed, if steady.

Summary

1.   Stand 12 to 18 inches from table.

2.   Bend at hips; hold onto table.

3.   Slowly lift one leg straight backwards.

4.   Hold position.

5.   Slowly lower leg.

6.   Repeat with other leg.

7.   Add modifications as you progress.

Side Leg Raise

Do leg raise as part of your regularly scheduled strength exercises, and add these modifications as you progress: Hold table with one hand, then one fingertip, then no hands; then do exercise with eyes closed, if steady.

Summary

1.   Stand straight, directly behind table or chair, feet slightly apart.

2.   Hold table for balance.

3.   Slowly lift one leg to side, 6-12 inches.

4.   Hold position.

5.   Slowly lower leg.

6.   Repeat with other leg.

7.   Your back and knees are straight throughout exercise.

8.   Add modifications as you progress.

"Anytime, Anywhere" Balance Exercises

These types of exercises also improve your balance. You can do them almost anytime, anywhere, and as often as you like, as long as you have something sturdy nearby to hold onto if you become unsteady.

Examples

• Walk heel-to-toe. Position your heel just in front of the toes of the opposite foot each time you take a step. Your heel and toes should touch or almost touch.

- Stand on one foot (while waiting in line at the grocery store or at the bus stop, for example). Alternate feet.

- Stand up and sit down without using your hands.

How to Improve Your Flexibility

Stretching exercises are thought to give you more freedom of movement to do the things you need to do and the things you like to do. Stretching exercises alone will not improve your endurance or strength.

How Much, How Often

- Stretch after you do your regularly scheduled strength and endurance exercises.

- If you can't do endurance or strength exercises for some reason, and stretching exercises are the only kind you are able to do, do them at least 3 times a week, for at least 20 minutes each session. Note that stretching exercises, by themselves, don't improve endurance or strength.

- Do each stretching exercise 3 to 5 times at each session.

- Slowly stretch into the desired position, as far as possible without pain, and hold the stretch for 10 to 30 seconds. Relax, then repeat, trying to stretch farther.

Safety

- If you have had a hip replacement, check with the doctor who did your surgery before doing lower body exercises.

- If you have had a hip replacement, don't cross your legs or bend your hips past a 90-degree angle.

- Always warm up before stretching exercises (do them after endurance or strength exercises, for example; or, if you are doing only stretching exercises on a particular day, do a little bit of easy walking and arm-pumping first). Stretching your muscles before they are warmed up may result in injury.

- Stretching should never cause pain, especially joint pain. If it does, you are stretching too far, and you need to reduce the stretch so that it doesn't hurt.

- Mild discomfort or a mild pulling sensation is normal.

- Never "bounce" into a stretch; make slow, steady movements instead. Jerking into position can cause muscles to tighten, possibly resulting in injury.

- Avoid "locking" your joints into place when you straighten them during stretches. Your arms and legs should be straight when you stretch them, but don't lock them in a tightly straight position. You should always have a very small amount of bending in your joints while stretching.

Progressing

You can progress in your stretching exercises; the way to know how to limit yourself is that stretching should never hurt. It may feel slightly uncomfortable, but not painful. Push yourself to stretch farther, but not so far that it hurts.

Examples of Stretching Exercises

Hamstrings

Stretches muscles in back of thigh. Sit sideways on a bench or other hard surface (such as two chairs placed side by side) without leaning back against anything and with your back and shoulders straight. Your left leg should be resting on the bench, toes pointing up. Your right leg should be resting over the side of the bench, with your right foot flat on the floor. If your left knee is bent, stretch to get it to lie flat on the bench. If you feel a stretch at this point, hold the position for 10 to 30 seconds. If your left leg is flat on the bench and you don't feel a stretch, lean forward slowly from the hips (not the waist) until you do, keeping your back and shoulders straight the entire time (note: omit this part if you have had a hip replacement—don't lean forward, unless your surgeon or physical therapist approves). Stop and hold this position for 10 to 30 seconds. Reverse the position so that you stretch your right leg in the same way. Repeat 3 to 5 times on each side.

Summary

1. Sit sideways on bench.

2. Keep one leg stretched out on bench, straight.

3. Keep other leg off of bench, with foot flat on floor.

4. Straighten back.

5. Lean forward from hips (not waist) until you feel stretching in leg on bench, keeping back and shoulders straight. Omit this step if you have had a hip replacement, unless surgeon/therapist approves.

6. Hold position.

7. Repeat with other leg.

Alternative Hamstring Stretch

Stretches muscles in the back of the thigh. Stand behind a chair, with your legs straight. Hold the back of the chair with both hands. Bend forward from your hips (not your waist), keeping your entire back and shoulders straight the whole time, until your upper body is parallel to the floor. Don't "hump" any part of your back or shoulders at any time. Hold position for 10 to 30 seconds. You should feel a stretch in the backs of your thighs. Repeat 3 to 5 times.

Summary

1. Stand behind chair, holding the back of it with both hands.

2. Bend forward from the hips, keeping back and shoulders straight at all times.

3. When upper body is parallel to floor, hold position.

Calves

Stretches lower leg muscles in two ways: with knee straight and knee bent. While standing, place your hands on a wall, with arms outstretched, elbows straight. Keeping your left knee slightly bent, toes of right foot slightly turned inward, move your right foot back one or two feet, with your right heel and foot flat on the floor. You should feel a stretch in your right calf muscle, but you shouldn't feel uncomfortable. If you don't feel a stretch, move your right foot farther back until you do. Keep your right knee straight and hold that position for 10 to 30 seconds. Continuing to keep your right heel and foot on the floor, bend your right knee and hold for another 10 to 30 seconds. Repeat with opposite leg. Repeat 3 to 5 times on each side.

Summary

1. Stand with hands against wall, arms straight.

2. Step back 1-2 feet with one leg, heel and foot flat on floor.

3. Hold position.

4. Bend knee of stepped-back leg, keeping heel and foot flat on floor.

5. Hold position.

6. Repeat with other leg.

Ankles

Stretches front ankle muscles. Remove your shoes. Sit toward the front edge of a chair and lean back, using pillows to support your back. Slide your feet away from the chair, in front of you, so your legs are outstretched. With your heels still on the floor, point your toes away from you until you feel a stretch in the front part of your ankles. If you don't feel a stretch, lift your heels slightly off the floor while doing this exercise. Hold the position briefly. Repeat 3 to 5 times.

Summary

1. Sit in chair.

2. Stretch legs out in front of you.

3. Bend ankles to point feet toward you.

4. Bend ankles to point feet away from you.

5. If you don't feel the stretch, repeat with your feet slightly off the floor.

Triceps Stretch

Stretches muscles in back of upper arm. Hold one end of a towel in your right hand. Raise your right arm; then bend your right elbow so that the towel drapes down your back. Keep your right arm in this position, and continue holding onto the towel. With your left hand, reach behind your lower back and grasp the other end (the bottom end) of the towel. Gradually grasp higher and higher up the towel with your left hand, as high as you can. As you do this, you will find that it also pulls your right arm down. Continue until your hands touch, or as close to that as you can comfortably go. Reverse positions.

Summary

1. Hold towel in right hand.

2. Raise and bend right arm to drape towel down back.

3. Grasp bottom end of towel with left hand.

4. Climb left hand progressively higher up towel, which also pulls your right arm down.

5. Reverse positions.

Wrist Stretch

Press your hands together, elbows down. Raise your elbows as nearly parallel to the floor as possible, while keeping your hands together. Hold for 10 to 30 seconds. Repeat 3 to 5 times.

Summary

1. Place hands together, in praying position.

2. Slowly raise elbows so arms are parallel to floor, keeping hands flat against each other.

3. Hold position for 10 to 30 seconds.

4. Repeat 3 to 5 times.

Quadriceps

Stretches muscles in front of thighs. Lie on your left side, on the floor. Your hips should be lined up so that the right one is directly above the left one. Rest your head on a pillow or your left hand. Bend your right knee, reach back with your right hand, and hold onto your right heel. If you can't reach your heel with your hand, loop a belt over your right foot. Pull slightly (with your hand or with the belt) until the front of your right thigh feels stretched. Hold the position for 10 to 30 seconds. Reverse position and repeat with other leg. Repeat 3 to 5 times on each side. If the back of your thigh cramps during this exercise, stretch your leg and try again, more slowly.

Summary

1. Lie on side.

2. Rest head on pillow or hand.

3. Bend knee that is on top.

4. Grab heel of that leg.

5. Gently pull that leg until front of thigh stretches.

6. Hold position.

7. Reverse position and repeat.

Double Hip Rotation

(Don't do this exercise if you have had a hip replacement, unless your surgeon approves.) Stretches outer muscles of hips and thighs. Lie on your back, knees bent, and feet flat on floor. Keeping your shoulders on the floor, with your knees bent and together, gently lower both knees to one side as far as possible without forcing them. Hold the position for 10 to 30 seconds, then bring knees back to center and repeat on opposite side. Repeat 3 to 5 times on each side.

Summary

1. Don't do this exercise if you have had a hip replacement, unless your surgeon approves.

2. Lie on floor, knees bent

3. Keep shoulders on floor at all times.

4. Keeping knees together, lower legs to one side.

5. Hold position.

6. Return legs to upright position.

7. Repeat toward other side.

Single Hip Rotation

Stretches muscles of pelvis and inner thigh. Lie on your back and bend your knees. Let your right knee slowly lower to the right, keeping your left leg and your pelvis in place. Hold the position for 10 to 30 seconds. Bring your right knee slowly back to place. Repeat the exercise with your left leg. Repeat 3 to 5 times on each side. Keep your shoulders on the floor throughout the exercise.

Summary

1. Lie on floor.

2. Bend knees.

3. Let one knee slowly lower to side.

311

4. Hold position.

5. Bring knee back up.

6. Keep shoulders on floor throughout exercise.

7. Repeat with other knee.

Shoulder Rotation

Stretches shoulder muscles. Lie on the floor with a pillow under your head, legs straight. If your back bothers you, place a rolled towel under your knees. Stretch your arms straight out to the side, on the floor. Your upper arms will remain on the floor throughout this exercise. Bend at the elbow so that your hands are pointing toward the ceiling. Let your arms slowly roll backwards from the elbow. Stop when you feel a stretch or slight discomfort, and stop immediately if you feel a pinching sensation or a sharp pain. Slowly raise your arms, still bent at the elbow, to point toward the ceiling again. Then let your arms slowly roll forward, remaining bent at the elbow, to point toward your hips. Stop when you feel a stretch or slight discomfort. Alternate pointing above your head, then toward the ceiling, then toward your hips in this manner. Begin and end with the pointing-above-the-head position. Hold each position 10 to 30 seconds. Keep your shoulders flat on the floor throughout. Repeat 3 to 5 times.

Summary

1. Lie flat on floor, pillow under head.

2. Stretch arms out to side.

3. Bend elbows to crook lower arms downward, at right angle.

4. Hold position.

5. Bend elbows to crook lower arms upward, at right angle.

6. Hold position.

7. Keep shoulders flat on floor throughout.

Neck Rotation

Stretches neck muscles. Lie on the floor with a thick book under your head, then slowly turn your head from side to side, holding position for 10 to 30 seconds on each side. Your head should not be tipped forward or backward, but should be in a comfortable position. You can keep your knees bent to keep your back comfortable during this exercise. Repeat 3 to 5 times.

Summary

1. Lie on back.

2. Turn head from side to side, holding position each time.

About Floor Exercises

Most of the remaining exercises are done on the floor and stretch some very important muscle groups. If you are afraid to lie on the floor to exercise because you think you won't be able to get back up, consider using the buddy system to do these. Adopt a buddy who will be able to provide assistance if you need it.

Knowing the right way to get into a lying position on the floor and the right way to get back up also may be helpful to you. If you have had a hip replacement, check with your surgeon before using the following method. If you have osteoporosis, check with your doctor first.

To Get into a Lying Position

*   Stand next to a very sturdy chair that won't tip over (put chair against wall for support if you need to).

*   Put your hands on the seat of the chair.

*   Lower yourself down on one knee.

*   Bring the other knee down.

*   Put your left hand on the floor and lean on it as you bring your left hip to the floor.

*   Your weight is now on your left hip.

*   Straighten your legs out.

*   Lie on your left side.

*   Roll onto your back.

*   **Note:** You don't have to use your left side. You can use your right side, if you prefer.

To Get up from a Lying Position

*   Roll onto your left side.

Table 18.2. Exercise Schedule

Get at least this much exercise each week:

Sunday	Monday	Tuesday	Wednesday	Thursday	Friday	Saturday
	Endurance	Strength/ balance, all muscle groups	Endurance	Strength/ balance, all muscle groups	Endurance	
Stretching			Stretching			Stretching

… OR, you can exercise up to this often each week (more than this could cause injuries):

Monday	Tuesday	Wednesday	Thursday	Friday	Saturday	Sunday
Endurance	Endurance	Endurance	Endurance	Endurance	Endurance	Endurance
Strength/ balance upper body	Strength/ balance lower body	Strength/ balance upper body	Strength/ balance upper body	Strength/ balance lower body	Strength/ balance upper body	Strength/ balance lower body
Stretching	Stretching	Stretching	Stretching	Stretching	Stretching	Stretching
Anytime, anywhere balance	Anytime, anywhere balance	Anytime, anywhere balance	Anytime, anywhere balance	Anytime, anywhere balance	Anytime, anywhere balance	Anytime, anywhere balance

- Use your right hand, placed on the floor at about the level of your ribs, to push your shoulders off the floor.

- Your weight is on your left hip.

- Roll forward, onto your knees, leaning on your hands for support.

- Lean your hands on the seat of the chair you used to lie down.

- Lift one of your knees so that one leg is bent, foot flat on the floor.

- Leaning your hands on the seat of the chair for support, rise from this position.

- **Note:** You don't have to use your left side; you can reverse positions, if you prefer.

How Much Exercise Should I Get Each Week?

When you first start out, you might have trouble keeping up with even the minimum amount of exercise we suggest in Table 18.2. Start out with a schedule that your body can tolerate and that you think you really can manage, and build up from there.

Note that the schedules are arranged so that you are never doing strength exercises of the same muscle groups on any two days in a row. If you want to do strength exercises every day, alternate muscle groups. For example, do strength exercises of your upper-body muscles on Monday, Wednesday, and Friday and of your lower-body muscles on Tuesday, Thursday, and Saturday. Or you can do strength exercises of all of your muscle groups up to every other day.

Begin exercising gradually. Once you have worked your way up to a regular schedule, get at least this much exercise each week.

How Am I Doing?

There are ways to tell when it's time to move ahead in your activities, and we have mentioned some of them. For example, when you can lift a weight more than 15 times, you know it's time to add more weight in your strength exercises. And when endurance activities no longer feel somewhat hard to you, it's time to exercise a little longer, then to add a little more difficulty, like walking up steeper hills.

As you progress, you can do some simple tests, shown here, that will tell you just how far you have come. These tests also can help

315

you assess how fit you are right now, before you have started exercising. After that, try them again every month. Record your scores each time, so you can compare them and see your improvement the next time you test yourself

You might be interested in doing these tests for at least a couple of reasons. For one, most people make rapid progress soon after they start exercising, and you might find the improvement you see in your scores after just a month encouraging.

For another, these tests are a good way of letting you know if you really are progressing. Although it's normal for your improvement to slow down at times, your test scores should get better overall (unless you have reached your goal and are maintaining your current level).

If you are not in condition to do these tests right now, keep working on your current exercises and activities until you are. Whether you are testing or actually exercising, your pace should never make you feel dizzy, lightheaded, or nauseated, and you shouldn't feel pain. If you have a chronic medical condition, or are at risk of developing one, follow the guidelines under "Is It Safe for Me to Exercise?" before testing yourself.

Endurance

See how far you can walk in exactly 6 minutes. Write down how far you walked (in feet, blocks, laps, miles, number of times you walked up and down a long hallway, or whatever is convenient for you). Do this test every month. As your endurance improves, you should find that you can walk farther in 6 minutes.

Lower-Body Power

This test measures your progress in lower-body power. Time yourself as you walk up a flight of stairs (at least 10 steps) as fast as you safely can. Record your score. Repeat the test, using the same stairs, one month later. It should take you less time.

Strength

In the back of this chapter, you will find a chart for recording how much weight you lift, and how many times you lift that weight, each time you do your strength exercises. We have provided another chart that helps you see how you are progressing in your strength. It shows how much more weight you can lift and how many more times you can lift it, compared to the amount you could lift a month ago.

Balance

Time yourself as you stand on one foot, without support, for as long as possible (stand near something sturdy to hold onto, in case you lose your balance). Record your score. Repeat the test while standing on the other foot. Test yourself again in one month. The amount of time you can stand on one foot should increase.

What Should I Eat?

Your body needs fuel for exercises and physical activities, and that fuel comes from food. Eating the right nutrients from a balanced diet helps build muscle and energy. But just what does "balanced diet" mean? What should you eat, and exactly how much of it should you eat?

In Chapter 13, Figure 13.2 presents the United States Department of Agriculture's food pyramid. If you use it as a guideline, you will be following a balanced diet. It tells you how many servings of each kind of food you should eat each day. We have also included a list that tells you what, exactly, counts as one serving of each kind of food.

If you use the food pyramid as a guideline, you may also be helping to prevent or delay some of the diseases associated with growing older. For example, by cutting down on fats, you will be reducing your risk of getting cardiovascular diseases like high blood pressure. By increasing the amount of fruits and vegetables you eat, you will be lowering your risk of getting some types of cancer. Looking at the guidelines, you will see that the biggest part of the calories you take in each day should come from grains, and the smallest amount should come from fats, oils, and sweets. The guidelines put heavy emphasis on vegetables and fruits, and less on meat and dairy products.

Some older adults are on restricted diets because of certain health conditions. Kidney disease is just one example of a condition that often requires restrictions of certain foods or fluids. If your doctor or nutritionist has asked you to follow a special diet, please follow his or her advice.

What Is "A Serving"?

Grains

    1 slice of bread
    ½ cup of cooked rice or pasta
    ½ cup of cooked cereal
    1 ounce of ready-to-eat cereal

Fruits

> 1 piece of fruit
> 1 melon wedge
> 3/4 cup fruit juice
> ½ cup canned fruit
> 1/4 cup dried fruit

Vegetables

> ½ cup of chopped raw or cooked vegetables
> 1 cup of leafy raw vegetables

Milk, Yogurt, and Cheese

> 1 cup of milk or yogurt
> 1½ to 2 ounces of cheese

Example: a 1-inch cube of hard cheese weighs about ½ ounce

- **Note:** Buy low-fat or skim dairy products to avoid harmful fats.

- **Note:** Some people have trouble digesting lactose, the sugar in milk products. If you have this problem, try eating yogurt with active cultures, low-fat cheese, or lactose-reduced milk. Pills and drops that help digest lactose also are available.

Meat, Poultry, Fish, Dry Beans, Eggs, and Nuts

> ½ cup of cooked beans, 1 egg, or 2 tablespoons of peanut butter make up 1/3 of a serving of this food group.
> 2½ to 3 ounces of cooked lean meat, poultry, or fish make up one serving of this food group.

Examples: a slice of cooked, lean meat or poultry that is about 1/4 inch thick and measures 3 inches by 4 inches weighs about 2 ounces; a cooked, lean hamburger patty that weighs 3 ounces is about 3 inches across and ½-inch thick—about the size of a large mayonnaise jar lid.

- **Note:** Before cooking, a patty this size weighs about 4 ounces.

- **Note:** Half of a skinless, cooked chicken breast weighs about 3 ounces.

- **Note:** Egg whites are a good source of protein, but egg yolks are high in fat and cholesterol. Consider discarding the yolk.

- **Note:** Nuts are a good source of protein, but are high in fat.

Fats, Oils, and Sweets

The fewer fats, oils, and sweets you eat the better.

The Big Picture

Often, people decide to exercise and eat a balanced diet because they want to control their weight. For many people, these healthy habits do result in weight loss, but that's only part of the big picture. Exercise and a healthy diet may not make you thin, but even if they don't, they can help make you healthier. For example, a study showed that obese men who were physically fit had a much lower death rate than normal-weight men who weren't physically fit.

That doesn't mean that being overweight is fine; obesity carries with it many health risks. What it does show is how important physical fitness is.

Exercise and a healthy diet are just one part of becoming physically fit. Think about other lifestyle changes you can make, too. For example, smoking contributes to a variety of serious diseases and can keep you from exercising. So does excessive alcohol. Together, habits like exercise, a balanced diet, and giving up smoking will help you achieve what we wish for you: the best of health.

It's Really Not Hard to Eat a Balanced Diet

Do you look at the USDA food guidelines and think, "How in the world will I be able to eat that much every day? I'd have a hard time just eating the 6 to 11 servings of grain I'm supposed to eat daily!" Take a look at the sample menu below, and you might change your mind. This menu provides the minimum amount recommended for each of the food groups. You might find that you are already eating a balanced diet and that you even have room to add more grains or fruits and vegetables.

Breakfast

- Western-style omelet (use egg whites or egg replacers and low-fat cheese)
- Oven-baked hashbrown potatoes

- Whole-grain toast and jelly
- Small glass of fruit juice

Lunch

- Broiled salmon patty on a toasted whole-grain bun
- Spinach
- Rice
- Fruit salad with low-fat or nonfat yogurt dressing

Dinner

- Pasta with tomato and onion sauce, topped with low-fat parmesan cheese (lean meatballs optional)
- Garlic bread
- Salad with low-fat or nonfat dressing
- Low-fat ice cream or frozen yogurt

Supplements: Costly and Not Necessarily Helpful

Supplements are helpful for some older adults who can't eat all the nutrients they need—nutrients like vitamins and minerals. Recently, however, some new kinds of supplements have been appearing in stores even though they haven't been shown to improve health and their safety remains unproven.

A balanced diet is the best way for most older exercisers to get the nutrients they need. But some people in the marketing industry are doing a good job of convincing older people that they need expensive nutritional supplements, some of which haven't been shown to be helpful or safe and some of which most older people may not even need. Some of these claims give older adults the impression that certain supplements can restore youthful energy and strength.

For example, one persuasive clerk at a popular health-food store recently told an older shopper interested in exercise that she should buy certain supplements that cost about $70 a month to increase her energy and her ability to build muscles. The supplements included a protein powder and a vitamin-mineral pill containing the same ingredients as generic-brand vitamins, available at a fraction of the cost at drug stores, and some other substances not proven to build muscles or energy in older people.

This 75-year-old shopper had eaten an excellent diet based on the USDA food pyramid for years, and really didn't need these supplements.

No one likes to spend money needlessly, but for older adults on a limited income—social security, for example—unnecessary expenditures can deprive them of things they really do need (the money to buy whole foods rich in nutrients, for example). What's more, too much protein puts extra demands on the kidneys and can lower calcium levels. Although protein, vitamin, and mineral supplements are helpful to older people who truly need them, excessive doses can have harmful side effects

A clerk at another health-food store told the same shopper that, if she planned to start exercising, she should buy a powder made of protein, vitamins, and minerals that cost $19 for a 10-serving bottle. Taken once a day, that comes out to about $60 a month. One of the reasons she needed this supplement, the clerk told her, was that it contained the mineral potassium, and "older people require more of that."

Taken as directed on the label, the supplement wouldn't have harmed our intrepid shopper. But the clerk's scientific-sounding advice might have. Overdoses of potassium can cause an irregular heart beat and even death.

For most older adults, standard FDA-approved multivitamin-mineral supplements that contain potassium are just fine if taken as directed. It would be virtually impossible for most people to overdose on potassium by eating foods that contain this essential mineral naturally. Some people really do need potassium supplements, as prescribed by a doctor, only, for very specific medical conditions and in very specific, carefully monitored amounts. The point we are making here is that anyone can make scientific-sounding claims, but it doesn't necessarily mean that those claims are true or safe. This caution is especially important for people who are on diets with special restrictions—people with kidney disease, congestive heart failure, or diabetes, for example.

Buyer, beware—and check with your doctor before spending your hard-earned money on supplements that promise to restore youthful energy and strength.

Appendices to Chapter 18

Appendix A: Target Heart Rate

Target heart rate (THR) is a common way of judging how hard you should exercise during endurance activities. It tells you how fast the average person should try to make his or her heart beat during endurance sessions. It's not always the best way for older adults to decide how hard to exercise, though, because many have long-standing medical conditions or take medications that change their heart rate. We recommend using the Borg scale shown under "Examples of Exercises to Do at Home" instead. However, some older exercisers who are in basically good health and who like taking a "scientific" approach to their endurance activities may find the THR method useful. Others should check with their doctors first.

For those of you who can use THR, the chart on the next page shows an estimate of how fast you should try to make your heart beat, once you have gradually worked your way up to it. "Gradually" is an important word here. Going immediately from an inactive lifestyle to exercising at the rate shown in the chart is not advised.

One way to reach your THR gradually is to take your pulse during an endurance-type activity that is already a part of your life (walking, for example). Do it at the pace you normally do it, and record your heart rate. From session to session (or over several sessions), increase how hard you work, so that your pulse rate gradually gets faster, over time.

Eventually, you can try to get your heart rate up to 70 to 85 percent of its maximum ability (the rate shown in the chart). Making it beat faster than this is not advised.

Note: The goal is not for your heart rate to be faster all the time—just when you do your endurance activities. In fact, you should find that, as your heart becomes more efficient from endurance exercise, your resting pulse rate is slower than it was before you took up this healthy habit.

To take your pulse, press the tips of your index and middle fingers against the inside of the opposite wrist, just below the mound at the base of your thumb, and count how many pulsations you feel in a 10-second period. Multiplying this number by 6 will give you your heart rate. (Note: Don't count your pulse for an entire minute. During the minute that you have stopped exercising to take your pulse, your heart will have slowed down, and you won't get an accurate reading.)

DO NOT Use the THR Method If

- You take medications that change your heart rate, if you have a pacemaker for your heart, if you have an irregular heart rhythm called "atrial fibrillation," or if you have any other condition that affects your pulse rate. All of these situations can give you inaccurate readings. For example, many older adults take medications in a class called "beta blockers" for high blood pressure or some heart conditions (your doctor can tell you if your heart or blood-pressure medicine is a beta blocker, or if you have other conditions or medications that will affect your pulse rate during exercise). Some eyedrops used to treat glaucoma also contain beta blockers.

- Your heart rate is a reflection of how hard your body is working. Beta blockers tend to keep your heart rate slower, so no matter how hard you push yourself, you might never reach the heart rate you are trying for. You might end up exerting yourself too much, as you try in vain to reach a heart rate that your beta blockers won't allow. Being on beta blockers doesn't mean you can't exercise vigorously; it just means you can't rely on the chart below, or on your pulse rate, to judge how hard you are working.

- One way to find out the heart rate you should strive to maintain during endurance exercise is through a treadmill test performed by a health professional. However, getting access to a treadmill test is not practical for some people, and it isn't necessary for most older adults who are in basically good health. It's something to consider if you're over 65 or if you have access to a treadmill test through a health professional.

Table 18.3. Target Heart Rate

Age	Desired Range for Heart Rate During Endurance Exercise (*beats per minute*)
40	126-153
50	119-145
60	112-136
70	105-128
80	98-119
90	91-111
100	84-102

Figure 18.1.
Sample "Weekly Schedule" form.

Weekly Schedule

Week of _____

You might want to make copies of this form. Leave this one blank, so you can copy it as needed. Using a pencil, write in the exercises and activities you plan to do. Create a schedule you think you really can manage. You can change your plan as your fitness improves and you are able to do more.

	Endurance	Strength/Balance	Flexibility	Notes
Sunday				
Monday				
Tuesday				
Wednesday				
Thursday				
Friday				
Saturday				

*Figure 18.2.
Sample "Daily
Record—
Encurance and
Flexibility" form.*

Daily Record

Week of _____

Endurance and Flexibility

You might want to make copies of this form. Leave this one blank, so you can copy it as needed.
This form is for keeping track of the activities and exercises you do each day.

	Sunday	Monday	Tuesday	Wednesday	Thursday	Friday	Saturday
activity ↑							
Endurance: *List the activity you did and how long you did it.*							
how long?							
Flexibility. *Check the box of each stretching exercise you did:*							
Hamstrings							
Alternate hamstring							
• **Calves**							
• **Ankles**							
• **Triceps**							
• **Wrists**							
• **Quadriceps**							
• **Double Hip Rotation**							
• **Single Hip Rotation**							
• **Shoulder Rotation**							
• **Neck Rotation**							

325

Figure 18.3.
Sample "Daily Record— Balance" form.

Daily Record

Anytime, Anywhere Balance

You might want to make copies of this form. Leave this one blank, so you can copy it as needed. Check the box of each exercise you did.

Week of _____

	Sunday	Monday	Tuesday	Wednesday	Thursday	Friday	Saturday
Anytime, anywhere balance. *Check the box of each exercise you did:*							
Stand on one foot Left							
Right							
Stand and sit without using hands							
Walk heel-to-toe							

Daily Record

Strength/Balance

You might want to make copies of this form. Leave this one blank, so you can copy it as needed.
This form is for keeping track of the activities and exercises you do each day.

Week of _____

		Sunday	Monday	Tuesday	Wednesday	Thursday	Friday	Saturday
Arm Raise	reps							
	lbs							
Chair Stand	# of Stands							
Bicep Curl	reps							
	lbs							
Plantar Flexion	reps							
	lbs							
Triceps Extension	reps							
	lbs							
Dip	# of Dips							
Knee Flexion	reps							
	lbs							
Hip Flexion	reps							
	lbs							
Shoulder Flexion	reps							
	lbs							
Knee Extension	reps							
	lbs							
Hip Extension	reps							
	lbs							
Side Leg Raise	reps							
	lbs							

Figure 18.4.
Sample "Daily Record— Strength/ Balance" form.

327

Figure 18.5.
Sample
"Monthly
Progress
Record—
Endurance,
Lower Body,
and Balance"
form.

Monthly Progress Record

Endurance, Lower Body, and Balance

Year _____

You might want to make copies of this form. Leave this one blank, so you can copy it as needed.
Fill out this form on the same day of each month. Compare your scores to see your improvement.

	January	February	March	April	May	June	July	August	September	October	November	December
Endurance *Measure how far you are able to walk in 6 minutes. Use the same track and the same unit of measure each time.*												
Lower-Body Power *Time how fast you can walk up a flight of stairs. Use the same stairs. Use the same stairs—at least 10 steps—each time.*												
Balance *Time yourself as you stand on one foot, then the other, without support, for as long as you can.*												

*Figure 18.6.
Sample "Monthly
Progress
Record—
Strength/Bal-
ance" form.*

Monthly Progress Record

Strength/Balance

You might want to make copies of this form. Leave this one blank, so you can copy it as needed.
Fill out this form on the same day of each month. Compare your scores to see your improvement.

Year _____

		January	February	March	April	May	June	July	August	September	October	November	December
Arm Raise	reps												
	lbs												
Chair Stand	# of Stands												
Bicep Curl	reps												
	lbs												
Plantar Flexion	reps												
	lbs												
Triceps Extension	reps												
	lbs												
Dip	# of Dips												
Knee Flexion	reps												
	lbs												
Hip Flexion	reps												
	lbs												
Shoulder Flexion	reps												
	lbs												
Knee Extension	reps												
	lbs												
Hip Extension	reps												
	lbs												
Side Leg Raise	reps												
	lbs												

329

Appendix C: Resources

Below are examples of some nonprofit organizations that offer exercise programs for older adults or information about such programs. Most offer literature about exercise. Usually, single copies of pamphlets are free, but most organizations charge for bulk orders. Be sure to ask about the credentials of anyone leading an exercise program. If you have any doubts, check with your doctor to ensure that the exercises offered are suitable for you.

American Academy of Orthopedic Surgeons
6300 North River Road
Des Plaines, IL 60018-4262
Toll-Free: 1-800-824-BONES (2663)
Phone: 847-823-7186
Fax: 847-823-8125
Internet: http://www.aaos.org
E-Mail: custserv@aaos.org

Professional association of surgeons who care for the body's musculoskeletal system. Ask for free publications about how to safely do exercises like walking or stretching if you have arthritis, osteoporosis, or other musculoskeletal conditions, or if you have had a joint replacement.

American College of Sports Medicine
401 W. Michigan St.
Indianapolis, IN 46202-3233
Phone: 317-637-9200
Fax: 317-634-7817
Internet: http://www.acsm.org

Scientific and medical association of sports physicians, exercise scientists, and other health professionals with an interest in exercise. Trains and certifies people to work with older adults. Send self-addressed, stamped envelope for free brochures. Be sure to specify that you want material on exercise for older adults.

American Diabetes Association

1701 Beauregard Street
Alexandria, VA 22314
Phone: 703-549-1500
Internet: http://www.diabetes.org

Offers free pamphlets about exercise for people of all ages who have diabetes. Request "Exercise and Diabetes," "Starting to Exercise," and "20 Steps to Safe Exercise."

American Heart Association

National Center
7272 Greenville Ave.
Dallas, TX 75231-4596
Toll-Free: 1-800-AHA-USA1
Internet: http://www.americanheart.org

Offers free pamphlets about exercise for people of all ages.

American Physical Therapy Association

1111 North Fairfax St.
Alexandria, VA 22314-1488
Toll-Free: 1-800-999-2782
Internet: http://www.apta.org

Request "For the Young at Heart" (free exercise brochure).

Arthritis Foundation

P.O. Box 7669
Atlanta, GA 30309
Toll-Free: 1-800-283-7800
Internet: http://www.arthritis.org

Free pamphlet provides guidelines on how to protect joints during exercise; includes range-of-motion exercises for joint mobility, and others.

The Cooper Institute for Aerobics Research

12330 Preston Road
Dallas, TX 75230
Toll-Free: 800-635-7050
Fax: 972-341-3225
Internet: http://www.cooperinst.org
E-Mail: products@cooperinst.org

Provides information about physical activity and other health topics.

50-Plus Fitness Association
P.O. Box 20230
Stanford, CA 94309
Phone: 650-323-6160
Internet: http://www.50plus.org

Nonprofit organization that promotes fitness and active lifestyles for people 50 and older through a variety of activities, including walks, fitness events, seminars, and newsletters. Membership costs $35.00 a year (people of any age may join). Provides information for people interested in starting a 50-Plus chapter in their locale. Videos and s on fitness for older people also available; costs vary.

Jewish Community Centers
(also appears as Young Men's Hebrew Association or Young Women's Hebrew Association.)
Check phone for local listing; if unable to find, call the national head-quarters at the phone number below:
Phone: 212-532-4949
Internet: http://www.jcca.org

Services differ from location to location; most offer a variety of exercise and physical activity programs for older adults. All denominations welcome.

Mature Fitness Awards USA
1850 W. Winchester Rd., Suite 213
Libertyville, IL 60048
Phone: 847-816-8660
Fax: 847-816-8662
Website: http://www.acpinc.com/seniors/mfausa
E-Mail: seniorprograms@aol.com

Offers 25 activities for older adults, from beginning exercisers to long-time fitness enthusiasts; many of the activities are appropriate for (or can be adapted for) disabled participants. Adults age 50 and older who engage in regular physical activity may receive awards through this program. Write for a registration form and activity log.

National Association for Health and Fitness/Network of State and Governor's Councils

201 S. Capitol Avenue, Suite 560
Indianapolis, IN 46225
Phone: 317-237-5630
Fax: 317-237-5632
Internet: http://www.physicalfitness.org

Sponsors physical-fitness events for older adults; these events vary by state. Ask for address and phone number of your state's association.

National Heart, Lung and Blood Institute

NHLBI Information Center
P.O. Box 30105
Bethesda, MD 20824-0105
Phone: 301-592-8573
Internet: http://www.nhlbi.nih.gov

Part of the National Institutes of Health. Offers free publications, on exercise, diet, and cholesterol.

National Institute of Arthritis and Musculoskeletal and Skin Diseases (NIAMS)

NIAMS Information Clearinghouse
1 AMS Circle
Bethesda, MD 20892-3675
Phone: 301-495-4484
Fax copies on request (301) 881-2731 (follow instructions and enter "10301" for the publication number)
Internet: http://www.nih.gov/niams/healthinfo

Part of the National Institutes of Health. Provides free information about exercise and arthritis; large print copies available on request.

National Institute on Aging

National Institutes of Health
Bldg. 31, Rm. 5C27
31 Center Drive, MSC 2292
Bethesda, MD 20892-2292
Toll Free Phone: 800-222-2225; Toll Free TTY: 800-222-4225
Internet: http://www.nih.gov/nia

Part of the National Institutes of Health. Call or write to receive free publications about health and fitness for older adults.

National Osteoporosis Foundation
1232 22nd St., NW
Washington, DC 20037
Phone: 202-223-2226
Fax: 202-223-2237
Internet: http://www.nof.org

Voluntary organization that promotes study and treatment of osteoporosis. Call to request free copy of "The Role of Exercise in the Prevention and Treatment of Osteoporosis," "Guidelines for Safe Movement," and "Fall Prevention."

The President's Council on Physical Fitness and Sports
DHHS/OS/OPHS
200 Independence Ave., SW
HHH Bldg. Room 738-H
Washington, DC 20201
Phone: 202-690-9000
Internet: http://www.os.dhhs.gov

Provides "Pep Up Your Life," a free exercise let for older adults, in partnership with the American Association of Retired Persons.

Presidential Sports Award/Amateur Athletic Union
Walt Disney World Resort
P.O. Box 10000
Lake Buena Vista, FL 32830-1000
Phone: 407-934-7200
Internet: http://www.aausports.org

Call or write to receive a log on which to record your physical activities or sports activities. When you accomplish your goals, return the log with $8 to cover materials and shipping. You will receive a personalized certificate of achievement from the President of the United States, a congratulatory letter from the co-chairpersons of the President's Council on Physical Fitness and Sports, and an embroidered emblem that can be sewn onto a blazer or sweater Other wearable Presidential Sports Award items can be ordered, at additional cost, by calling 800-780-4048. (All sales support the Amateur Athletic Union/Presidential Sports Award.)

United States Department of Agriculture Center for Nutrition Policy and Promotion
Internet: http://www.usda.gov/cnpp

To see an explanation of the food guide pyramid on the Internet, visit the website and choose "food guide pyramid," then choose "interactive food guide pyramid." The website also offers large-print version of food guide pyramid.

YMCA and YWCA
Check phone for local listings.

Services vary from location to location; many offer exercise programs for older adults, including endurance exercises, strength exercises, water exercises, and walking.

Appendix D: Acknowledgements

The National Institute on Aging, part of the National Institutes of Health, brought together some of the nation's best-informed experts on the topic of exercise for older adults to discuss the writing of this information. They include:

Panel co-chairpersons: **Chhanda Dutta, Ph.D.**, and **Marcia Ory, Ph.D.**; Health Scientist Administrators; National Institute on Aging, National Institutes of Health.

David Buchner, M.D., M.P.H.; Professor, Department of Health Services, University of Washington

Marie Elaine Cress, Ph.D.; Associate Professor, Department of Exercise Science and Gerontology Center, University of Georgia

William Evans, Ph.D.; Director of Nutrition, Metabolism, and Exercise Laboratory at Donald W. Reynolds Department of Geriatrics, University of Arkansas for Medical Sciences

Maria Fiatarone Singh, M.D.; Associate Professor, School of Nutrition and Science Policy, Tufts University

Alan Jette, Ph.D.; Dean, Sargent College of Health and Rehabilitation Sciences, Boston University

Thomas R. Prohaska, Ph.D.; Director, Center for Research on Health and Aging, University of Illinois at Chicago

Anita Stewart, Ph.D.; Professor in Residence, Institute for Health & Aging, University of California San Francisco

We also extend special thanks to Steven N. Blair, P E. D., Director of Research at the Cooper Institute for Aerobics Research; and to Roger Fielding, Ph.D., Assistant Professor of Health Sciences and Brookdale National Fellow at the Sargent College of Health and Rehabilitation Sciences, Boston University, for their contributions.

Each of these experts is a major force in research devoted to improving the health and independence of older adults through exercise. We are grateful to them and to other leaders in the field whose work is reflected in these pages for sharing their expertise.

We are also grateful to Jerome L. Fleg, M.D., and Edward G. Lakatta, M.D., of the Gerontology Research Center, the American College of Sports Medicine; the American Heart Association; the American Physical Therapy Association; the National Center for Medical Rehabilitation and Research; the National Heart, Lung and Blood Institute; the National Institute of Arthritis and Musculoskeletal and Skin Diseases; the National Institute of Child Health and Human Development, the Office of Disease Prevention, of the National Institutes of Health; the National Aeronautics and Space Administration; the Public Health Service Office on Women's Health; and the author, Susan Cahill.

Chapter 19

The Benefits of Aerobic Exercise for People with Disabilities

Following spinal cord injury and other physical disabilities, individuals often reduce physical activity and experience deconditioning. As a result of inactivity, problems with cardiorespiratory fitness and increases in serum cholesterol and triglyceride levels may occur, increasing the risk of coronary disease. Abnormalities in thyroid function have also been reported in people with disabilities. This study was designed to determine the effects of an upper-extremity exercise training device on anthropometric characteristics, cardiovascular conditioning, and endocrine/metabolic parameters in people with lower-extremity disability.

Twelve subjects (11 men, 1 woman) participated in this pilot study; 3 subjects had quadriplegia, 7 had paraplegia, 1 had a cerebrovascular accident, and 1 had a bilateral above-knee amputation. Subjects ranged in age from 25 to 58 years. They used the wheelchair aerobic fitness trainer (WAFT), which offers resistance to arm pedaling through computer-controlled electronic particle brakes. The subjects receive feedback from the computer, including target versus actual wheel speed, resistance setting, total distance, and expended kilocalories.

Each subject completed a maximal graded exercise test on the WAFT with increases in exercise intensity every 2 minutes that progressed from 55% to 90% of maximal heart rate. The maximal heart

From *Physical Therapy*, December 1999, vol. 79, issue 12, p. 1229. © 1999 American Physical Therapy Association, Inc.; reprinted with permission.

rate was based on age using the formula 220 minus age. Mean exercise intensity was 177 watts (range= 47-384 W) with a duration of 20 to 30 minutes. Testing was followed by a 10-minute cool-down. Training consisted of 2 to 3 exercise sessions per week for 10 weeks, and, at each session, the subjects were encouraged to increase the duration of exercise up to a maximum of 30 minutes. Methods for advancing the subjects through training were not discussed. Information regarding consistency of attendance, intensity of training, and use of feedback during training was not provided.

Baseline and post-training measurements included weight; blood pressure; heart rate; skinfold caliper measures (triceps, quadriceps); mid-arm circumference; abdominal circumference; and levels of fasting serum glucose, cholesterol, triglycerides, and lipoprotein fractions. Serum thyroxine and radioactive triiodthyronine uptake were also tested prior to and following training. In 8 subjects, peak oxygen utilization (VO_2max) was measured by the open circuit method. Following the study, the subjects were asked to judge the effect of training on their feelings of well-being.

All subjects reported improved feelings of well-being as a result of the training. Training produced a significant decrease in resting heart rate and an increase in VO_2max. Blood pressure did not change substantially. Mid-arm circumference increased significantly, and upper arm fat area (calculated from the circumference and skin-fold measures) decreased. Abdominal circumference and quadriceps skinfold thickness did not change significantly nor did mean arm power.

Fasting serum cholesterol levels decreased significantly with training, but there was no change in the levels of fasting serum glucose, triglycerides, or high-density lipoprotein (HDL) cholesterol. The serum free thyroxine index increased significantly, but there was no change in serum thyroid-stimulating hormone.

The authors suggested that the increase in the free thyroxine index after training may be caused by increased sympathetic activity associated with exercise, and the decrease in serum cholesterol may be linked with increases in free thyroxine. They further speculated that improved thyroid function might improve myocardial contractility and neuromuscular function, which might improve VO_2max. The authors suggested that the lack of improvement in HDL cholesterol levels with training might be attributed to the short duration of training and the fact that HDL levels were measured 48 to 72 hours after the exercise sessions (that is, HDL levels had returned to baseline levels before they were measured). Nevertheless, they argued that the

WAFT appears to be a useful tool for cardiovascular conditioning for patients with lower-extremity disabilities.

Source: Exercise Effect with the Wheelchair Aerobic Fitness Trainer on Conditioning and Metabolic Function in Disabled Persons: A Pilot Study. Midha M, Schmitt JK, Sclater M (Spinal Cord Injury Service and General Internal Medicine Sections, Hunter Holmes McGuire Veterans Administration Medical Center, Richmond, Va), *Arch Phys Med Rehabil.* 1999;80:258-261.

—Karen McCulloch, PT, NCS,
University of North
Carolina at Chapel Hill,
Chapel Hill, NC

Chapter 20

Women's Fitness

Contents

Section 20.1

Post-Pregnancy Benefits of Aerobics

From *USA Today* (Magazine), February 1996, vol. 124, no. 2609, p. 5(2). © 1996 Society for the Advancement of Education; reprinted with permission.

Women trying to lose weight and cut body fat after a pregnancy will enjoy more success if they choose aerobic exercise over other types of physical activity. Ohio State University researchers found that new mothers who did high-intensity aerobic workouts lost two to 10 pounds after 15 weeks of exercise. Those who did warm-up and toning exercises such as sit-ups and stretches lost zero to eight pounds. More significantly, the total body fat of the aerobic exercisers decreased as much as seven percent, compared with a loss of about two percent in the others.

"It's not known how many women have a problem with retention of weight and body fat after pregnancy," explains Mary Kay Mitchell, associate professor of nutrition. "Estimates range from 12% to 25%. But women who do have trouble shedding those extra pounds perceive it as an enormous problem."

The study involved 27 women who had given birth from three to 11 weeks before the program began. None were "heavy-duty" exercisers before pregnancy, and most had gained the typical 25 to 30 pounds during pregnancy.

The women were split into two groups: 15 joined a "high-intensity" workout group and participated in hour-long aerobic dance classes at a local fitness center twice a week. They walked and jogged another half-hour each week. The remaining 12 exercised at home and were given a videotape of the warm-up and toning exercises that the first group did before aerobics classes. They were told to perform those exercises with the videotape for at least 20 minutes three times a week. None of the women were put on diets, but they were asked to record what they ate on six days during the 15-week study.

The researchers noted something they didn't expect to find as well. The camaraderie that developed among the women in the aerobics class seemed to motivate them to exercise more regularly than those who exercised at home. "You'd be amazed at the networking that went on," notes doctoral student Diane Habash, who worked on the study. "The class atmosphere really seemed to make a difference. They could really commiserate about no sleep or crying babies or sick kids, and they enjoyed getting together, so they made it a point to be there. I think this is something that needs more study—it might also have an effect on postpartum depression."

Section 20.2

Boning up with Vitamins and Exercise

From *Saturday Evening Post*, May 1999, vol. 271, issue 3, p. 20. © 1999 Benjamin Franklin Literary and Medical Society Inc. Reprinted with permission.

Most Americans don't consume enough calcium to protect themselves from the bone-weakening disease osteoporosis, the National Academy of Science warned in1998 when it increased the recommended intake of the mineral to between 1,000 and 1,300 milligrams per day.

But calcium consumption is just part of the picture for preventing and treating this debilitating disease, which affects more than 28 million Americans, 80 percent of them women. Exercise also is essential for building bone in youth and preventing bone loss with age.

"You can eat lots of protein and not gain any muscle unless you strength-train," notes Tufts University physiologist Miriam Nelson. Similarly, "exercise will kick-start the calcium to make bones stronger and denser."

Vitamin D also is important because it aids the absorption of calcium, notes Nelson, who says good sources of vitamin D are fortified dairy products and 15 minutes of exposure to sunlight daily. However, the skin can't manufacture vitamin D in people wearing sunscreen or during winter months in latitudes above 42 degrees north, such as Boston or Milwaukee.

Two kinds of exercise are recommended for bone health: weight-bearing activities and resistance exercise.

Weight-bearing activities are those in which you work your bones and muscles against gravity. Walking, stair climbing, dancing, running, and racket sports are all weight-bearing activities with differing degrees of impact. In general, the higher the impact, the more the activity strengthens bones. This is why the bones in the racket arms of tennis players are denser than the bones in their other arms.

Resistance exercise, such as working out with free weights or weight machines, is a particularly effective bone strengthener. Nelson's study, published in the *Journal of the American Medical Association*, showed that postmenopausal women who performed two 40-minute strength-training sessions each week for a year gained one percent in bone density, while women in a sedentary control group lost 2 to 2.5 percent.

"People who do weight-bearing activities have bone density that is up to 10 percent higher than people who don't exercise," notes Gail Dalsky, an assistant professor of medicine at the University of Connecticut Health Center. "People who do resistance exercise have bone density up to 30 percent higher."

If your goal is bone health, Dalsky says, "it's important to use a heavy weight that you can only lift between eight to ten times. Doing lots of repetitions with a very light weight won't do much for your bones."

The exercise prescription for optimum bone health may differ depending on your life stage, notes Felicia Cosman, a New York endocrinologist who serves as clinical director of the National Osteoporosis Foundation (NOF). She offers these recommendations:

- **Youth through age 30:** Bone is built during this period, with peak bone mass achieved between ages 20 and 30. To help youngsters reach their full potential, they should get 30 to 60 minutes of physical activity most days of the week. For optimum bone health, choose sports that involve jumping and running, such as basketball, volleyball, and soccer. Activities that promote a "thin aesthetic," such as gymnastics and dance, also can be beneficial, except when a female athlete's menstrual periods become irregular. Unhealthy weight control practices used by some girls in these sports can lead to irregular periods that put them at increased risk of osteoporosis early in life.

- **30s and 40s:** Bone loss may begin to occur in some parts of the skeleton at a rate of up to one percent per year. To help maintain bone, do at least 30 minutes of weight-bearing exercise three to five days a week and about 30 minutes of resistance exercise two to three days a week.

- **Menopause (around ages 45 to 55) and up to eight years beyond:** Bone loss is most rapid at this time, with women losing up to 20 percent of their bone mass during this time. Hormone replacement therapy or other "anti-resorptive" medications are particularly effective at this time in protecting against bone loss. To help make the decision about medication, women with osteoporosis risk factors (such as family history) should get a bone density test at menopause. While exercise is not a substitute for medications at this time, it is still helpful to continue with weight-bearing and resistance exercises.

- **Age 60 and above:** Men and women tend to lose bone mass at a similar rate during this period. People who have been sedentary should start exercising gradually with a walking program, working up to walking 30 minutes or more, most days of the week. Twice-weekly sessions of resistance exercise may also be beneficial.

In this age group, the combination of calcium and vitamin D is particularly effective at preventing bone loss, which is one reason why the National Academy of Sciences just tripled the recommended intake of vitamin D for people over age 70 to 600 international units (IU) per day. The academy's calcium recommendation is 1,200 milligrams a day, while the Osteoporosis Foundation's is even higher: 1,500 mg. daily. (One eight-ounce glass of milk provides about 300 mg. of calcium and 100 IU of vitamin D.)

People with low bone density in the spine—which can be indicated by height loss or "dowager's hump"—should avoid activities that involve bending forward and twisting, such as bowling or golf, notes University of Connecticut's Dalsky. "These activities can put undue stress on the vertebrae," she says, "and literally be the straw that breaks their back."

Resources

- "Boning Up on Osteoporosis"—a comprehensive 70-page booklet about prevention, diagnosis, and treatment—is available for $4 by writing the National Osteoporosis Foundation, 1232 22nd St. NW, Washington, DC 20037.

- *Strong Women Stay Young* by Miriam Nelson, with Sarah Wernick, Bantam Books, 1997, $23.95.

- The Osteoporosis and Related Bone Diseases National Resource Center, funded by the National Institutes of Health, offers free information for consumers and healthcare providers. Call 800-624-BONE.

—by Carol Krucoff

Section 20.3

An Active Menopause: Using Exercise to Combat Symptoms

From *The Physician and Sportsmedicine*, July 1996.
© 1996 The McGraw-Hill Companies. Reproduced with permission of McGraw-Hill, Inc.

Menopause, which occurs at an average age of 52 years, is defined as a woman's final menstrual period. This event results from lack of endometrial stimulation by estrogen as the ovarian follicles become depleted. For 5 to 10 years preceding menopause and for 5 to 10 years following it, a woman is hormonally different from the way she was before and the way she will be after this climacteric interval.

Premenopausal women (prior to the climacteric or perimenopausal years) usually experience cyclic production of estrogen and progesterone, with high concentrations of estrogen prior to each ovulation and high concentrations of estrogen and progesterone during the luteal phase, after ovulation. Postmenopausal women (following the climacteric or perimenopausal years) usually have low levels of estrogen and progesterone, with little fluctuation and no cyclicity. Perimenopausal women commonly have fluctuating levels of estrogen that lack cyclicity and predictability.

Symptoms are common among perimenopausal and postmenopausal women. Some symptoms and problems are due to hormonal changes of the menopausal transition, while others result from the aging process and adverse lifestyle factors (e.g., sedentary behavior, cigarette smoking, poor diet). It is often impossible to isolate these etiologic factors in evaluating and counseling individual women.

Benefits of Exercise

Specific types of exercise can be used to treat many problems experienced by menopausal women, and those who exercise regularly tend to report fewer menopausal symptoms and problems than sedentary women.

Vasomotor Symptoms

The cause of vasomotor symptoms (hot flashes) is not yet known. However, these symptoms can be very uncomfortable and can lead to chronic sleep deprivation, as well as mood and behavior changes. Vasomotor symptoms are less common among physically active postmenopausal women than among sedentary controls, but exercise has not been shown to relieve such symptoms.[1] Estrogen remains the most effective treatment for vasomotor symptoms.

Bone Loss

Bone loss results from deficiencies of estrogen, exercise, and dietary calcium. The rate of bone loss in women accelerates at menopause because of the marked reduction in serum estrogen concentrations. It is preferable to prevent bone loss before it occurs, rather than to treat osteopenia or osteoporosis. Strategies for prevention of bone loss include hormone replacement therapy, calcium supplementation (unless dietary sources are adequate), and exercise.

Both weight training and aerobic exercise enhance and maintain bone density. Postmenopausal women require 1,500 mg of calcium daily if they are not taking exogenous estrogen therapy and 1,000 mg of calcium daily if they are. Estrogen therapy prevents bone loss better than calcium supplementation or resistance exercise does; however, the combination of hormone replacement therapy and resistance exercise leads to a greater increase in bone density than does hormone replacement therapy alone and it is likely that the combination of estrogen, calcium, and exercise is even more beneficial.[2]

Cardiovascular Disease

Cardiovascular disease risks rise with age among both sexes as a result of aging, other risk factors, and the cumulative effects of an adverse lifestyle. In women, cardiovascular disease risks rise sharply after menopause because estrogen deficiency induces lipid and vascular changes. Many of the adverse effects of aging and menopause on lipids are reversed by aerobic exercise.[3] Aerobic exercise promotes cardiovascular fitness and reduces risks of cardiovascular disease and cardiovascular mortality. Estrogen replacement therapy leads to a reduction in mortality from coronary heart disease and other causes.[4]

Urogenital Atrophy

Urogenital atrophy results from estrogen deficiency and is best treated with estrogen therapy, administered by any route. Exercise does not affect urogenital atrophy.

Depression and Sleep Disturbances

Some mood and sleep disturbances are related to estrogen deficiency; vasomotor symptoms can impair sleep and induce chronic sleep deprivation, which can cause mood disorders. Estrogen therapy improves sleep quality and enhances mood for many women with these symptoms. Regular aerobic exercise improves cognitive function, enhances mood, and promotes daytime alertness and nocturnal sleepiness. If mood and sleep disturbances are not relieved by estrogen therapy and/or exercise, antidepressant or other psychotropic medication should be prescribed, depending on the specific diagnosis.

Weight Gain

Weight gain and accumulation of fat from aging and inactivity are common among perimenopausal and postmenopausal women. Aerobic and resistance exercise, which increase energy expenditure and lean-body mass, are the most effective ways to treat this problem.

Muscle Weakness

Another common accompaniment of the aging process is loss of muscle tissue and strength. Many older women lack sufficient strength to remain functional and independent. Resistance exercise is the most effective way to increase and maintain muscle strength.

Hormone Replacement Therapy

Hormone replacement therapy includes both estrogen and progestogen. Nearly all of the benefits result from estrogen alone. Progestational therapy should be added for endometrial protection in any woman who has a uterus but should not be prescribed for any woman who has had a hysterectomy.

Benefits

As described, estrogen therapy relieves vasomotor symptoms, prevents bone loss, reduces cardiovascular disease risk, relieves urogenital atrophy, and improves mood and sleep quality.

Contraindications and Risks

In general, estrogen should not be prescribed for women who have breast or endometrial cancer, a history of thromboembolic disease, active hepatic dysfunction, or undiagnosed vaginal bleeding. Rare exceptions to these contraindications should be considered and managed on an individual basis. Relative contraindications include hormonally induced headaches and myomata uteri.

Hormone replacement therapy has not been associated with weight gain, despite nonscientific beliefs to the contrary.[5] The major risk of hormone replacement therapy is the inconvenience of vaginal bleeding, which can often be minimized, eliminated, or regulated. If progestational therapy is adequate, the risk of endometrial cancer is less than in untreated women.

A Commitment to Exercise

All women should be encouraged to exercise regularly, and older women often need instruction in specific, individualized programs. A plan that includes both aerobic and resistance training can help to prevent or relieve problems that are common among menopausal women, such as cardiovascular disease, obesity, muscle weakness, osteoporosis, depression, and sleep disturbances. It is the responsibility of physicians caring for these women to educate them appropriately and monitor their compliance.

Emphasizing the exercise component for women who are undergoing menopause can dramatically improve their quality of life. The short-term goal of exercise therapy is minimizing menopause symptoms, and the long-term goal is enabling women to remain independent and self-sufficient.

References

1. Hammar M, Berg G, Lindgren R: Does physical exercise influence the frequency of postmenopausal hot flushes? *Acta Obstet Gynecol Scand* 1990;69(5):409-412.

2. Notelovitz M, Martin D, Tesar R, et al: Estrogen therapy and variable-resistance weight training increase bone mineral in surgically menopausal women. *J BoneMiner Res* 1991;6(6):583-590.

3. Taylor PA, Ward A: Women, high-density lipoprotein cholesterol, and exercise. *Arch Intern Med* 1993;153(10):1178-1184.

4. Ettinger B, Friedman GD, Bush T, et al: Reduced mortality associated with long-term postmenopausal estrogen therapy. *Obstet Gynecol* 1996;87(1):6-12.

5. Kritz-Silverstein D, Barrett-Connor E: Long-term postmenopausal hormone use, obesity, and fat distribution in older women. *JAMA* 1996;275(1):46-49.

Suggested Reading: Shangold M, Mirkin G: *Women and Exercise: Physiology and Sports Medicine, ed 2*. Philadelphia, FA Davis, 1994

— by Mona M. Shangold

Dr. Shangold is director of the Center for Sports Gynecology and Women's Health in Philadelphia. She is a fellow of the American College of Sports Medicine and the American College of Obstetricians and Gynecologists.

Section 20.4

Exercising Your Pelvic Muscles

National Institutes of Health, NIH Publication No. 97-4188, January 1997.

Why Exercise Pelvic Muscles?

Life's events can weaken pelvic muscles. Pregnancy, childbirth, and being overweight can do it. Luckily, when these muscles get weak, you can help make them strong again.

Pelvic floor muscles are just like other muscles. Exercise can make them stronger. Women with bladder control problems can regain control through pelvic muscle exercises, also called Kegel exercises.

Pelvic Fitness in Minutes a Day

Exercising your pelvic floor muscles for just 5 minutes, three times a day can make a big difference to your bladder control. Exercise strengthens muscles that hold the bladder and many other organs in place.

The part of your body including your hip bones is the pelvic area. At the bottom of the pelvis, several layers of muscle stretch between your legs. The muscles attach to the front, back, and sides of the pelvis bone.

Two pelvic muscles do most of the work. The biggest one stretches like a hammock. The other is shaped like a triangle. These muscles prevent leaking of urine and stool.

How do you exercise your pelvic muscles? Find the right muscles. This is very important. Your doctor, nurse, or physical therapist will help make sure you are doing the exercises the right way. You should tighten the two major muscles that stretch across your pelvic floor. They are the "hammock" muscle and the "triangle" muscle. Here are three methods to check for the correct muscles. You can make these pelvic floor muscles stronger with a few minutes of exercise every day.

1. Try to stop the flow of urine when you are sitting on the toilet. If you can do it, you are using the right muscles.

2. Imagine that you are trying to stop passing gas. Squeeze the muscles you would use. If you sense a "pulling" feeling, those are the right muscles for pelvic exercises.

3. Lie down and put your finger inside your vagina. Squeeze as if you were trying to stop urine from coming out. If you feel tightness on your finger, you are squeezing the right pelvic muscle.

Don't squeeze other muscles at the same time. Be careful not to tighten your stomach, legs, or other muscles. Squeezing the wrong muscles can put more pressure on your bladder control muscles. Just squeeze the pelvic muscle. Don't hold your breath.

Repeat, but don't overdo it. At first, find a quiet spot to practice—your bathroom or bedroom—so you can concentrate. Lie on the floor. Pull in the pelvic muscles and hold for a count of 3. Then relax for a count of 3. Work up to 10 to 15 repeats each time you exercise.

Healthy sphincter muscles can keep the urethra closed. Do your pelvic exercises at least three times a day. Every day, use three positions: lying, sitting, and standing. You can exercise while lying on the floor, sitting at a desk, or standing in the kitchen. Using all three positions makes the muscles strongest.

Be patient. Don't give up. It's just 5 minutes, three times a day. You may not feel your bladder control improve until after 3 to 6 weeks. Still, most women do notice an improvement after a few weeks.

Exercise aids. You can also exercise by using special weights or biofeedback. Ask your health care team about these exercise aids.

Hold the Squeeze 'Til after the Sneeze

You can protect your pelvic muscles from more damage by bracing yourself. Think ahead, just before sneezing, lifting, or jumping. Sudden pressure from such actions can hurt those pelvic muscles. Squeeze your pelvic muscles tightly and hold on until after you sneeze, lift, or jump. After you train yourself to tighten the pelvic muscles for these moments, you will have fewer accidents.

Points to Remember

- Weak pelvic muscles often cause bladder control problems.
- Daily exercises can strengthen pelvic muscles.
- These exercises often improve bladder control.

- Ask your doctor or nurse. Are you squeezing the right muscles?
- Tighten your pelvic muscles before sneezing, lifting, or jumping. This can prevent pelvic muscle damage.

My Pelvic Muscle Exercise Log

Sunday
- I exercised my pelvic muscles ____ times.
- I spent ____ minutes exercising.
- At each exercise session, I squeezed my pelvic muscles ____ times.

Monday
- I exercised my pelvic muscles ____ times.
- I spent ____ minutes exercising.
- At each exercise session, I squeezed my pelvic muscles ____ times.

Tuesday
- I exercised my pelvic muscles ____ times.
- I spent ____ minutes exercising.
- At each exercise session, I squeezed my pelvic muscles ____ times.

Wednesday
- I exercised my pelvic muscles ____ times.
- I spent ____ minutes exercising.
- At each exercise session, I squeezed my pelvic muscles ____ times.

Thursday
- I exercised my pelvic muscles ____ times.
- I spent ____ minutes exercising.
- At each exercise session, I squeezed my pelvic muscles ____ times.

Friday
- I exercised my pelvic muscles ____ times.
- I spent ____ minutes exercising.
- At each exercise session, I squeezed my pelvic muscles ____ times.

Saturday
- I exercised my pelvic muscles ____ times.
- I spent ____ minutes exercising.
- At each exercise session, I squeezed my pelvic muscles ____ times.

For More Information

National Kidney and Urologic Diseases Information Clearinghouse
3 Information Way
Bethesda, MD 20892 3580
E-mail: nkudic@aerie.com

The National Kidney and Urologic Diseases Information Clearinghouse is a service of the National Institute of Diabetes and Digestive and Kidney Diseases, of the National Institutes of Health, under the U.S. Public Health Service. Established in 1987, the clearinghouse provides information about diseases of the kidneys and urologic system to people with these disorders and to their families, health care professionals, and the public. The clearinghouse answers inquiries; develops, reviews, and distributes publications; and works closely with professional and patient organizations and government agencies to coordinate resources about kidney and urologic diseases. Publications produced by the clearinghouse are reviewed carefully for scientific accuracy, content, and readability.

Let's Talk about Bladder Control for Women is a public health awareness campaign conducted by the National Kidney and Urologic Diseases Information Clearinghouse (NKUDIC), an information dissemination service of the National Institute of Diabetes and Digestive and Kidney Diseases (NIDDK), National Institutes of Health. 1-800-891-5388.

Part Four

Exercise and Specific Medical Conditions

Chapter 21

AIDS (Acquired Immune Deficiency Syndrome) and Exercise

Contents

Section 21.1

Nutrition and Exercise with HIV

Even though you have HIV, you don't have to lose weight. Good nutrition and exercise can improve your health and slow down your HIV infection.

Q: What problems could make it hard for me to eat a healthy diet?

A: You might have trouble eating if you have sores in your mouth, diarrhea, nausea or just a poor appetite. If you have trouble eating and exercising, talk to your doctor.

Q: What are some good tips for eating right?

A: A few simple steps can help you make sure your food is healthy and safe:

- Wash your hands with soap and water before you eat so you won't get an infection from germs on your hands.

- Wash fruits and vegetables before you eat them or cook them.

- Wash your hands with soap and water after you touch raw fish, chicken or meat so you won't get an infection from germs on your hands.

- Be sure that meat, eggs and fish are well cooked before you eat them.

Here are some ways to put good nutrition into your diet:

- Have high-calorie drinks like milkshakes. Adding powdered milk can increase the nutrition in other drinks.

- Drink 8 to 10 glasses of filtered water each day.

- Keep nutritious snacks on hand.

- Eat high-calorie foods if you're losing weight.

- Call your doctor if you lose 5 pounds or more when you didn't want to.

- Talk to your doctor about taking a multivitamin every day. Take your multivitamin with a meal so your stomach won't get upset.

Q: *What can I do if I'm having trouble eating?*

A: There are several things you can do:

- If you don't have an appetite, try to eat your favorite foods. Instead of eating three big meals each day, eat six to eight small meals. Drink high-calorie protein shakes with your meals or between meals.

- If you have diarrhea, don't eat fried foods and other high-fat foods like potato chips. Don't eat high-fiber foods. Instead, eat bland foods like bread, rice and applesauce. Ask your doctor about taking nutritional supplements, like Ensure.

- If you have mouth sores, avoid citrus fruits like oranges and grapefruit. Avoid very hot or cold foods. Don't eat spicy foods. Try not to eat hard foods like chips and pretzels. Use a straw to drink liquids.

- If you have nausea and vomiting, avoid drinking any liquid with your meals. Eat six to eight small meals each day instead of three large meals. Eat foods with a mild flavor. Eat foods at a medium temperature, not hot or cold. Drink nutritional supplements and sports drinks.

- Sit and relax for 30 minutes after you eat.

Q: *How can I increase my strength?*

A: An aerobic exercise like walking will help make you stronger. It's good to begin exercising slowly. Little by little, increase the amount of exercise. For example, you might start walking for 20 minutes three times a week. Then, after you get a little stronger, you can increase the walking time to 30 minutes four times a week. Talk with your doctor before you start.

Weight lifting is also a good way to increase your strength. Start by trying to do a weight lifting exercise 10 times. This is called a "repetition." More than one repetition is called a "set." Try to do two sets of 10 repetitions. Rest for 90 seconds between each set.

You don't need to have fancy exercise equipment to do weight lifting. You can use soup or juice cans, books and other objects you have in the house. Start by lifting a weight that's comfortable for you and doesn't cause too much strain.

In the first week, do one or two different weight lifting exercises for each body part once or twice in the week. Start with a small weight in each hand, like 10 to 15 ounces (a can of soup or a can of beans), depending on the exercise. Each week increase the number of exercises you do and the number of times you exercise. Rest for 1 to 2 days between exercise sessions. When you're feeling sick, either exercise less or stop for a while.

Dumbbell Bench Press
(for your chest, shoulders and the back of your arms)

Lie on a bench on your back. Hold a dumbbell in each hand, with your hands lined up with your shoulders. Have the palms of your hands facing down (toward your toes). Lower the dumbbells until your elbows are below the bench. Don't relax your arms at the bottom of this movement. As soon as your elbows are as low as they can go, move your arms up again to the starting position. Don't "lock" your elbows at the top of the movement. (This means, don't make your arms be exactly straight—leave a tiny little bend in your elbows.) Remember: You can use cans of soup instead of dumbbells in these exercises.

Crunches
(for your abdomen)

Lie on your back on the floor. Keep your feet on the floor and your knees bent. Fold your arms across your chest. Now raise just your head and shoulders from the floor. This is a small and slow movement, like a curl. Your back stays on the floor. Slowly lower your head and shoulders back to the floor. When you are curling your head up, keep your chin up and your eyes looking at the ceiling. You can add resistance to this exercise by holding a weight on your chest.

Upright Row
(for your shoulders, upper back and the front of your arms)

Hold a dumbbell in each hand. Let your arms be almost straight and resting on the front of your thighs. Your palms should face toward your legs. Now pull the dumbbells up to the level of your shoulders. Your elbows should go up first. When your elbows are about even with your ears, lower the dumbbells to your thighs again. Keep your knees bent just a tiny bit. Don't let yourself lean backwards.

Lunge
(for the front and back of your legs and your buttocks)

Hold a dumbbell in each hand. Keep your arms down at your sides. Your palms should face your legs. Your feet should be even with your shoulders. Take a large step forward with your left leg. Lower your right knee until it's one inch above the floor. Now straighten your left leg and step back to the starting position. Repeat on the other leg. Remember that the movement is up and down, not really forward. Keep your back straight and your head up. Don't let yourself lean forward.

Section 21.2

Exercise Does Not Spur AIDS Course

From *Science News,* May 9, 1998, vol. 153, no. 19, p. 299(1). Reprinted with permission from *Science News*, the weekly newsmagazine of science, © 1998 by Science Services, Inc.

People infected with HIV, the virus responsible for AIDS, tend to develop muscle wasting. Though their surviving muscle can be strengthened with exercise, many AIDS sufferers have been reluctant to pump iron for fear that the muscle injury accompanying this training might initiate an immune response that would cause HIV to replicate.

A new study indicates that such worries may be unfounded. Ronenn Roubenoff of the Tufts University School of Medicine in Boston and his colleagues recruited 21 men and 4 women infected with HIV. They underwent a 15-minute step-climbing activity. Once every 5 seconds throughout the trial they stepped onto and off of a 30-centimeter-high platform. While it was rigorous work, all of the volunteers finished it (although they reported feeling sore for days afterward).

Comparing the results of laboratory tests performed during the week after the exercise trial to those before, "we did see activation of the immune system, muscle damage, and activation of muscle protein turnover—all things that we know are part of the response to exercise," Roubenoff says. "What we didn't see was a rise in (HIV). In fact, there was a statistically significant, but not biologically significant, decline."

Studies by others have shown that if one stimulates the immune system—for example, by vaccinating people who have HIV—"you can get a walloping increase" in the number of HIV-infected cells, he notes. Doctors were concerned that HIV-positive people who move from inactivity to exercise, as weekend athletes or gardeners do, might experience a similar increase. "But this level of exercise doesn't seem to be that strong a stimulus," Roubenoff says. "That's reassuring," he notes, because earlier research by his team has shown that any follow-up exercise will have a far smaller impact on immunity.

—by Janet Raloff

Section 21.3

Exercise Benefits Men with HIV Wasting Disease

Reprinted from *AIDS Weekly Plus*, April 26, 1999. © 1999 Charles W. Henderson.

Men who suffer from HIV wasting syndrome can benefit significantly from a combination of exercise and regular, moderate doses of male hormones, according to a new clinical study led by a University of California San Francisco researcher.

The study team found the combined therapy produced an increase in lean-body mass and muscle strength, regardless of whether a patient was undergoing treatment with HIV anti-retroviral drugs known as protease inhibitors.

"This is an important point because weight gain after initiation of protease inhibitor therapy usually takes place through the accumulation of body fat, but our goal in patients with HIV-related weight loss is to build up the lean tissue," said lead study investigator Marc Hellerstein, MD, PhD, UCSF associate professor of medicine who treats patients at San Francisco General Hospital Medical Center.

The other key finding is that only a small amount of male hormones, or androgens, was necessary to produce positive results. "Much larger doses of androgens are often used by body-builders to develop muscular tissues, but such amounts have unproven long-term safety," said Hellerstein, who also is an associate professor of nutritional sciences at UC Berkeley.

The research results were reported in the April 14, 1999, issue of the *Journal of the American Medical Association*.

There were 22 study patients, all of whom took part in a weight-lifting exercise regimen that was supervised by a trainer and received the male hormone, testosterone, by injection. In addition, one group of 11 patients received oxandrolone, a synthetic hormonal agent belonging to the class of androgens called anabolic steroids. Another 11 patients received a placebo. The study was double-blind. Both placebo and oxandrolone were taken in tablet form. Of the total study population,

13 patients were taking protease inhibitors as a treatment for HIV infection. They were represented evenly in both groups.

Study findings showed that both groups had increases in lean body mass, weight, and strength, but the gains were substantially greater in the oxandrolone-supplemented group. These results were the same whether or not patients were undergoing protease inhibitor therapy.

Previous research done elsewhere in healthy men had found that a very high dose of testosterone combined with exercise produced greater increases in lean tissue and in muscle strength than either treatment by itself.

"These results presented our team with valuable data, but the long-term safety and behavior consequences of very high doses of testosterone are unknown, so we developed a protocol that would incorporate a lower dose of androgen therapy that included testosterone and an anabolic steroid," Hellerstein said.

At the beginning of the UCSF study, participants ranged in age from 40-42 years and in weight from about 151-161 pounds. Other characteristics included HIV positive status, normal testosterone levels, and an average weight loss of 8-9 percent during the previous two years but stable weight during the preceding three months.

Research findings from the oxandrolone and placebo groups, respectively, were: average weight gain, 14.7 pounds versus 9.3, and rate of lean body mass gain per week, 2.0 pounds versus 1.0. The oxandrolone group also showed an increase in muscle strength (chest, triceps, leg) over the placebo group by a measurement of .04 percent.

Patients in both groups showed a similar decrease in body fat and increase in bone mineral content.

While physical overtraining may suppress immune function, the exercise program incorporated in the study showed "no evidence of worsening immunologic or virologic status," according to the researchers.

The study lasted eight weeks and was carried out in conjunction with the Western Human Nutrition Research Center in San Francisco, operated by the U.S. Department of Agriculture. Study subjects spent two 10-day periods as inpatients at the Center, where metabolic and other tests were conducted.

Placebo tablets and oxandrolone tablets were provided by Bio-Technology General Corporation. The research was supported in part by grants from the U.S. National Institutes of Health, Bio-Technology General Corporation, and a sport consortium of the National Collegiate Athletic Association, United States Olympic Committee, and National Football League.

Section 21.4

Exercise Decreases Depression for AIDS Patients

Reprinted from *AIDS Weekly Plus*, July 22, 1996, p. 7(2). © 1996, Charles W. Henderson.

HIV-positive men and women become less depressed, less angry, and less fatigued after a regular program of aerobic and resistive exercise.

Barbara Smith of the Ohio State University School of Nursing, Columbus, Ohio, reported findings from a clinical trial of the effects of exercise at the XI International Conference on AIDS, held July 7-12, 1996, in Vancouver, British Columbia, Canada.

The 60 HIV-positive study subjects averaged 38 years of age, weighed 177 pounds, had 350 CD4 cells, were stable on antiretrovirals and antidepressants, and led a sedentary lifestyle (aerobic power (VO_2 max) 35 on average).

"We really wanted to go after the couch potatoes," quipped Smith.

Experimental subjects engaged in 12 weeks of supervised exercise, three days per week for 60 minutes. Subjects exercised on treadmills at a workload of 60 to 80 percent of individual VO_2 maximum and completed two sets of 12 repetitions on three upper body and three lower body resistive exercise machines. Control subjects engaged in 12 weeks of usual activity and were exercised during weeks 13 to 24.

Only three subjects were lost to follow-up. Smith credited the excellent subject retention to the use of personal trainers.

No differences were found between the two groups on measures of immune status.

Significant differences were found between the exercise group and the control group on the psychological measures. Depression, anger, and fatigue were all found to decrease in the experimental group.

"The Beck Depression Inventory scores were cut in half over twelve weeks' participation in our exercise program," reported Smith.

Chapter 22

Arthritis and Exercise

This chapter answers general questions about arthritis and exercise. The amount and form of exercise recommended for each individual will vary depending on which joints are involved, the amount of inflammation, how stable the joints are, and whether a joint replacement procedure has been done. A skilled physician or physical therapist who is knowledgeable about the medical and rehabilitation needs of people with arthritis can design an exercise plan for each patient.

What Is Arthritis?

Arthritis is a general term that refers to many rheumatic diseases that can cause pain, stiffness, and swelling in joints and other connective tissues. These diseases can affect supporting structures such as muscles, tendons, and ligaments and may also affect other parts of the body. Some common types of arthritis are osteoarthritis, rheumatoid arthritis, systemic lupus erythematosus, gout, juvenile rheumatoid arthritis, ankylosing spondylitis, and psoriatic arthritis. Osteoarthritis is the most common.

Q: Should people with arthritis exercise?

A: Yes. Studies have shown that exercise helps people with arthritis in many ways. Exercise reduces joint pain and stiffness and increases

National Arthritis and Musculoskeletal and Skin Diseases Information Clearinghouse (NAMSIC), Document No. PP2/97, 1997. Available at www.nih.gov/niams.

flexibility, muscle strength, and endurance. It also helps with weight reduction and contributes to an improved sense of well-being.

Q: How does exercise fit into a treatment plan for people with arthritis?

A: Exercise is one part of a comprehensive arthritis treatment plan. Treatment plans also may include rest and relaxation, proper diet, medication, and instruction about proper use of joints and ways to conserve energy (that is, not waste motion) as well as the use of pain relief methods.

Q: What types of exercise are most suitable for someone with arthritis?

A: Three types of exercise are best for people with arthritis:

- Range-of-motion exercises help maintain normal joint movement and relieve stiffness. This type of exercise helps maintain or increase flexibility.

- Strengthening exercises help keep or increase muscle strength. Strong muscles help support and protect joints affected by arthritis.

- Aerobic or endurance exercises improve cardiovascular fitness, help control weight, and improve overall function. Weight control can be important to people who have arthritis because extra weight puts extra pressure on many joints. Some studies show that aerobic exercise can reduce inflammation in some joints.

Q: How does a person with arthritis start an exercise program?

A: People with arthritis should discuss exercise options with their doctors. Most doctors recommend exercise for their patients. Many people with arthritis begin with easy, range-of-motion exercises and low-impact aerobics. People with arthritis can participate in a variety of, but not all, sports and exercise programs. The doctor will know which, if any, sports are off-limits. The doctor may have suggestions about how to get started or may refer the patient to a physical therapist. It is best to find a physical therapist who has experience working with people who have arthritis. The therapist will design an appropriate home exercise program and teach clients about pain-relief methods, proper body mechanics (placement of the body for a given task, such as lifting a heavy box), joint protection, and conserving energy.

Step Up to Exercise: How to Get Started

- Discuss exercise plans with your doctor.

- Start with supervision from a physical therapist or qualified athletic trainer.

- Apply heat to sore joints (optional; many people with arthritis start their exercise program this way).

- Stretch and warm up with range-of-motion exercises.

- Start strengthening exercises slowly with small weights (a 1 or 2 pound weight can make a big difference).

- Progress slowly.

- Use cold packs after exercising (optional; many people with arthritis complete their exercise routine this way).

- Add aerobic exercise.

- Consider appropriate recreational exercise (after doing range-of-motion, strengthening, and aerobic exercise). Fewer injuries to arthritic joints occur during recreational exercise if it is preceded by range-of-motion, strengthening, and aerobic exercise that gets your body in the best condition possible.

- Ease off if joints become painful, inflamed, or red and work with your doctor to find the cause and eliminate it.

- Choose the exercise program you enjoy most and make it a habit.

Q: What are some pain-relief methods?

A: There are known methods to stop pain for short periods of time. This temporary relief can make it easier for people who have arthritis to exercise. The doctor or physical therapist can suggest a method that is best for each patient. The following methods have worked for many people.

Moist heat supplied by warm towels, hot packs, a bath, or a shower can be used at home for 15 to 20 minutes three times a day to relieve symptoms. A health professional can use short waves, microwaves, and ultrasound to deliver deep heat to non-inflamed joint areas. Deep heat is not recommended for patients with acutely inflamed joints. Deep heat is often used around the shoulder to relax tight tendons prior to stretching exercises.

369

Cold supplied by a bag of ice or frozen vegetables wrapped in a towel helps to stop pain and reduce swelling when used for 10 to 15 minutes at a time. It is often used for acutely inflamed joints. People who have Raynaud's phenomenon should not use this method.

Hydrotherapy (water therapy) can decrease pain and stiffness. Exercising in a large pool may be easier because water takes some weight off painful joints. Community centers, YMCAs, and YWCAs have water exercise classes developed for people with arthritis. Some patients also find relief from the heat and movement provided by a whirlpool.

Mobilization therapies include traction (gentle, steady pulling), massage, and manipulation (using the hands to restore normal movement to stiff joints). When done by a trained professional, these methods can help control pain and increase joint motion and muscle and tendon flexibility.

TENS(transcutaneous electrical nerve stimulation) and biofeedback are two additional methods that may provide some pain relief, but many patients find that they cost too much money and take too much time. TENS machines cost between $80 and $800. The inexpensive units are fine. Patients can wear them during the day and turn them off and on as needed for pain control.

Relaxation therapy also helps reduce pain. Patients can learn to release the tension in their muscles to relieve pain. Physical therapists may be able to teach relaxation techniques. The Arthritis Foundation has a self-help course that includes relaxation therapy and also sells relaxation tapes. Health spas and vacation resorts sometimes have special relaxation courses.

Acupuncture is a traditional Chinese method of pain relief. A medically qualified acupuncturist places needles in certain sites. Researchers believe that the needles stimulate deep sensory nerves that tell the brain to release natural painkillers (endorphins). Acupressure is similar to acupuncture, but pressure is applied to the acupuncture sites instead of using needles.

Q: How often should people with arthritis exercise?

A: Range-of-motion exercises can be done daily and should be done at least every other day. Strengthening exercises also can be done daily and should be done at least every other day unless you have severe pain or swelling in your joints. Endurance exercises should be done for 20 to 30 minutes three times a week unless you have severe pain or swelling in your joints.

Q: What type of strengthening program is best?

A: This varies depending on personal preference, the type of arthritis involved, and how active the inflammation is. Strengthening one's muscles can help take the burden off painful joints. Strength training can be done with small free weights, exercise machines, isometrics, elastic bands, and resistive water exercises. Correct positioning is critical, because if done incorrectly, strengthening exercises can cause muscle tears, more pain, and more joint swelling.

Q: Are there different exercises for people with different types of arthritis?

A: There are many types of arthritis. Experienced doctors, physical therapists, and occupational therapists can recommend exercises that are particularly helpful for a specific type of arthritis. Doctors and therapists also know specific exercises for particularly painful joints. There may be exercises that are off-limits for people with a particular type of arthritis or when joints are swollen and inflamed. People with arthritis should discuss their exercise plans with a doctor. Doctors who treat people with arthritis include rheumatologists, general practitioners, family doctors, internists, and rehabilitation specialists (physiatrists).

Q: How much exercise is too much?

A: Most experts agree that if exercise causes pain that lasts for more than 1 hour, it is too much. People with arthritis should work with their physical therapist or doctor to adjust their exercise program when they notice any of the following signs of too much exercise:

- Unusual or persistent fatigue
- Increased weakness
- Decreased range of motion
- Increased joint swelling
- Continuing pain (pain that lasts more than 1 hour after exercising)

Q: Should someone with rheumatoid arthritis continue to exercise during a general flare? How about during a local joint flare?

A: It is appropriate to put joints gently through their full range of motion once a day, with periods of rest, during acute systemic flares or local joint flares. Patients can talk to their doctors about how much rest is best during general or joint flares.

Q: *Are researchers studying exercise and arthritis?*

A: Researchers are comparing the development of musculoskeletal disabilities, including arthritis, in long-distance runners and non-runners. Preliminary results show that running does not increase the likelihood of developing osteoarthritis.

Researchers also are looking at the effects of muscle strength on the development of osteoarthritis. Other researchers continue to look for and find benefits from exercise to patients with rheumatoid arthritis, spondyloarthropathies, systemic lupus erythematosus, and polymyositis.

Q: *Where can people find more information on arthritis and exercise?*

A: More information can be had from the following sources:

Arthritis Foundation
1330 West Peachtree Street
Atlanta, GA 30309
Phone: 404-872-7100
Toll-Free: (800) 283-7800
Or, call your local chapter (listed in the telephone directory).
http://www.arthritis.org.

This is the major voluntary organization devoted to arthritis. The Foundation publishes a free pamphlet on exercise and arthritis and a monthly magazine for members that provides up-to-date information on all forms of arthritis. Local chapters organize exercise programs for people who have arthritis, including People with Arthritis Can Exercise (PACE) and an aquatic exercise program held in swimming pools. The Foundation also can provide physician and clinic referrals.

PACE Catalog Center
Arthritis Foundation
P.O. Box 1616
Alpharetta, GA 30009
(800) 207-8633

This center sells PACE exercise videotapes at two levels, basic and advanced. Each videotape is approximately 30 minutes long and includes a warm-up section, a gentle or moderate exercise routine, and a rhythmic movement sequence to help improve endurance. The videotapes are available for $19.50 per tape, plus shipping charges.

Spondylitis Association of America (SAA)
14827 Ventura Blvd.
Suite 222
Sherman Oaks, CA 91403
(818) 981-1616
(800) 777-8189
http://www.spondylitis.org

This nonprofit, voluntary organization helps people who have ankylosing spondylitis and related conditions. SAA sells books, posters, videotapes, and audiotapes about exercises for people who have arthritis of the spine.

American College of Rheumatology/Association of Rheumatology Health Professionals
1800 Century Place, Suite 250
Atlanta, GA 30345
(404) 633-3777
Fax: (404) 633-1870
http://www.rheumatology.org

This association provides referrals to physical therapists who have experience designing exercise programs for people with arthritis. The organization also provides exercise guidelines developed by the American College of Rheumatology.

Acknowledgments

The NIAMS gratefully acknowledges the assistance of Jeanne Hicks, M.D., and Naomi Lynn Gerber, M.D., both of the Rehabilitation Medicine Department, and Stanley R. Pillemer, M.D., Office of the Director, NIAMS, at the National Institutes of Health, in the preparation and review of this chapter.
The National Arthritis and Musculoskeletal and Skin Diseases Information Clearinghouse (NAMSIC) is a public service sponsored by the NIAMS that provides health information and information sources. The NIAMS, a part of the National Institutes of Health (NIH), leads the Federal medical research effort in arthritis and musculoskeletal

and skin diseases. The NIAMS sponsors research and research train-ing throughout the United States as well as on the NIH campus in Bethesda, MD, and disseminates health and research information. PP 2/97

Chapter 23

Asthma during Exercise

Exercise is a common cause or trigger of asthma symptoms. For some people, exercise may be their only trigger. Exercise can trigger asthma symptoms in up to 80 percent of people with asthma. Fortunately, treatment and monitoring of exercise-induced asthma can allow most people with asthma to participate in physical activity and sports and achieve their highest potential.

How Will I Know If I Have Exercise-Induced Asthma?

For some individuals, exercise-induced asthma usually occurs within three to eight minutes of starting activity or exercise. For most, exercise-induced asthma occurs after stopping exercise. The most common symptoms of exercise-induced asthma are coughing, wheezing, shortness of breath and/or chest tightness. It is important to recognize the difference between poor conditioning and exercise-induced asthma. In well-conditioned athletes, symptoms of exercise-induced asthma may only occur with the most vigorous activity or exercise.

Think about how you feel when you exercise or participate in physical activities and share this information with your health care provider. It may be helpful to perform a test called an exercise challenge to diagnose exercise-induced asthma. An exercise challenge is usually performed in your doctor's office or the hospital. During an exercise challenge, you will walk or run on a treadmill or ride an exercise bicycle and perform repeated breathing tests. Using this information, your health care provider will be able to understand if exercise can make your asthma symptoms worse.

How Is Exercise-Induced Asthma Treated?

Fortunately, there is a simple and effective way of treating exercise-induced asthma. By using a prescribed "pre-treatment," people with asthma should be able to participate safely and successfully in exercise, sports and physical activities.

A pre-treatment can prevent exercise from triggering asthma symptoms. Many people with well-controlled asthma who experience asthma symptoms during exercise respond well to the use of an inhaled, short-acting bronchodilator medication, such as albuterol (Proventil®, Ventolin®) or pirbuterol (Maxair®). This medication is usually prescribed 10 to 15 minutes before exercise and quickly opens the airways to prevent asthma symptoms. Discuss the use of a pre-treatment with your health care provider.

Some people with exercise-induced asthma respond well to other medications. Health care providers may recommend using cromolyn sodium (Intal®) or nedocromil sodium (Tilade®) as a pre-treatment. In all cases, work with your health care provider to decide the treatment that is right for you.

Regardless of which medicine(s) you use, it is always important to use good technique with your inhaled medications. Without good technique, the medication may not reach your airways, and therefore cannot help prevent exercise-induced asthma. Using a spacer or open mouth technique can improve delivery of the medication to the airways. Review your inhaler technique with your health care provider at your next visit.

Monitoring Exercise-Induced Asthma with a Peak Flow Meter

The peak flow meter can be a useful tool in monitoring exercise-induced asthma. A peak flow meter is a portable, hand-held device that measures how well you are breathing. When the airways are narrowed by asthma, the peak flow number will drop. A significant drop in your peak flow number may be a signal that you need additional medication or maybe a short rest during exercise.

A peak flow meter can be an objective way to make decisions about participation in sports, gym class, recess or other activities. In many situations physical education teachers, coaches and employers are confused about asthma and exercise or physical activity. Some prohibit individuals from participation while others push those with asthma to keep up with their peers without proper monitoring or treatment. A peak flow meter combined with monitoring asthma symptoms can help take the confusion out of this situation.

What Sports Are Best for People with Exercise-Induced Asthma?

Sports or activities with intermittent periods of activity are least likely to cause asthma symptoms. Activities followed by brief rest periods can allow the person to regain control of his or her breathing. Activities such as baseball, softball, volleyball, tennis, downhill skiing, golf and some track and field events all have intermittent rest periods.

Sports that require continuous activity, such as swimming, cycling, distance running and soccer also can be enjoyed by people with exercise-induced asthma. Participation in any sport often requires use of a pre-treatment before exercise and close monitoring. Along with appropriate treatment and close monitoring, a good warm-up and cooldown period is beneficial.

It is important to realize that people with exercise-induced asthma can participate in any sport. In fact, it is estimated that exercise-induced asthma affects one in ten athletes. At the 1984 summer Olympic games in Los Angeles, 67 of the 597 members (or 11%) of the American team tested positive for exercise-induced asthma. These 67 athletes won a total of 41 medals!

Note: This information is provided to you as an educational service of National Jewish Medical and Research Center. It is not meant to be a substitute for consulting with your own physician.

Chapter 24

Cancer Patients and Exercise

Contents

Section 24.1

Exercise Good for Some Cancer, Heart Patients

From *Science News*, May 3, 1997, vol. 151, no. 18, p. 269(1). Reprinted with permission from *Science News*, the weekly newsmagazine of science, © 1997 by Science Services, Inc.

Getting over chemotherapy? Hobbled by heart failure? That's no excuse. Haul out those sweats, pull on those sneakers—and get some exercise.

Surprising and callous though it seems, doctors may soon be giving patients such advice. Two new studies, though small in scope, suggest that exercise is as important for people with congestive heart failure and those recovering from chemotherapy as it is for healthy people.

Without any firm evidence, doctors have cautioned such patients against vigorous exercise, fearing that physical activity would make matters worse. Most studies probing the safety and usefulness of exercise in people with cancer or congestive heart disease have yielded untrustworthy or inconclusive results.

In the new studies, however, two groups of researchers working independently found that such individuals can increase their stamina, stave off fatigue, and boost their muscles' oxygen-carrying capacity by riding stationary bicycles and walking. The studies could have an enormous impact on cancer and cardiovascular rehabilitation efforts, expanding existing programs and spawning new ones. Sadly, there is no shortage of clients.

About 70 percent of cancer patients report that the one-two punch of a malignancy and aggressive treatment saps their strength and energy. Most cancer rehabilitation programs offer only physical therapy aimed at specific problems such as those caused by amputations.

Fernando C. Dimeo, a rehabilitation and sports medicine specialist at Freiburg University Medical Center in Germany, and his colleagues decided to step into the cancer rehabilitation arena with a pilot study of 32 patients, half of whom participated in an active exercise program. The rest served as controls. After chemotherapy ended, but before the exercise regimen began, the two groups were evenly matched—achieving the limit of their tolerance for exercise on treadmills paced at about 6 kilometers per hour.

After 7 weeks, those in the exercise group had increased their exercise tolerance to 8 km per hour, compared to 7 km per hour for the control group. In addition, they had significantly higher concentrations of hemoglobin in their blood, indicating that their oxygen-carrying capacity had risen substantially.

"Cancer patients should be counseled to increase their level of exercise in the recovery phase after high-dose chemotherapy," the investigators report in the May 1, 1997 *Cancer*.

"To my knowledge, this is the first study that has solidly documented this," says Harmon Eyre of the American Cancer Society in Atlanta. "Even though it's a small study, I think it's pretty impressive."

People with congestive heart failure, whose hearts are already so impaired that they pump just one-third the normal volume of blood, fared about as well as the cancer patients. Until now, cardiac rehabilitation through exercise was considered too risky for these people because their damaged heart muscles are often thin-walled and weak. This cautious approach gained currency after a 1988 Canadian study—using a medical application of sonar—showed that exercise in cardiac patients appeared to damage the heart.

Using a more precise method called magnetic resonance imaging (MRI), a study of 25 men with congestive heart failure now shows that exercise does not damage the heart. Twelve of the men undertook a 2-month regimen of daily walks and regular 45-minute sessions on a stationary bike; 13 others did not exercise.

The investigators then used MRI to measure the thickness of the men's heart walls, which showed no evidence of damage from the exercise. "The results are indisputable," says Jonathan Myers of Stanford University. His team's study, reported in the April 15 *Circulation*, also showed that physical activity improved exercise capacity by 26 percent. The 13 sedentary patients showed no such gain.

Bernard Chaitman, chief of cardiology at Saint Louis University Health Sciences Center, says that a 26 percent improvement may permit people to carry out their normal activities rather than remain bedridden.

Evidence is also mounting that exercise can help keep people from getting cancer as well as heart disease. A study of 20,624 women by Inger Thune and her colleagues at the University of Tromso in Norway, published in the May 1, 1997 *New England Journal of Medicine*, found that those who worked out regularly cut their breast cancer risk by 72 percent.

— by Steve Sternberg

Section 24.2

Exercise May Alleviate Effects of Chemotherapy

Fatigue and impaired physical performance are common side effects of cancer treatment, affecting up to 70 percent of all patients undergoing radiation treatment or chemotherapy. These problems are due, in part, to inactivity during hospitalization and the acute phase of treatment. Dimeo and colleagues evaluated the effects of aerobic exercise on the loss of physical performance in patients undergoing high-dose chemotherapy followed by autologous peripheral blood stem cell transplant. The impact of aerobic activity on the incidence and severity of complications during this treatment was also reviewed.

Eighty patients between the ages of 18 and 60 years with solid cancerous tumors were considered for enrollment in the study. Of that group, 70 were randomly assigned to one of two groups. Thirty-three patients were assigned to a regular exercise protocol during treatment, while the remaining 37 were assigned to the control group with no intervention. One week before starting chemotherapy, all patients underwent a treadmill stress test to determine baseline physical performance.

Patients in the training group followed a daily regimen in which they "biked" on a bed ergometer for one minute in order to reach at least 50 percent of their cardiac reserve, then rested for one minute. This exercise-rest regimen was performed 15 times, so patients were training for 30 minutes a day. In addition, complete blood cell counts and serum chemistry measurements were obtained each day 12 hours after training. On the day of discharge, patients in both groups underwent resting electrocardiography, echocardiography and a treadmill stress test. Hematologic and nonhematologic toxicities also were assessed at this time.

At the beginning of the study, the baseline physical performance of both groups was the same. After hospitalization with no exercise, patients in the control group had a 27 percent higher loss of physical function than those in the exercise group. Hemoglobin and hematocrit levels were similar for both groups at the beginning and end of the study, but the training group had a shorter duration of neutropenia and thrombocytopenia. In addition, patients in the treatment group reported less severe pain and diarrhea, less need for analgesics and a shorter average hospital stay than those in the control group. During the exercise program no injuries to the patients were reported.

The authors conclude that initiation of an aerobic exercise program immediately after high-dose chemotherapy is safe and may prevent severe loss of physical performance. Exercise may also decrease some of the toxic side effects associated with chemotherapy.

Source: Dimeo F. et al. Effects of aerobic exercise on the physical performance and incidence of treatment-related complications after high-dose chemotherapy. *Blood* 1997 November 1;90:3390-4.

Section 24.3

Exercise Reduces Risk of Breast Cancer

Vigorous and even moderate exercise may affect the menstrual cycle, perhaps by suppressing gonadotropin-releasing hormone and lowering a woman's cumulative exposure to estrogen and progesterone. Energy balance and caloric restriction might also inhibit carcinogenesis. Thune and colleagues[1] conducted a survey to investigate the relationship between everyday exercise and the risk of breast cancer in women. Norwegian women from 35 to 49 years of age and a random sample of 10 percent of women from 20 to 34 years of age in three counties were invited to participate in the study. A total of 25,624 women were surveyed from 1974 to 1978 and from 1977 to 1983. All of these women were asked to complete a questionnaire and bring it with them when they attended a screening clinical examination.

Participants were also asked to complete a food frequency questionnaire that was used to calculate energy and fat intake. The women were asked to self-report their physical activity during leisure and work hours using a scale of 1 to 4. A grade of 1 was assigned to those whose leisure time was spent reading, watching television or in other sedentary activities and to those whose work was described as sedentary. A grade of 2 was given to women who spent at least four hours per week walking, bicycling or engaging in other types of physical activity or had jobs that involved a great deal of walking. A grade of 3 was given to women who spent at least four hours a week exercising to keep fit and participating in recreational activities, and whose jobs involved both walking and lifting. A grade of 4 was given to women who engaged in regular, vigorous training or participated in competitive sports several times a week or whose jobs required heavy manual labor. Women were followed for a mean of 14 years. Women who developed cancer or who died within the first year of the study were excluded from the analyses.

Breast cancer was diagnosed in 351 women. Two thirds of women reported participating in moderate activity during leisure time. Fifteen percent exercised regularly. Only 14 percent reported being sedentary at work. Energy intake was positively correlated with physical activity. The association was more pronounced with work activity than with leisure time activity. After adjustment for the factors of age, body mass index, height, parity and county, greater activity during leisure time was associated with a reduced risk of breast cancer. In women who exercised regularly, the risk reduction was greater in premenopausal women and in women younger than 45 years of age. Women who exercised at least four hours a week during their leisure time had a 37 percent reduction in the risk of breast cancer. The risk of breast cancer was lowest in lean women (body mass index less than 22.8) who exercised at least four hours per week. Risk was also reduced in women with higher levels of activity at work, again with a more pronounced effect among premenopausal than postmenopausal women. The authors conclude that physical activity during both leisure time and work reduced the overall risk of breast cancer in women, particularly among premenopausal and younger postmenopausal women.

1.   Thune I, et al. Physical activity and the risk of breast cancer. *N Engl J Med* 1997; 336:1269-75.

—by Kathryn M. Andolsek

Chapter 25

Aerobic Exercise and Chronic Fatigue Syndrome

Exercise may cause a disproportionate degree of fatigue in patients with chronic fatigue syndrome. Testing usually demonstrates normal muscle function, but physical deconditioning may play a role in the etiology of this exaggerated fatigability since patients with chronic fatigue syndrome frequently reduce their level of exercise. Graded aerobic exercise has been demonstrated to improve function and reduce symptoms in patients with conditions similar to chronic fatigue syndrome (such as the postpoliomyelitis syndrome). Fulcher and White (Fulcher KY, White PD. Randomised controlled trial of graded exercise in patients with the chronic fatigue syndrome. *British Medical Journal* 1997;314:1647-52.) studied the effects of a 12-week graded aerobic exercise program and a 12-week program of flexibility and relaxation therapy in patients attending a chronic fatigue syndrome outpatient clinic in England.

Sixty-six patients met Oxford criteria for chronic fatigue syndrome; 33 patients each were assigned to the exercise group and the flexibility and relaxation therapy group. The mean age of the patients was 37 years, and the average duration of symptoms was 2.7 years. Patients completed a general health questionnaire, visual analog scales that measured physical, mental and total fatigue, and a treadmill walking test. The maximal voluntary contraction of the quadriceps muscle of the dominant leg was also assessed in each patient. Baseline measurements of function were identical between the two groups.

The two programs each involved a weekly class for 12 weeks, plus exercises at home on at least five days per week. For those in the aerobic exercise group, the daily exercise program was an individualized exercise prescription designed to help the patient reach 40 percent of peak oxygen consumption (approximately 50 percent of the maximum heart rate) for up to 30 minutes. Patients used ambulatory heart rate monitors to evaluate heart rate. Patients in the flexion and relaxation group learned and practiced the techniques in the weekly class and were asked to perform these exercises at home once a day for five days each week for up to 30 minutes each session. All of the patients kept activity and symptom diaries. After patients completed the flexibility program, they were invited to join the aerobic exercise program. Twenty-two of these patients subsequently began participating in the aerobic exercise program.

Patients were reassessed after 12 weeks, including a structured clinical interview with a psychiatrist who was blinded as to the treatment intervention. The principal outcomes of interest were the patients' self-assessments of well-being and function. The patients' self-perceptions were assessed by a mailed questionnaire again after three months and one year after the study ended.

Sixteen of the 29 patients who initially joined and completed the exercise program rated themselves as either "much" or "very much" improved, compared with only eight of the 30 patients completing the flexibility and relaxation program. Two patients (one from each group) stopped treatment because they felt worse. Significant differences in functional improvement were noted between the groups in terms of median peak oxygen consumption, increased isometric strength and perceived submaximal exertion score. Patients' self-assessments of fatigue, functional capacity and fitness were significantly better after the exercise program than after the flexibility program. Physiologic improvements were maintained or exceeded the 12-week level at the three-month follow-up in the 47 patients assessed.

One year after the program, 35 (74 percent) of the 47 patients who participated in the exercise program still rated themselves as improved. Thirty-two (68 percent) had continued to exercise regularly and 31(66 percent) had returned to work or school. Information at one-year follow-up was available for seven patients who only participated in flexibility and relaxation therapy. The remaining patients had discontinued therapy, switched to the exercise program or were lost to follow-up. Two of the seven patients who were contacted reported feeling better.

The authors conclude that a graded exercise program is more effective than a flexibility and relaxation program in enabling patients with chronic fatigue syndrome to achieve improvement in well-being and functional capacity. Very few patients discontinued the exercise program, and most patients continued with the exercise after the completion of the 12-week class.

—by Anne D. Walling

Chapter 26

Chronically Ill Patients and Exercise

Exercise has the potential to benefit virtually all who can participate. Often overlooked, however, are patients with serious chronic conditions. For them, standard exercise programs may be exhausting, painful or literally impossible due to their physical disabilities. Moreover, such patients often have little or no interest in exercising, with many avoiding even mild physical activity such as strolling. Yet these patients comprise a large group that encompasses a wide range of ages and medical conditions (Table 26.1).[1-44] The physician can use an individualized exercise prescription to help chronically ill patients begin and maintain a low-intensity program that minimizes the risk and maximizes the benefits of this adjuvant therapy (Table 26.2).

Chronically ill patients need to learn about the long-term medical benefits they can expect from exercising, such as reduced blood pressure, improved lipid levels, reduced risk of osteoporosis and lower mortality risk. What seems more important to many of them, however, is learning about the functional and psychologic improvements that become apparent almost immediately after they begin to increase their level of physical activity. These include reduced fatigue, improved endurance, increased muscular strength for performing everyday tasks, enhanced sense of well-being and reduced perceived stress.

Chronically ill patients are more receptive to the idea of exercising when the physician shows concern for their special limitations.

It is important to emphasize that each exercise prescription is safe and appropriate for the particular patient's disease state, cardiopulmonary limitations and degree of muscular weakness.

Table 26.1. Medical Conditions with a Key Reference Regarding the Benefits of Regular Exercise for Prevention or Therapy

Acquired immunodeficiency syndrome[1]
Aging: physical frailty[2]
Ankylosing spondylitis[3]
Arthritis (rheumatoid arthritis)[4]
    osteoarthritis[5]
Cancer
    breast[6]
    colon[7]
    prostate[8]
    terminal cancer[9]
Cardiac transplant[10]
Congestive heart failure[11]
Coronary heart disease[12]
Chronic fatigue[13]
Chronic obstructive pulmonary disease[14]
Chronic pain[15]
Diabetes mellitus
    Type I[16]
    Type II[17]
Hemophilia[18]
Hyperlipidemia
Total cholesterol[19]
    High-density lipoprotein[20]
    Low-density lipoprotein

Total triglycerides[23]
    Very low-density lipoprotein triglycerides[23]
Hypertension[24]
Low back pain[25]
Mental health
    anxiety[26]
    depression[27]
Migraine headaches[28]
Multiple sclerosis[29]
Myasthenia gravis[30]
Obesity[31]
Osteoporosis
    premenopausal[32]
    postmenopausal[33]
Parkinson's disease[34]
Peripheral vascular disease[35]
Physical disability[36]
Post-polio syndrome[37]
Premenstrual syndrome[38]
Reduced muscle mass[39]
Renal transplant[40]
Sickle cell anemia[41]
Sleep disorders[42]
Stroke[43]
Urinary incontinence[44]

Table 26.2. Overview of the Exercise Prescription for Minimizing Risk and Maximizing Benefits in Chronically III Patients

Medical benefits
    Increased functional capacity
    Increased strength and endurance
    Improved medical status

Factors increasing the risks of exercise
    Age
    Unstable heart disease
    Intensity of effort

Components of training
    Frequency: regular
    Intensity: low
    Duration: accumulation of 30 minutes per day
    Mode: walking or equivalent activity
    Progression: very gradual

Injury prevention
    Adequate warm-up period
    Adequate cool-down period
    Low-intensity activity
    Adequate hydration
    Proper olothing and chooc

Compliance
    Reasonable goals
    Regular reassessment
    Definition of exercise benefits
    Low-impact activities
    Discussing the benefits of exercise

Emphasizing the Safety of Exercise

Patients need to be reassured that they can exercise safely. Thus, the physician should provide a written summary of general guidelines emphasizing a conservative approach to exercise (Table 26.3).

Table 26.3. General Guidelines for the Exercise Prescription for Chronically Ill Patients

Exercise daily if not fatigued

Start with a warm-up period lasting at least three minutes.

Exercise at a target heart rate of no more than 20 beats over the resting heart rate, or at normal walking pace.

Accumulate 20 to 30 minutes of exercise per day in one or several sessions.

Perform aerobic exercise (e.g., walking), as well as resistance and stretching exercises when prescribed.

Finish with a cool-down period lasting at least three minutes.

NOTE: Report any unusual symptom to the doctor.

It is widely assumed that only young, asymptomatic patients should begin an exercise program without first undergoing exercise stress testing. The main purpose of such testing is to identify underlying cardiovascular conditions that could be exacerbated by exercise.[45] However, exercise stress testing is often impractical and is probably not cost-effective for chronically ill patients. These patients are rarely fit enough to endure the exercise stress that is required to produce an adequate rate-pressure product. Moreover, the intensity of effort prescribed for them at the outset of exercise therapy is very low—usually at, or just above, their normal walking speed.

If a patient's medical history is known and pre-exercise screening shows a medically stable condition with no major contraindications to exercise, stress testing prior to the initiation of exercise therapy is probably unnecessary.[45] However, the patient should be advised to watch for signs of cardiovascular problems and to report them to the physician immediately. After a chronically ill patient has exercised for several months and wishes to increase the intensity of effort, it may be appropriate to consider an exercise stress test.[45]

Because chronically ill patients begin exercise at very low intensity levels, they have a low risk of musculoskeletal injuries. The risk of injury can be further minimized by informing patients about the principles of injury prevention (e.g., proper biomechanics of ambulation) and the need for cushioned, supportive footwear.

Patients should be reminded to maintain adequate hydration. They may also need to be reminded to use standard environmental protections, such as sunscreen lotions, light-colored clothing in hot weather and layered clothing in inclement weather.

Motivation, Adherence, and Compliance

Lack of time is one reason that patients often give for not starting or staying with an exercise program. Other reasons include the following: lack of an exercise partner; dislike of the physical activity; physical limitations due to arthritis or other medical conditions; lack of muscle coordination; obesity; fear of ridicule, injury, accident or criminal threat; inclement weather; laziness; lack of exercise facilities; lack of equipment; feeling fatigued and feeling "too old."

The patient's initial objections to exercise need to be identified and addressed. Measures to improve compliance with an exercise prescription are listed in Table 26.4.

Table 26.4. Guidelines to Improve Compliance with Exercise Therapy

Create reasonable short-term and long-term goals.

Establish a firm initial commitment (e.g., a written contract).

Use reinforcing and cognitive strategies (e.g., have the patient make "appointments" to exercise at specific times and on specific days).

Begin the patient's program with a very low level of intensity.

Periodically review both the general benefits of exercise and the patient's progress toward achieving specific goals.

Exercise Elements and Variables

An ideal exercise prescription includes four elements: aerobic exercise, musculoskeletal strength training, flexibility training, and warm-up and cool-down procedures. Exercise variables include type, frequency, intensity and time. These exercise elements and variables should be discussed with the patient.

Aerobic Exercise

Aerobic exercise is central to most exercise prescriptions, because it has the greatest impact on health.[45] Aerobic activity is any isotonic movement of large muscle groups that is sustained long enough to qualify as endurance or cardiovascular activity. Examples are walking and cycling.

Musculoskeletal Strength Training

Musculoskeletal strength training has both isotonic and isometric components. This type of training can be done using weight-training machines or, more appropriately to many patients, improvised devices such as unopened soup cans or plastic jugs filled with sand or water. The minimum should be eight to 10 different exercises that build strength in major muscle groups. Each exercise should be performed in a set of eight to 12 repetitions using a heavy enough weight to result in voluntary fatigue.

Flexibility Training

Flexibility training includes both range-of-motion and stretching exercises.

Warm-Up and Cool-Down Procedures

The beginning and ending stages of exercise are very important. By starting a physical activity very slowly (warming up), patients minimize their sense of fatigue and their risk for cardiovascular complications. By ending exercise slowly (cooling down), they allow their heart rate to return safely to a resting rate. The warm-up and cool-down periods each should last at least three minutes.

Type of Exercise

The type of exercise depends on the facilities and equipment that are available, as well as the patient's preferences and limitations. Walking is excellent for most chronically ill patients. This activity is easy, inexpensive, largely self-explanatory and enjoyable.

Frequency of Exercise

To maximize progress and compliance, the frequency of exercise should be a minimum of three times per week, but preferably daily. Daily sessions result in higher long-term compliance, because they accelerate progress (reinforcing the value of the activity) and because exercise eventually becomes habitual.

Intensity of Exercise

Intensity is the exercise variable that is dramatically reduced to fit the needs of the chronically ill patient. In walking, for example, the competitive race walker covers a mile in less than seven minutes, and the accomplished fitness walker goes the same distance in 12 to 15 minutes. However, at the start of the exercise program, the chronically ill patient may require 30 minutes or more to walk one-half mile.

Duration of Exercise

Because intensity is reduced for the chronically ill patient, particularly at the start of the exercise prescription, exercise duration, or time, must be prolonged to achieve significant health improvement. Typically, 20 to 30 minutes of exercise per day is the minimum exercise time prescribed for patients with chronic illnesses. This time may be covered in one session or accumulated in several shorter periods throughout the day.

Levels of Training

The three levels of aerobic exercise training are as follows: adjuvant health training, which is used to assist medical treatment; health training, which is a means to improve health risk factors, and fitness training, which is a means to achieve fitness goals. The so-called FIT factors (frequency, intensity and time) for each of these training levels are given in Table 26.5.

Chronically ill patients may begin their exercise program at the adjuvant health training level with a prescription for mild aerobic exercise therapy. Then they may progress to the health training level to achieve greater therapeutic results. Ultimately, a few chronically ill patients may request a move to the fitness training level in order to achieve still more benefits.

Level 1

Adjuvant health training begins with a very low intensity of effort. In chronically ill patients, a safe exercise target heart rate can be 20 beats over the resting pulse. Since this rate is usually reached with the normal walking speed of these patients, it can be achieved almost immediately without concern about heart rate monitoring.

The frequency of exercise can be daily, because the intensity of effort is so low. In addition, patients can easily adjust the duration of exercise. For example, at the outset when patients are the weakest, they can divide an exercise session into several shorter sessions, with the goal of working toward accumulating 20 to 30 minutes of activity per day. Despite interruptions, the desired energy expenditure can be achieved using this approach.

Exercise prescriptions vary for individual patients. An example of level 1 aerobic exercise might be walking at a slow pace, perhaps one to two miles per hour.

Table 26.5. Aerobic Exercise Levels.

FIT factors	Level 1: adjuvant health training(*)
Frequency	Five to seven days per week
Intensity	20 beats or more per minute above the resting heart rate
Time	20 to 30 minutes
FIT factors	Level 2: health training(**)
Frequency	Five to seven days per week
Intensity	40 to 70 percent of the maximum heart rate
Time	30 to 60 minutes
FIT factors	Level 3: fitness training(***)
Frequency	Three or four days per week
Intensity	85 percent of the maximum heart rate
Time	30 to 60 minutes

(*)—Chronically ill patients start at level 1 training.
(**)—Some chronically ill patients progress to level 2 training.
(***)—Only a few chronically ill patients progress to level 3 training.
Maximum heart rate is determined through a graded exercise test or is estimated by subtracting the patient's age from 220.

Level 2

Health training represents more vigorous activity than level 1 exercise. Nonetheless, many chronically ill patients are capable of, and benefit from, "graduating" to level 2 exercise. Benefits at this level can be striking, based on the principle that maximum oxygen uptake begins to markedly increase when exercise is undertaken at 60 percent or more of an individual's maximum heart rate.

An example of level 2 exercise is walking at a moderate to brisk pace, perhaps three to four miles per hour.

Level 3

While fitness training is too rigorous for most chronically ill patients, there are notable exceptions. An example of level 3 exercise might be running at a speed of eight minutes per mile.

Assessing Progress

In assessing progress, the physician can also focus on caloric expenditure (Table 26.6). According to the American Heart Association, a person must expend at least 700 calories per week to achieve minimum physical conditioning and health benefits, and as many as 2,000 calories per week to achieve optimum health.[45]

Table 26.6. Calories expended in 30 minutes for three body weights.

Perceived speed	Miles per hour	MET(*)	55 kg (121 lb)	70 kg (154 lb)	80 kg (176 lb)
Slow	1.7	2.3	63	81	92
	2.0	2.5	69	88	100
Moderate	2.5	2.9	80	102	116
	3.0	3.3	91	116	132
Brisk	3.4	3.6	99	126	144
	3.7	3.9	107	137	156

(*)MET = metabolic equivalent (oxygen consumption). The MET is a unit used to estimate the metabolic cost (oxygen consumption) of physical activity. One MET equals the resting metabolic rate of approximately 3.5 mL (O.sub.2) (kg.sup.-1) (min.sup.1).

Initially, chronically ill patients in level 1 exercise therapy may expend only 400 to 700 calories per week. However, as these patients gain in strength and self-confidence, and as they increase their exercise intensity and time, their caloric expenditures should soon reach the weekly minimum of 700 calories.

Intermittent Protocol for Aerobic Exercise

A successful aerobic exercise plan for chronically ill patients is the intermittent protocol (Table 26.7). This approach usually allows weak patients to burn more calories than they could expend in continuous exercise. Typically, patients begin at week 1 with two to five minutes of aerobic exercise, such as walking, followed by one to two minutes of reduced intensity during which they walk more slowly or, if necessary, sit. The short periods of more vigorous activity followed by recovery can be repeated throughout an exercise session, with the goal of accumulating 30 minutes or more of the more vigorous activity.

An exercise prescription can safely progress by increasing the duration of exercise periods by one minute per week. After patients work up to two 15-minute periods of activity at an easy intensity with only a brief rest in between, they can start over at the beginning of the progression, this time at a moderate intensity. Later they can begin the progression again at a brisk pace, which may be their eventual maintenance intensity.

Many types of exercise lend themselves to the intermittent protocol. Examples include walking in shopping malls, where recovery periods can be the time needed to look over one store window, or walking on a track and using a slower pace on curves.

Monitoring the Course of Exercise Therapy

The course of exercise therapy for the chronically ill patient has three phases: an initial conditioning phase, a phase to improve conditioning and a maintenance phase.

The initial conditioning phase usually requires one to three months. During this phase, the focus is on having the patient develop a daily, or at least a regular, exercise habit. For patients who choose walking as their exercise, this may require less effort than normal ambulation to overcome psychologic as well as physical barriers.

Ideally, a staff member from the physician's office should make weekly calls to the patient, especially during the first month of an exercise prescription, to monitor medical status, to check on possible changes in medications and to assist in solving problems that may interfere with compliance. The common complaints of muscle stiffness and soreness can be handled by advising rest or a different activity until symptoms diminish.

After the patient has completed one or two months of aerobic exercise training, a clinical follow-up examination can be helpful. At this time, the physician can assess the patient's progress and determine whether medication levels need to be adjusted, since exercise training can have a pronounced effect on metabolism and cardiorespiratory parameters. For example, patients receiving insulin or antihypertensive medications usually can reduce their dosage after they begin exercising regularly, especially if they are losing weight as well.

If the patient is making satisfactory progress, the exercise prescription can be adjusted to move the intensity level to the next stage (i.e., that of improving conditioning). At the same time, new elements can be added to the aerobic-centered prescription. These elements include resistance training with light weights to build muscular strength and flexibility training along with a combination of range-of-motion exercises and static positions to stretch muscle groups.

Ideally, resistance and flexibility training are performed immediately after an aerobic exercise session. At this time, blood flow to the muscles is at an increased level, a condition that generally reduces the risk of muscular injury during resistance and flexibility training.

Resistance training helps the chronically ill patient gain strength and lean tissue mass. Initially, the patient can work with a very light weight in each hand (perhaps an unopened soup can), so that, as much as possible, movements can be performed over a joint's entire range of motion. The resistance program can include standard upper-body resistance exercises, such as arm curls, chest presses and abdominal curls. These exercises can easily be adapted to the patient's ability by slightly increasing resistance levels as strength is gained.

Flexibility exercises should focus on the lower back, hamstring, gastrocnemius and soleus muscles. Increased flexibility in these areas generally improves function considerably. In one type of flexibility exercise, the patient attempts to move joints slowly through their range of motion. The purpose is to reduce limitations progressively. A second type of flexibility exercise is static stretching, which is the prolonged extension of muscles to their maximum length. The purpose of static exercise, which is performed in various stationary positions, is to progressively elongate muscles and related structures. Static stretching helps to prevent muscle injuries, stiffness and soreness.

401

Table 26.7. Intermittent exercise program for severely deconditioned patients.

Week	Warm-up period	Easy, moderate, brisk walk	Recovery period	Number of repeats	Total time	Cool-down period
Week 1	Walk slowly for five minutes	Two to five minutes	One to two minutes	Six to 15 times	25 to 30 minutes	Walk slowly for five minutes
Week 2	Walk slowly for five minutes	Three to six minutes	One to two minutes	Five to 10 times	25 to 30 minutes	Walk slowly for five minutes
Week 3	Walk slowly for five minutes	Four to seven minutes	One to two minutes	Four to eight times	28 to 32 minutes	Walk slowly for five minutes
Week 4	Walk slowly for five minutes	Five to eight minutes	One to two minutes	Four to six times	30 to 32 minutes	Walk slowly for five minutes
Week 5	Walk slowly for five minutes	Six to nine minutes	One to two minutes	Three to five times	27 to 30 minutes	Walk slowly for five minutes
Week 6	Walk slowly for five minutes	Seven to 10 minutes	One to two minutes	Three to four times	28 to 30 minutes	Walk slowly for five minutes
Week 7	Walk slowly for five minutes	Eight to 11 minutes	One to two minutes	Three to four times	33 to 34 minutes	Walk slowly for five minutes

Week 8	Walk slowly for five minutes	Nine to 10 minutes	One to two minutes	Three to four times	27 to 30 minutes	Walk slowly for five minutes
Week 9	Walk slowly for five minutes	10 to 11 minutes	One to two minutes	Three times	30 to 33 minutes	Walk slowly for five minutes
Week 10	Walk slowly for five minutes	11 to 12 minutes	One to two minutes	Three times	33 to 36 minutes	Walk slowly for five minutes
Week 11	Walk slowly for five minutes	12 to 13 minutes	One to two minutes	Three times	36 to 39 minutes	Walk slowly for five minutes
Week 12	Walk slowly for five minutes	13 to 14 minutes	One to two minutes	Two to three times	30 to 39 minutes	Walk slowly for five minutes
Week 13	Walk slowly for five minutes	14 to 15 minutes	One to two minutes	Two times	28 to 30 minutes	Walk slowly for five minutes
Week 14	Walk slowly for five minutes	15 minutes	One to two minutes	Two times	30 minutes	Walk slowly for five minutes
Week 15	Walk slowly for five minutes	Maintain or start over at a faster pace				

Additional follow-up examinations can be performed every three or four months. At these visits, the physician can discuss how and whether the exercise prescription needs to be revised so that progress continues or a maintenance phase is established.

Final Comment

Physicians and other health care professionals have a unique opportunity to encourage chronically ill patients to exercise. Once patients understand the benefits of exercise and the obstacles to compliance have been identified and cleared, the best approach is to provide an individualized exercise prescription. Most importantly, the exercise prescription should be tailored to the needs and capabilities of the patient, so that the regimen is easy and safe to follow. The end result can be a significant improvement in health.

The author thanks William Laitner and Barbara N. Campaigne, Ph.D., for their helpful critique and editorial comments, and Linda Beguhn for her assistance in the preparation of the manuscript.

References

1. MacArthur RD, Levine SD, Birk TJ. Supervised exercise training improves cardiopulmonary fitness in HIV-infected persons. *Med Sci Sports Exerc* 1993;25:684-8.

2. Fiatarone MA, O'Neill EF, Ryan ND, Clements KM, Solares GR, Nelson ME, et al. Exercise training and nutritional supplementation for physical frailty in very elderly people. *N Engl J Med* 1994;330:1769-75.

3. Bakker C, Hidding A, van der Linden S, van Doorslaer E. Cost effectiveness of group physical therapy compared to individualized therapy for ankylosing spondylitis. A randomized controlled trial. *J Rheumatol* 1994;21:264-8.

4. Harkcom TM, Lampman RM, Banwell BF, Castor CW. Therapeutic value of graded aerobic exercise training in rheumatoid arthritis. *Arthritis Rheum* 1985;28:32-9.

5. Fisher NM, Pendergast DR. Effects of a muscle exercise program on exercise capacity in subjects with osteoarthritis. *Arch Phys Med Rehabil* 1994; 75:792-7.

6. Bernstein L, Henderson BE, Hanisch R, Sullivan-Halley J, Ross RK. Physical exercise and reduced risk of breast cancer in young women. *J Natl Cancer Inst* 1994;86:1403-8.

7. Longnecker MP, Gerhardsson le Verdier M, Frumkin H, Carpenter C. A case-control study of physical activity in relation to risk of cancer of the right colon and rectum in men. *Int J Epidemiol* 1995;24:42-50.

8. Lee IM, Paffenbarger RS Jr, Hsieh CC. Physical activity and risk of prostatic cancer among college alumni. *Am J Epidemiol* 1992;135:169-79.

9. Yoshioka H. Rehabilitation for the terminal cancer patient. *Am J Phys Med Rehabil* 1994;73:199-206.

10. Kavanagh T, Yacoub MH, Mertens DJ, Kennedy J, Campbell RB, Sawyer P. Cardiorespiratory responses to exercise training after orthotopic cardiac transplantation. *Circulation* 1988;77:162-71.

11. Kostis JB, Rosen RC, Cosgrove NM, Shindler DM, Wilson AC. Nonpharmacologic therapy improves functional and emotional status in congestive heart failure. *Chest* 1994;106:996-1001.

12. Lavie CJ, Milani RV. Effects of cardiac rehabilitation programs on exercise capacity, coronary risk factors, behavioral characteristics, and quality of life in a large elderly cohort. *Am J Cardiol* 1995;76:177-9.

13. McCully KK, Sisto SA, Natelson BH. Use of exercise for treatment of chronic fatigue syndrome. *Sports Med* 1996;21:35-48.

14. Strijbos JH, Postma DS, van Altena R, Gimeno F, Koeter GH. A comparison between an outpatient hospital-based pulmonary rehabilitation program and a home-care pulmonary rehabilitation program in patients with COPD. A follow-up of 18 months. *Chest* 1996;109:366-72.

15. Davis VP, Fillingim RB, Doleys DM, Davis MP. Assessment of aerobic power in chronic pain patients before and after a multi-disciplinary treatment program. *Arch Phys Med Rehabil* 1992; 73:726-9.

16. Campaigne BN, Gilliam TB, Spencer ML, Lampman RM, Schork MA. Effects of a physical activity program on metabolic control and cardiovascular fitness in children with insulin-dependent diabetes mellitus. *Diabetes Care* 1984;7:57-62.

17. Lehmann R, Vokac A, Niedermann K, Agosti K, Spinas GA. Loss of abdominal fat and improvement of the cardiovascular risk profile by regular moderate exercise training in patients with NIDDM. *Diabetologia* 1995;38:1313-9.

18. Greene WB, Strickler EM. A modified isokinetic strengthening program for patients with severe hemophilia. *Dev Med Child Neurol* 1983;25:189-96.

19. Sopko G, Jacobs DR Jr, Jeffery R, Mittelmark M, Lenz K, Hedding E, et al. Effects on blood lipids and body weight in high risk men of a practical exercise program. *Atherosclerosis* 1983;49:219-29.

20. Lavie CJ, Milani RV. Effects of cardiac rehabilitation and exercise training in obese patients with coronary artery disease. *Chest* 1996;109:52-6.

21. Lavie CJ, Milani RV. Effects of cardiac rehabilitation and exercise training on low-density lipoprotein cholesterol in patients with hypertriglyceridemia and coronary artery disease. *Am J Cardiol* 1994; 74:1192-5.

22. Lampman RM, Schteingart DE. Effects of exercise training on glucose control, lipid metabolism, and insulin sensitivity in hypertriglyceridemia and non-insulin dependent diabetes mellitus. *Med Sci Sports Exerc* 1991;23:703-12.

23. Kiens B, Lithell H. Lipoprotein metabolism influenced by training-induced changes in human skeletal muscle. *J Clin Invest* 1989;83:558-64.

24. Martin JE, Dubbert PM, Cushman WC. Controlled trial of aerobic exercise in hypertension. *Circulation* 1990;81:1560-7.

25. Johannsen F, Remvig L, Kryger P, Beck P, Warming S, Lybeck K, et al. Exercises for chronic low back pain: a clinical trial. *J Orthop Sports Phys Ther* 1995;22:52-9.

26. King AC, Taylor CB, Haskell WL. Effects of differing intensities and formats of 12 months of exercise training on psychological outcomes in older adults. *Health Psychol* 1993;12:292-300 [Published erratum appears in *Health Psychol* 1993,12:405].

27. North TC, McCullagh P, Tran ZV. Effect of exercise on depression. *Exerc Sport Sci Rev* 1990;18:379-415.

28. Darling M. The use of exercise as a method of aboffing migraine. *Headache* 1991;31:616-8.

29. Petajan JH, Gappmaier E, White AT, Spencer MK, Mino L, Hicks RW. Impact of aerobic training on fitness and quality of life in multiple sclerosis. *Ann Neurol* 1996;39:432-41.

30. Lohi EL, Lindberg C, Andersen O. Physical training effects in myasthenia gravis. *Arch Phys Med Rehabil* 1993;74:1178-80.

31. Lampman RM, Schteingart DE, Foss ML. Exercise as a partial therapy for the extremely obese. *Med Sci Sports Exerc* 1986;18:19-24.

32. Dilsen G, Berker C, Oral A, Varan G. The role of physical exercise in prevention and management of osteoporosis. *Clin Rheumatol* 1989;8(Suppl 2):70-5.

33. Prince RL, Smith M, Dick IM, Price RI, Webb PG, Henderson NK, et al. Prevention of postmenopausal osteoporosis. A comparative study of exercise, calcium supplementation, and hormone-replacement therapy. *N Engl J Med* 1991;325:1189-95.

34. Kuroda K, Tatara K, Takatorige T, Shinsho E Effect of physical exercise on mortality in patients with Parkinson's disease. *Acta Neurol Scand* 1992;86:55-9.

35. Regensteiner JG, Steiner JF, Hiatt WR Exercise training improves functional status in patients with peripheral arterial disease. *J Vasc Surg* 1996;23:104-15.

36. Davidoff GN, Lampman RM, Westbury L, Deron J, Finestone HM, Islam S. Exercise testing and training of persons with dysvascular amputation: safety and efficacy of arm ergometry. *Arch Phys Med Rehabil* 1992;73:334-8.

37. Agre JC. The role of exercise in the patient with post-polio syndrome. *Ann N Y Acad Sci* 1995;753: 321-34.

38. Prior JC, Vigna Y, Alojada N. Conditioning exercise decreases premenstrual symptoms. A prospective controlled three month trial. *Eur J Appl Physiol* 1986;55:349-55.

39. Evans WJ. Reversing sarcopenia: how weight training can build strength and vitality. *Geriatrics* 1996;51(5):46-7,51-3.

40. Miller TD, Squires RW, Gau GT, Ilstrup DM, Frohnert PP, Sterioff S. Graded exercise testing and training after renal

transplantation: a preliminary study. *Mayo Clin Proc* 1987;62:773-7.

41.　Alcorn R, Bowser B, Henley EJ, Holloway V. Fluidotherapy and exercise in the management of sickle cell anemia. A clinical report. *Phys Ther* 1984;64:1520-2.

42.　Edinger JD, Morey MC, Sullivan RJ, Higginbotham MB, Marsh GR, Dailey DS, et al. Aerobic fitness, acute exercise and sleep in older men. *Sleep* 1993;16:351-9.

43.　Hesse S, Bertelt C, Schaffrin A, Malezic M, Mauritz KH. Restoration of gait in nonambulatory hemiparetic pahents by treadmill training with partial body-weight support. *Arch Phys Med Rehabil* 1994;75:1087-93.

44.　Wells TJ, Brink CA, Diokno AC, Wolfe R, Gillis GL. Pelvic muscle exercise for stress urinary incontinence in elderly women. *J Am Geriatr Soc* 1991;39:785-91.

45.　Fletcher GF, Balady G, Froelicher VF, Hartley LH, Haskell WL, Pollock ML. Exercise standards. A statement for healthcare professionals from the American Heart Association. *Circulation* 1995,91:580-615.

— by Richard M. Lampman, Ph.D.

Richard M. Lampman, Ph.D. is director of research for the Department of Surgery at St. Joseph Mercy Hospital, Ann Arbor, Mich., and adjunct associate professor in the Department of Physical Medicine and Rehabilitation at the University of Michigan Medical School, also in Ann Arbor. Dr. Lampman earned his doctoral degree from the University of Michigan. Previously he served as research scientist and director of cardiac rehabilitation in the Division of Cardiology at the University of Michigan Medical Center.

Chapter 27

Taking Care of Your Diabetes Every Day

The four things you have to do every day to lower high blood sugar are:

1. Eat healthy food
2. Get regular exercise
3. Take your diabetes medicine
4. Test your blood sugar.

Experts say most people with diabetes should try to keep their blood sugar level as close as possible to the level of someone who does not have diabetes. This may not be possible or right for everyone. Check with your doctor about the right range of blood sugar for you.

You will get plenty of help in learning how to do this from your health care providers. Your main health care providers are your doctor, nurse, and dietitian. (A dietitian is someone who is specially trained to help people plan their meals.)

The next sections of this document will tell you more about the four main ways you take care of your diabetes: Eat healthy food, get regular exercise, take your diabetes medicine, and test your blood sugar.

Bring a family member or friend with you when you see your doctor. Ask lots of questions. Before you leave, be sure you understand everything you need to know about taking care of your diabetes.

National Institute of Diabetes and Digestive and Kidney Diseases (NIDDK), National Diabetes Information Clearinghouse, available at http://www.niddk.nih.gov/health/diabetes/dylb/chap2.htm.

Eat Healthy Food

People with diabetes do not need special foods. The foods on your diabetes eating plan are the same foods that are good for everyone in your family! Try to eat foods that are low in fat, salt, and sugar and high in fiber, such as beans, fruits and vegetables, and grains. Eating right will help you:

1. Reach and stay at a weight that is good for your body.
2. Keep your blood sugar in a good range.
3. Prevent heart and blood vessel disease.

Your daily eating plan should include foods from these groups:

- Milk and milk products, such as yogurt.
- Meat, chicken or other poultry, fish, beans, cheese, and eggs.
- Fruits and vegetables.
- Bread, cereal, rice, noodles, and potatoes.

People with diabetes should have their own eating plans. Ask your doctor to give you the name of a dietitian who can work with you to develop an eating plan for you and your family. Your dietitian can help you plan meals to include foods that you and your family like to eat and that are good for you.

Action Steps

If you USE insulin:

- Give yourself an insulin shot before you eat.
- Eat at about the same time and the same amount of food every day.
- Don't skip meals, especially if you have already given yourself an insulin shot because your blood sugar may go too low.

If you DON'T USE insulin

- Follow your meal plan.
- Don't skip meals, especially if you take diabetes pills because your blood sugar may go too low. Skipping a meal can make you eat too much at the next meal. It may be better to eat several small meals during the day instead of one or two big meals.

Get Regular Exercise

Exercise is good for your diabetes. Walking, swimming, dancing, riding a bicycle, playing baseball, and bowling are all good ways to exercise. You can even get exercise when you clean house or work in your garden. Exercise is especially good for people with diabetes because:

1. Exercise helps keep weight down.
2. Exercise helps insulin work better to lower blood sugar.
3. Exercise is good for your heart and lungs.
4. Exercise gives you more energy.

Before you begin exercising, talk with your doctor. Your doctor may check your heart and your feet to be sure you have no special problems. If you have high blood pressure or eye problems, some exercises like weight-lifting may not be safe. Your doctor or nurse will help you find safe exercises.

Try to exercise regularly. Exercise at least three times a week for about 30 to 45 minutes each time. If you have not exercised in a while, begin slowly. Start with 5 to 10 minutes, and then work up to more time.

If you haven't eaten for over an hour or if your blood sugar is less than 100-120, eat or drink something like an apple or a glass of milk before you exercise.

When you exercise, carry a snack with you in case of low blood sugar. Wear or carry an identification tag or card saying that you have diabetes.

Regular exercise such as walking and bicycling can help keep your blood sugar in a good range.

Action Steps

If you USE insulin

- Exercise after eating, not before.
- Test your blood sugar before, during, and after exercising. Don't exercise when your blood sugar is over 240.
- Don't exercise right before you go to sleep, because it could cause low blood sugar during the night.

If you DON'T USE insulin

- See your doctor before starting an exercise program.

- Test your blood sugar before and after exercising if you take diabetes pills.

Take Your Diabetes Medicine Every Day

Insulin and diabetes pills are the two kinds of medicines used to lower blood sugar.

If You Use Insulin

You need insulin if your body has stopped making insulin or if it doesn't make enough insulin. Everyone with insulin-dependent diabetes needs insulin, and many people with noninsulin-dependent diabetes need insulin.

Insulin cannot be taken as a pill. You will have to give yourself shots every day. Some people give themselves one shot a day. Some people give themselves two or more shots a day. You need to take your insulin every day. Never skip a shot, even if you are sick.

Insulin is injected with a needle. Your doctor will tell you what kind of insulin to use, how much, and when to give yourself a shot. Talk to your doctor before changing the type or amount of insulin you use or when you give your shots. Your doctor or the diabetes educator will show you how to draw up insulin in the needle. They will also show you the best places on your body to give yourself a shot. Ask someone to help you with your shots if your hands are shaky or you can't see well.

Good places on your body to give shots are:

- The outside part of your upper arms.
- Around your waist and hips.
- The outside part of your upper legs.
- Avoid areas with scars and stretch marks.
- Ask your doctor or nurse to check your skin where you give your shots.

You may be a little afraid at first to give yourself a shot. But most people find that the shots hurt less than they expected. The needles are small and sharp and do not go deep into your skin. Always use your own needles and never share them with anyone else. Your doctor or diabetes educator will tell you how to throw away used needles safely.

Keep extra insulin in your refrigerator in case you break the bottle you are using. Do not keep insulin in the freezer or in hot places like the glove compartment of your car. Also, keep it away from bright light. Too much heat, cold, and bright light can damage insulin.

If You Take Diabetes Pills

If your body makes insulin, but the insulin doesn't lower your blood sugar, you may have to take diabetes pills. Diabetes pills only work in people who have some insulin of their own. Some pills are taken once a day, some are taken more often. Ask your doctor when you should take your pills.

Diabetes pills are safe and easy to take. Be sure to tell your doctor if your diabetes pills make you feel bad or if you have any other problems. Remember, diabetes pills do not lower blood sugar all by themselves. You will still have to follow an eating plan and exercise to help lower your blood sugar.

Sometimes, people who take diabetes pills may need insulin shots for a while. This may happen if you get very sick, need to go to a hospital, or become pregnant. You may need insulin shots if the diabetes pills no longer work to lower your blood sugar.

You may be able to stop taking diabetes pills if you lose weight. Losing even a little bit of weight can sometimes help to lower your blood sugar.

If You Don't Use Insulin or Take Diabetes Pills

Many people with noninsulin-dependent diabetes don't have to use insulin or take diabetes pills. However, everyone with diabetes needs to follow his or her doctor's advice about eating and getting enough exercise.

Ask your doctor when you should take your pills or insulin. Tell your other doctors that you take insulin or diabetes pills.

Test Your Blood Sugar Every Day

You need to know how well you are taking care of your diabetes. You need to know if you are lowering your high blood sugar. The best way to find out is to test your blood to see how much sugar is in it. If your blood has too much or too little sugar in it, your doctor may need to change your eating, exercise, or medicine plan.

Some people test their blood once a day. Others test their blood three or four times a day. Your doctor may want you to test before eating, before bed, and sometimes in the middle of the night. Ask your doctor how often and when you should test your blood sugar.

413

How to Test Your Blood Sugar

To test your blood, you need a small needle called a lancet. You also need special blood testing strips that come in a bottle. Your doctor or diabetes educator will show you how to test your blood. Here are the basic steps to follow:

1. Prick your finger with the lancet to get a drop of blood.

2. Place the blood on the end of the strip.

3. After a minute or so, the strip changes color. Match the color of the strip to a color chart on the bottle or box that the strips came in. This will give you a round number for your blood sugar, like 80 or 140. To get a more exact figure, you may want to use a blood sugar testing machine called a meter. If you use a meter, follow the first two steps listed above. Then:

4. Put the strip into the meter. The meter will give you an exact number for your blood sugar.

Pricking your finger with a lancet may hurt a little. It's like sticking your finger with a pin. Use the lancet only once and be careful when you throw away used lancets. Ask your doctor or nurse how to throw them away safely.

You can buy lancets, strips, and meters at a drug store. Some of these items are costly, especially the blood testing strips. Lancets do not cost very much, and meters are often on sale. There are many different kinds of meters available in drug stores. If you decide to buy one, ask your doctor or diabetes educator for advice on what kind to buy. Take your blood testing items with you when you see your doctor or nurse so that you can learn how to use them correctly.

Other Tests for Your Diabetes

Urine Tests

You may need to test your urine ketones when you are sick or if your blood sugar is over 240 before eating a meal. A urine test will tell you if you have "ketones" in your urine. Your body makes ketones when there is not enough insulin in your blood. Ketones can make you very sick. Call your doctor right away if you find ketones when you do a urine test. You may have a sickness called "ketoacidosis."

Ketoacidosis is serious. If not treated, it can cause death. Signs of ketoacidosis are vomiting, weakness, fast breathing, and a sweet smell on the breath. Ketoacidosis is more likely to develop in people with insulin-dependent diabetes.

You can buy strips for testing urine ketones at a drug store. Your doctor or diabetes educator will show you how to use them.

The Hemoglobin Alc Test

Another test for blood sugar, the hemoglobin A1c test, shows what your average blood sugar was for the past 3 months. It shows how much sugar is sticking to your red blood cells. The doctor does this test to see what level your blood sugar is most of the time.

See your doctor for a hemoglobin A1c test every 3 months. To do the test, the doctor or nurse takes a sample of your blood. The blood is tested in a laboratory. The laboratory sends the results to your doctor.

If most of the blood sugar tests you do yourself show that your blood sugar is around 150, the hemoglobin A1c test should be almost normal. If most of your tests show high levels of blood sugar, then the hemoglobin Alc test is usually high. Ask your doctor what your hemoglobin A1c test showed.

Keep Daily Records

Write down the results of your blood tests every day in a record book. You can use a small notebook or ask your doctor for a blood testing record book. You may also want to write down what you eat, how you feel, and how much you have exercised.

By keeping daily records of your blood and urine tests, you can tell how well you are taking care of your diabetes. Show your book to your doctor. The doctor can use your records to see if you need to make changes in your insulin shots or diabetes pills, or in your eating plan. Ask your doctor or nurse if you don't know what your test results mean.

Things to write down every day in your notebook are:

- if you had very low blood sugar

- if you ate more or less food than you usually do

- if you felt sick or very tired

- what kind of exercise you did and for how long

Action Steps

If you USE insulin, keep a daily record of:

- When you gave yourself an insulin shot.
- How much and what kind of insulin you gave in each shot.
- If you tested your urine and found ketones.

Stay Informed

These groups have more information about diabetes and exercise.

Diabetes educators. To find a diabetes educator near you, call or write:

American Association of Diabetes Educators
100 West Monroe Street, Suite 400
Chicago, IL 60603-1901
(800) 338-3633 or (312) 424-2426
Home Page: www.aadenet.org

Dietitians. To find a dietitian near you who can help you plan your meals, call or write:

The American Dietetic Association
216 West Jackson Boulevard
Chicago, IL 60606-6995
Nutrition Information Line: (800) 366-1655; Telephone: (312) 899-0040
Home Page: www.eatright.org

Programs about diabetes. To find programs about diabetes or to talk to other people who have diabetes, call or write:

American Diabetes Association
1701 North Beauregard Street
Alexandria, VA 22311
Telephone: (800) 232-3472 or (703) 549-1500
Home Page: www.diabetes.org

Juvenile Diabetes Foundation International
120 Wall Street, 19th Floor
New York, NY 10005
Telephone: (800) 533-CURE or (212) 785-9500
Home Page: www.jdfcure.org

Both of these organizations have magazines and other information for people with diabetes. The American Diabetes Association has a magazine called *Diabetes Forecast*. The Juvenile Diabetes Foundation International has a magazine called *Countdown*.

Both organizations also have local groups in many places where you can meet other people who have diabetes. Look in your telephone book to see if a local group is listed in your area.

Other Places to Get Help

Other special services for people with diabetes are:

Diabetes Exercise and Sports
1647 West Bethany Home Road #B
Phoenix, AZ 85015
Toll Free: (800) 898-IDAA
Telephone: (602) 433-2113
Home Page: www.diabetes-exercise.org

The Diabetic Traveler
P.O. Box 8223 RW
Stamford, CT 06905
Telephone: (203) 327-5832

Both of these organizations have newsletters and other information for people with diabetes who like to take part in sports and outdoor activities, or like to travel.

Other magazines and newsletters for people with diabetes are:

Diabetes Self-Management, published by:
R.A. Rapaport Publishing Company
P.O. Box 52889
Boulder, CO 80321
Telephone: 1-800-234-0923

Diabetes Interview, published by:
Diabetes Interview
3715 Balboa Street
San Francisco, CA 94121
Telephone: 1-800-473-4636

The National Diabetes Information Clearinghouse has more information about diabetes and places to get help with your diabetes. Call or write the clearinghouse at:

National Diabetes Information Clearinghouse
1 Information Way
Bethesda, MD 20892-3560
(301) 654-3327

Chapter 28

Lifestyle and Therapeutic Methods for Treating and Managing Fibromyalgia

Experts recommend a multi-faceted approach for treating fibromyalgia that involves exercise to reduce pain and strengthen muscles, regular sleep routines, drug therapies to improve sleep and other symptoms, and psychological tools for coping with the emotional disorders caused by the disease and for reducing stress that can exacerbate pain. One study compared three treatment options (biofeedback and relaxation techniques; exercise; and a combination of the other two) with a passive educational approach used as a control. After two years, the combination approach proved to be most beneficial and the passive control approach was the least. Another study also found that interdisciplinary treatment programs were effective in significantly improving pain in 42% of patients. Improvements in pain and other symptoms, including depression and sense of physical capability, persisted for at least six months, although patients tended to become fatigued again. The effectiveness of the treatments tended to depend on how depressed the patients were, the sense of their own disability, personal support networks, and if the cause was unknown.

The severity of the pain at the start of treatment had little to do with outcome. Patients must realize that such therapies are prolonged—in some cases, lifelong—and they should not be discouraged by relapses. Enlisting family, partners, and close friends, particularly with exercise and stretching programs, and becoming involved with support groups of fellow patients are very helpful. Patients must have realistic expectations about the long-term outlook and their own individual capabilities. Improvement is subjective, and some patients are pleased with only a 10% reduction in pain and other symptoms. It is important to understand that the condition can be managed and patients can live a full life.

Exercise

Many studies have indicated that exercise is the most effective component in managing fibromyalgia, and patients must expect to undergo a long-term exercise program. Some patients of fibromyalgia avoid exercise for fear it will exacerbate their pain. However, according to studies, any pain caused by exercising subsides within 30 minutes. Physical activity prevents muscle atrophy, increases a sense of well-being, and, over time, reduces fatigue and pain itself.

Aerobic Exercise. Regular low-impact aerobic exercises are the most helpful for raising the pain threshold, although it may take months to perceive benefits. A very gradual incremental program of activity, beginning with mild exercise and building over time, is important; patients who attempt strenuous exercise too early actually experience an increase in pain and are likely to become discouraged and quit. Every patient must be prepared for relapse and setbacks, which are nearly universal, but this should not dissuade the patient from exercising. Rather, patients should experiment with various forms of physical activity that can be tolerated using their available energy levels. Desirable exercises are walking, swimming, and the use of stationary bikes. Swimming and water therapy, which eliminate weight-bearing, appear to be excellent choices for getting started.

Some experts recommend the use of a training index for gauging progress and establishing a goal. This index is the product of three calculations: the duration of exercise in minutes, number of days per week that the patient exercises, and the percentage of maximum heart rate. People just beginning an exercise program should start with an index of 10 to 25 and aim over time for at least 42. As examples for achieving these goals, an initial index of 15 may be achieved with a maximum heart rate percentage of 60% during exercise performed for 5 minutes 5 times a week (.60 x 5 x 5); the later goal of an index of 42 could be achieved with a maximum heart rate percentage of 70% that occurs with 20-minute exercises three days a week (.70 x 20 x 3 = 42).

(Stretching exercises should be performed for about 10 minutes before aerobic exercise, but they are not considered part of the total exercise time that the patient uses in calculating the index goal.)

Determining Percentage of Maximum Heart Rate

1. Determine the maximum heart rate by subtracting one's age from 220.

2. Determine the heart rate by measuring the pulse either at the carotid artery on the neck or on the inside of the wrist during a workout. It's easiest to count pulse beats for 10 seconds, then multiply by six for the per-minute total.

3. Calculate the percentage of maximum heart rate by dividing the exercise heart rate by the maximum heart rate and multiply by 100.

Stretching Techniques. Much of the pain experienced by patients occurs where muscles join tendons or bones, particularly when the muscles are stretched. Stretching, or flexibility exercises, are part of the warm-up and cool-down routines of any regular program, but the stretching technique used for muscle relaxation and pain reduction must be performed by a person other than the patient, usually a family member or close friend. One such technique is known as "spray and stretch." Using this method, the tender points are located by pressing on the suspected areas, which are then targeted and sprayed with either ethyl chloride (Chloroethane) or Fluori-Methane, which are chemicals that cool the blood vessels in the skin. The patient must be in a comfortable position and the face covered if the spray is being used near the head. The spray bottle is held upside-down about 12 to 18 inches from the targeted area. The spray is not used as an anesthetic but to inactivate the tender points so that the patient's partner can slowly stretch the affected muscle. (Anesthetic skin creams do not appear to be effective for this treatment.) After the procedure, the muscle should feel looser, and the patient should have a greater range of motion with that muscle.

In some cases, injections of lidocaine, called "trigger-point injections," may be used for particularly painful tender points as an aid to stretching. The injection causes intense, transient pain in the trigger point, but after the medication has taken effect, the ability to stretch the muscle is greatly enhanced. After an injection, the spray may be used on the whole muscle to inactivate less severe tender points. In some cases, injections may be needed two or three times over six to eight weeks. There is some soreness afterward, which can be severe, and the benefits of the treatment may not be apparent immediately.

With use of either injections or the spray, the benefits may last from a few days to weeks. Neither the spray nor the injection is useful without muscle stretching.

Cognitive Therapy

Studies continue to show that when fibromyalgia patients increase their psychological capacity to deal with the specific conditions of their disorder and their lives, they are more apt to experience physical improvement. Behavioral cognitive therapy is an effective method for enhancing patients' belief in their own abilities and to develop methods for dealing with stressful situations. A specific goal of cognitive therapy is to change the distorted perceptions that patients have of the world and of themselves; for fibromyalgia patients, this means that they learn to think differently about their pain.

Many fibromyalgia patients live their lives in extremes. They first become heroes or martyrs, doggedly pushing themselves past the point of endurance until they collapse and withdraw. This inevitable backlash reverses their self-perception, and they then view themselves as complete failures, unable to cope with the simplest task. One important aim of cognitive therapy is to help such patients discover a middle route, whereby they can prioritize their responsibilities and drop some of the less important tasks or delegate them to others. Such behavior will eventually lead to a more manageable life and to less of an absolutist perspective on themselves and others. Using specific tasks and self-observation, patients gradually shift their fixed ideas that they are helpless against the pain that dominates their lives to the perception that pain is only one negative and, to a degree, a manageable experience among many positive ones.

Fulfilling experiences and many areas of control are still available. Cognitive therapy may be expensive and not covered by insurance. It should be noted that, in one center, educational discussion groups were as effective, or even more so, than a cognitive therapy program. Such results cannot necessarily be applied to all centers; therapeutic success varies widely depending on the skill of the therapist. The studies do indicate, however, that patients who cannot afford cognitive therapy may do as well with strong, intelligently managed support groups.

Maintaining a Healthy Lifestyle

Establishing Regular Sleep Routines. Sleep is essential, particularly since pain is aggravated by disturbed sleep. Improvement is low in those who are unable to sleep consistently and at night. Swing shift work, for example, is extremely hard on fibromyalgia patients.

Diet. Fibromyalgia patients should maintain a healthy diet low in animal fat and high in fiber, with plenty of fresh fruits and vegetables. There is no evidence that any specific dietary factor is effective in managing fibromyalgia; taken in moderation, vitamins and most nutritional supplements are probably not harmful, but megadoses of vitamins and even certain supplements may be toxic.

Stress Reduction Techniques

There is some evidence that people with fibromyalgia have a more stressful response to daily conflicts and encounters than those without the disorder. A number of relaxation and stress-reduction techniques have proven to be helpful in managing chronic pain.

Deep Breathing. Inhale slowly and deeply to the count of ten, making sure that the stomach and abdomen expand. Inhale through the nose and exhale slowly and completely, also to the count of ten. To help quiet the mind, concentrate fully on breathing and counting through each cycle. Repeat five to ten times and make a habit of doing the exercise several times each day, even when not feeling stressed.

Progressive Muscle Relaxation. After lying down in a comfortable position without crossing the limbs, concentrate on each part of the body, beginning with the top of the head and progressing downward to focus on all the muscles in the body. Be sure to include the forehead, ears, eyes, mouth, neck, shoulders, arms and hands, fingers, chest, belly, thighs, calves and feet. (Some individuals even imagine tensing and releasing internal muscles once the external review is complete.) A slow, deep breathing pattern should be maintained throughout this exercise. Tense each muscle as tightly as possible for a count of five to ten and then release it completely; experience the muscle as totally relaxed and lead-heavy. Continue until the feet are reached. In the beginning it is useful to have a friend or partner check for tension by lifting an arm dropping it; the arm should fall freely. Practice makes the exercise much more effective and produces relaxation much more rapidly.

Meditation. Meditation, used for many years in eastern cultures, is now widely accepted in this country as an effective relaxation technique. For example, one recent study reported that patients who performed *qigong*, an Oriental technique, reported reduced pain, fatigue, and sleeplessness and improved function, mood, and general health after eight weeks. The practiced meditater can achieve a reduction in heart rate, blood pressure, adrenaline levels, and skin temperature while meditating.

A number of organizations, both religious and nonreligious, teach meditation; the names of these organizations, along with instructional books, can be found at public libraries.

The goal of all meditative procedures, both religious and therapeutic, is to quiet the mind, essentially to relax thought. The first step is to be as physically comfortable as possible in a quiet place, preferably in a semi-dark room, isolated from noise or distraction. One should be sitting up with the eyes closed and concentrating on a simple image or sound. Some methods suggest imagining a point of light behind the forehead and between the eyes. Other techniques, such as transcendental mediation, assign "mantras," words that have particular chanting sounds, which are repeated silently. (Anyone can make up a word or a sound; the only condition is that the word or sound not be associated with a real thing, which can distract the meditater from the internal process.) When the mind begins to wander, the meditater gently brings concentration back to the central image or sound. Some recommend meditating for no longer than 20 minutes in the morning after awakening and then again in early evening before dinner. Even once a day is helpful. When successful, the meditater experiences deep relaxation and renewed energy. (One should probably not meditate before going to bed; some people who meditate before sleep wake up in the middle of the night, alert and unable to return to sleep.)

One technique requiring little adaptation of the daily schedule has been termed mini-meditation. The method involves heightening awareness of the immediate surrounding environment. One should first choose a routine activity when alone. For example, while washing dishes concentrate on the feel of the water and dishes; allow the mind to wander to any immediate sensory experience, such as sounds outside the window, smells from the stove, or colors in the room. If the mind begins to think about the past or future, abstractions or worries, redirect it gently back. This redirection of brain activity from thoughts and worries to the senses disrupts the stress response and prompts relaxation. It also helps promote an emotional and sensual appreciation of simple pleasures already present in a person's life.

Biofeedback. During biofeedback, electric leads are taped to a subject's head. The person is encouraged to relax using methods such as those described above. Brains waves are measured and an auditory signal is emitted when alpha waves are detected, a frequency that coincides with a state of deep relaxation. By repeating the process, subjects associate the sound with the relaxed state and learn to achieve relaxation by themselves.

Massage Therapy. Massage therapy is thought to stimulate the parasympathetic nervous system, which slows down the heart and relaxes the body. Rather than causing drowsiness, massage actually increases alertness; the reduction of stress and anxiety levels and the resulting relaxation, however, do contribute to better sleep. A number of massage therapies are available for relaxing muscles, including the following: (1) shiatsu, which applies intense pressure to parts of the body, can be painful but people report deep relaxation at the end; (2) reflexology manipulates hands and feet using Eastern techniques; (3) Swedish massage has been available for years and some experts believe is still the best method for relaxation.

Other Procedures

Because of the difficulties in treating fibromyalgia, many patients seek alternative treatments. Everyone should be wary of those who promise a cure or urge the purchase of expensive but useless and potentially dangerous treatments.

Acupuncture. Acupuncture may be effective for some patients. One study measured blood levels of the chemicals serotonin and substance P, which change in response to pain or its cessation. After acupuncture, the blood levels of these chemicals increased, which paralleled the reduction in fibromyalgia pain.

Magnet Therapy. Magnet therapy has received some attention and one study using magnets that were only slightly more powerful than refrigerator magnets showed some benefits.

Well-Connected Board of Editors

Harvey Simon, M.D., Editor-in-Chief
Massachusetts Institute of Technology; Physician, Massachusetts General Hospital

Masha J. Etkin, M.D., Gynecology
Harvard Medical School; Physician, Massachusetts General Hospital

John E. Godine, M.D., Ph.D., Metabolism
Harvard Medical School; Associate Physician, Massachusetts General Hospital

Daniel Heller, M.D., Pediatrics
Harvard Medical School; Associate Pediatrician, Massachusetts General Hospital; Active Staff, Children's Hospital

Irene Kuter, M.D., D. Phil., Oncology
Harvard Medical School; Assistant Physician, Massachusetts General Hospital

Paul C. Shellito, M.D., Surgery
Harvard Medical School; Associate Visiting Surgeon, Massachusetts General Hospital

Theodore A. Stern, M.D., Psychiatry
Harvard Medical School; Psychiatrist and Chief, Psychiatric Consultation Service, Massachusetts General Hospital

Carol Peckham, Editorial Director

Cynthia Chevins, Publisher

426

Chapter 29

Heart Health

Contents

Section 29.1

Physical Activity and Cardiovascular Health: Questions and Answers

Q: If I exercise, will I prevent heart disease?

A: Physical inactivity, along with cigarette smoking, high blood pressure, and high blood cholesterol, is one of the major modifiable risk factors for heart attack. There is no guarantee that you will not get heart disease; however, your chances of heart disease developing are lower if you avoid the risk factors.

Q: I have been inactive for years. Shouldn't I see a doctor before I start becoming physically active?

A: People middle-aged or older who are inactive and at high risk for heart disease or who already have a medical condition should seek medical advice before they start or significantly increase their physical activity. Most apparently healthy people of any age can safely engage in moderate levels of physical activity (e.g. moderate walking, gardening, yard work) without prior medical consultation.

Q: How much physical activity is enough?

A: If you are inactive, doing anything is better than nothing! Studies show that people who have a low fitness level are much more likely to die early than people who have achieved even a moderate level of fitness. If you want to exceed a moderate level of fitness, you need to exercise three or four times a week for 30 to 60 minutes at 50 to 80 percent of your maximum capacity.

Q: Is exercise safe?

A: The potential health benefits of exercise greatly outweigh the risk, although there is a very slight increased risk of death due to heart attack during vigorous exercise. Consult your doctor first if you have any concerns, have been sedentary, are overweight, are middle-aged or older or have a medical condition.

Q: Do I need to do vigorous exercise?

A: To achieve health benefits, no. Doing moderate-level activities often will help lower your health risks. If you want to attain a high level of cardiovascular fitness, you need to gradually work up to exercising at least three or four times a week for 30 to 60 minutes at 50 to 80 percent of your maximum capacity.

Q: Does exercise counteract the harmful effects of other risk factors?

A: Studies show that being physically fit lowers heart disease risk even in people who have other health problems such as high blood pressure and high blood cholesterol. To minimize risk, however, you should be physically fit and avoid the other major modifiable risk factors: cigarette smoke, high blood pressure and high blood cholesterol.

Q: Do women get the same benefits from exercise as men?

A: Most studies showing the positive effects of exercise have been done with men. The few studies that have included women have indicated that women may benefit even more than men from being physically fit. Early indications show the reduced rates of death by heart disease are higher for women who are physically fit than for men.

Women who do not exercise have twice the chance of dying from heart disease than women who do exercise, just as women who smoke double their chances of dying from heart disease than women who don't smoke. Women may live longer than men, but they don't necessarily live better. Elderly women who have not been physically active experience more disability in their daily function than women who have been active.

Q: I am a senior citizen. Is it too late for me to become physically active? Should I take special precautions?

A: More and more seniors are proving every day that they are not too old to exercise. In fact, the older you are, the more you need regular exercise. However, there are some special precautions you should take. If you have a family history of heart disease, check with your doctor first. Don't try to do too much too fast. Exercise at an intensity appropriate for you. Pick activities that are fun, that suit your needs and that you can do year-round. Wear comfortable clothing and footwear. Choose a well-lighted, safe place with a smooth, soft surface. Take more time to warm up and cool down before and after your workout. Stretch slowly. Don't rely on your sense of thirst; drink water on a fixed schedule.

Q: As a parent, how can I make sure that my children are physically fit?

A: Set a good example by practicing good heart-healthy habits yourself. Limit sedentary activities such as television, movies, videos and computer games to no more than two hours a day. Plan active family outings and vacations. Assign household chores (mowing lawns, raking leaves, scrubbing floors, etc.) that require physical exertion. Observe what sports and activities appeal to your children, then encourage their development with lessons or by joining teams. If it is safe to walk or bike rather than drive, do so. Use stairs instead of elevators and escalators. Make sure that your children's physical activities at school or in daycare are adequate. When your children are bored, suggest something that gets them moving—play catch or build a snowman!

The information contained in this American Heart Association (AHA) website is not a substitute for medical advice or treatment, and the AHA recommends consultation with your doctor or health care professional.

Section 29.2

Target Heart Rates

American Heart Association (AHA) Recommendation

Healthcare professionals recognize the importance of pacing your efforts when you exercise. The goal is not to tire too quickly, but still receive the benefits of being physically active. Pacing yourself is especially important if you have been inactive.

Target heart rates are effective in measuring initial fitness level and monitoring progress after you begin a fitness program. This approach requires measuring your pulse periodically as you exercise and staying within 50 to 75 percent of your maximum heart rate. This range is called your target heart rate.

What Is an Alternative to Target Heart Rates?

Some people are unable to measure their pulse, or do not want to take their pulse when exercising. Another alternative is to use a "conversational pace" to monitor your efforts if you are doing moderate activities like walking. If you can talk and walk at the same time, you are not working too hard. If you can sing and maintain your level of effort, you are probably not working hard enough. If you get out of breath quickly, you are probably working too hard—especially if you actually have to stop and catch your breath.

When Should I Use the Target Heart Rate?

If you want to participate in more vigorous activities like brisk walking and jogging, where the "conversational pace" approach may not work, then try using the target heart rate. It works for many people, and it is a good way for healthcare professionals to monitor your progress.

The following table shows estimated target heart rates for different age categories. Look for the age category closest to yours and read across to find your target heart rate.

Table 29.1. Target Heart Rates

Age	Target HR Zone 50-75 %	Average Maximum Heart Rate 100 %
20 years	100-150 beats per minute	200
25 years	98-146 beats per minute	195
30 years	95-142 beats per minute	190
35 years	93-138 beats per minute	185
40 years	90-135 beats per minute	180
45 years	88-131 beats per minute	175
50 years	85-127 beats per minute	170
55 years	83-123 beats per minute	165
60 years	80-120 beats per minute	160
65 years	78-116 beats per minute	155
70 years	75-113 beats per minute	150

Your maximum heart rate is approximately 220 minus your age. The figures above are averages and should be used as general guidelines.

Note: A few high blood pressure medications lower the maximum heart rate and thus the target zone rate. If you are taking high blood pressure medicine, call your physician and find out if your program needs to be adjusted.

How Should I Pace Myself?

When beginning an exercise program, aim at the lowest part of your target zone (50 percent) during the first few weeks. Gradually build up to the higher part of your target zone (75 percent). After six months or more of regular exercise, you might be able to exercise comfortably up to 85 percent of your maximum heart rate, if you wish, but you do not have to exercise that hard to stay in condition.

Chapter 30

Hypoglycemia: The Unwelcome Exercise Intruder

You're 20 minutes into your aerobic workout when you begin to notice some lightheadedness. Your heart begins to beat stronger than the intensity of your workout seems to warrant, and your sweat has turned cold and clammy. The cadence of your run on the treadmill has changed; you find your feet are moving sluggishly and feel heavy and awkward. You ask yourself, "What is going on here?"

If you have ever found yourself in this situation during a workout, checking your blood glucose would likely have provided you with an answer.

Hypoglycemia (low blood glucose) and hyperglycemia (high blood glucose) are the most significant potential risks associated with diabetes during exercise. Fortunately, when we understand a few key points about the metabolic changes that occur in the body during exercise, and a little about the diabetic disease process itself, we can usually avoid precipitous drops or dangerously high escalations in blood sugars during workouts.

The ability to precisely control your blood glucose, even in your everyday life, is dependent on a myriad of factors. Among the most important are the amount and type of insulin or oral medications taken to lower blood glucose, the number of calories you've consumed and the composition of such calories (for example, are they derived

Reprinted with permission from *Diabetes Forecast*, April 1999, vol. 52, issue 4, p. 31. © 1999 American Diabetes Association. For information on joining ADA and receiving *Diabetes Forecast*, call 1-800-806-7801.

from carbohydrates, fats, or proteins?), and the amount of physical activity and stress encountered during your daily routine.

Throwing exercise into the equation, however, requires us to consider additional factors. The type and duration of physical activity performed, the intensity of the workout, and timing of the insulin dose can each profoundly influence blood glucose levels. Your pre-exercise blood sugar levels, degree of physical fitness, and age also influence your blood glucose levels during exercise.

In this, the first part of a two-part series on exercise and blood glucose, we will explore the body's ability to control blood glucose levels when diabetes is not present. In our second column, we will detail the exact events occurring in diabetes that predispose a person with diabetes to hypoglycemia and hyperglycemia during exercise. We will also devise a plan to greatly reduce or prevent their future occurrence.

Without Diabetes

In those who don't have diabetes, blood glucose levels are naturally controlled and kept constant during periods of increased muscle work and energy demand such as exercise. This precise control is primarily dependent upon three major factors: insulin, two hormones that counter insulin's action (glucagon and epinephrine [adrenaline]), and the brain (which has the final say in regulating blood glucose).

While we all understand that insulin plays a key role in lowering blood glucose, it actually has a much more sophisticated metabolic function. Insulin takes the carbohydrates, fats, and proteins from the foods that we eat and finds bodily storage sites for them. Insulin promotes the storage of carbohydrates in the liver and muscles as glycogen (a complex chain of sugar molecules that can be broken down later into free glucose). It also helps store fats in adipose and muscle cells as triglycerides (which can be broken down later into free fatty acids, another great muscle fuel). Further, it promotes the storage of proteins in all forms of cells as amino acids. (Amino acids actually play a very limited role in providing energy; rather, they serve as vital building blocks for countless types of cellular structures.)

Glucagon and epinephrine counteract insulin's actions; these hormones sense the signals that are sent out when our muscles are demanding more fuel for exercise. Glucagon and epinephrine "awaken" storage sites, initiate breakdown of glycogen into glucose, and triglycerides into free fatty acids, and mobilize these breakdown products to serve as energy for the exercising muscle.

The brain's role in all of this complex circuitry is relatively simple. Mostly inactive in the resting state, the brain only gets involved during intense exercise when blood glucose or blood oxygen deviates from normal levels. Even subtle drops in blood glucose and, more importantly, oxygen, caused by the stress of exercise, cause the brain to override the entire system and initiate a surge of epinephrine and glucagon into the system. The surge of these hormones into the bloodstream causes more stored fuel to be released and lessens the need for oxygen in the muscles. As a result, oxygen is able to continue its service in sites where it is most needed, like the brain and heart.

With Diabetes

How does having diabetes alter this incredible physiologic process that occurs during exercise? Well, the good news is that it doesn't dramatically alter this process if it is tightly controlled!

Allow me to emphasize that again: It's essential to have your diabetes under good control before you begin to exercise. If you exercise during periods of hyperglycemia (blood glucose levels of 250 milligrams per deciliter or greater) or hypoglycemia, the entire metabolic process can go awry. (Hyperglycemia during exercise can result from taking either too little insulin or eating too much, and hypoglycemia can result from taking either too much insulin on the day that you exercise or not ingesting enough carbohydrates before you begin exercising.) That can wreak havoc on your workout and even threaten your safety.

I hope we have set an adequate foundation to begin to understand the potential and real risks of hypoglycemia and hyperglycemia associated with diabetes and exercising. I have always believed that knowledge is bliss. With this knowledge, we can minimize any chance of crazy blood sugars mining the workout that we all look forward to each passing day.

Before You Start

Although most people with diabetes can exercise safely, exercise involves some risks. To shift the benefit-to-risk ratio in your favor, take these precautions:

- Have a medical exam before you begin your exercise program, including an exercise test with EKG monitoring, especially if you have cardiovascular disease, you are over 35, you have high blood pressure or elevated cholesterol levels, you smoke, or you have a family history of heart disease.

- Discuss with your doctor any unusual symptoms that you experience during or after exercise such as discomfort in your chest, neck, jaw, or arms; nausea, dizziness, fainting, or excessive shortness of breath; or short-term changes in vision.

- If you have diabetes-related complications, check with your health care team about special precautions. Consider exercising in a medically supervised program, at least initially, if you have peripheral vascular disease, retinopathy, autonomic neuropathy, or kidney problems.

- Learn how to prevent and treat low blood glucose levels (hypoglycemia). If you take oral agents or insulin, monitor your blood glucose levels before, during, and after exercise.

- If you have type 1, and your blood glucose is above 250 milligrams per deciliter, check your urine for ketones. Don't exercise if ketones are present, because exercise will increase your risk of ketoacidosis and coma.

- Always warm up and cool down.

- Don't exercise outdoors when the weather is too hot and humid, or too cold.

- Pay special attention to proper footwear. Inspect your feet daily and always after you exercise.

This chapter provides general guidelines and advice regarding exercise and its role in the management of diabetes. This chapter is NOT intended to offer individualized medical or exercise advice. Those initiating, participating in, or altering an exercise program should do so with the assistance of a physician or health care team. The opinions expressed in this column are the author's, and do not necessarily correspond to the views of the institutions he is associated with.

—by Joel B. Braunstein

Joel B. Braunstein, MD, is a physician at the Department of Internal Medicine, Brigham and Women's Hospital Harvard Medical School Boston, Massachusetts.

Chapter 31

Mental Health and the Impact of Exercise

Many studies and scholarly articles praise the physical benefits of consistent exercise. Regular activity helps participants achieve and maintain healthy body weight and composition, raises beneficial cholesterol levels, assists in the treatment of Type 2 diabetes, and reduces the risk of osteoporosis, heart disease and some types of cancer. In addition, exercise helps reduce premenstrual distress, constipation, insomnia and varicose veins.

Participants also cite stress reduction and increased ability to cope in stressful situations, in addition to positive physical changes, as major reasons for exercising regularly. They feel better physically and emotionally, and are able to handle crises more effectively and rationally.

Although it is difficult to imagine any negative components of fitness, a few adverse psychological aspects exist. For example, rather than reducing stressful situations, exercise can manifest them and exacerbate a preexisting mental health disorder.

Mental Health Disorders

Mental health runs along a continuum, with health and wellness on one end and disabling emotional disorders on the other. In between are gradations in constant flux. An individual can feel relaxed and content one day and full of anxiety due to a stressful event the next.

Reprinted with permission from the Aerobics and Fitness Association of America. *American Fitness Magazine*, © 1996, vol. 14, no. 4, p. 24(6), July-August 1996.

During the course of our lives, we all undergo physical and mental stress, and each of us responds differently. How we respond emotionally to stressful situations is based upon a set of variables. These variables include frequency, intensity, duration, age of initial onset, and mode of the stressor, as well as family history and genetics.

Using these guidelines, mental health professionals can determine whether an emotional response to a stressful life situation is appropriate, or if the person may be experiencing an episode of psychopathology (abnormal or inappropriate behavior or thoughts). Investigating how long a person has had symptoms, how often they occur, intensity of feelings, thoughts or behaviors, age of initial onset, how the symptoms present themselves and whether there is a family history of mental health disorders or disturbances can help in making a diagnosis.

Often, a clue to a real disorder is the extent to which symptoms affect or rule a person's life. If many aspects of a person's life are affected by or revolve around symptoms or relief of symptoms, it bears more investigation.

It is important to remember everyone experiences varying degrees of emotional stress throughout life, and no one is exempt from pain, tragedy and heartache. Careful examination can help determine when a person has crossed the line from garden-variety stress and pain to a characterizable mental health disorder.

Many professionals in the mental health field refer to the *Diagnostic and Statistical Manual of Mental Disorders* when making diagnoses. The manual utilizes the variable approach in investigating symptomology, and furnishes clear guidelines for diagnoses.

Using the variable approach, psychologists determine whether the sadness a person is experiencing is an appropriate response to a recent loss or whether it may be one of the symptoms of major or clinical depression. Some of the diagnosable disorders include affective or mood disorders such as depression or manic depression, anxiety and adjustment disorders, psychotic disorders such as schizophrenia, and obsessive-compulsive and eating disorders.

The determination of a disorder has tremendous influence on treatment modality. Often, psychotherapists or psychiatrists suggest some form of exercise in conjunction with professional treatment depending on the type of the disorder.

Eating Disorders and Disordered Eating

The National Center for Health Statistics (NCHS) has estimated that by the first year of college, 5 to 18% of women and .4% of men have a history of bulimia or binge-eating patterns, and that as many as one in 100 females between the ages of 12 and 18 have anorexia. Individuals whose psychopathology is fueled and exacerbated by exercise include those with eating disorders, distorted body images and some obsessive-compulsives.

The NCHS does not address the growing number of people who experience disordered eating and exercise patterns (using exercise as a way to eliminate food or reduce anxiety associated with a mental health disorder). For those afflicted, exercise becomes an extension of their mental health disorder. The health club is a place where they punish themselves for not living up to their perception of thin and image of perfection. Often, they are women. The reasons and contributing factors are many: family or relationship disturbances, loss of a loved one, sexual trauma or abuse, societal influences or biochemical disturbances.

Psychological Benefits of Exercise

With up to 20% of the American population suffering a serious affective or mood disorder, depression being the most common, there has been a significant amount of research on the emotional advantages of exercise. Fortunately, there are more psychological benefits than costs.

A consensus statement from the National Institute of Mental Health (NIMH) in the early 1990s concluded there are positive psychological benefits to regular exercise. Exercise has been associated with a decreased level of mild to moderate depression, a lessening of anxiety levels, decline in stress, a reduction in neuroticism and an increase in self-esteem and well-being. Research also points to exercise increasing the production of important brain neurotransmitters associated with better mood and alertness by increasing blood flow to the brain and triggering the release of critical brain neurotransmitters such as serotonin, epinephrine, norepinephrine and dopamine.

Naturally occurring brain neurochemicals are often lower in those with clinical depression. In fact, antidepressant medications attempt to balance these chemicals by either increasing their production or decreasing the influence of other neurotransmitters in the brain. Therefore, exercise is an excellent adjunct in the treatment of depression.

Self-Esteem

Self-esteem is the value we place on our lives, skills, ability to function, cope, love and be loved. It's like a savings account. The amount of self-esteem in our account determines how we feel about ourselves and others, as well as how we get along with people. When our savings account is full, perhaps after a series of favorable events, we have the ability to fill other people's accounts, who in turn fill ours. We also have the ability to dip into other accounts with blaming, criticism or gossip, depleting not only their savings but our own.

There are ways to enhance self-esteem through physical activity that benefit participant and educator. The key is to understand fitness and wellness as a process and not a product, as a continuum and not an end point.

Fitness professionals need to provide an atmosphere that encourages individual improvement rather than competitiveness. For example, pointing out to a newcomer they did an excellent job rather than focusing on the group can go a long way in encouraging personal improvement.

It is important to understand the role of a fitness professional is to educate clients, not dazzle them with complicated movements. It is vital not only to teach a skill, but also educate clients about the role exercise plays in health and wellness and help them better understand how they can make fitness a lifetime commitment.

Individuals with low self-esteem often get ignored or neglected by those who develop exercise programs. Some are unable to take the risk of getting into a fitness program due to the fear of failure. These people would get a lot of psychological benefit. Developing remedial programs in health clubs in outreach formats can help many begin exercise programs and increase their self-worth.

Focusing on enjoyment level during physical activity as opposed to difficulty level can help with adherence, leading to improved self-image. We tend to stay longer in activities we like, hence increasing benefits.

There is a lot more to exercise than building muscles, increasing endurance and creating a strong heart. A regular exercise program boosts morale, strengthens the mind and contributes to a healthier, happier life.

—byAnne Clifford Bradley

Anne Clifford Bradley, ELM., CAES, is an educational psychologist, and AFAA certified aerobics instructor and personal trainer in Cape Cod, Massachusetts.

Chapter 32

Obesity:
The Role of Exercise in
Management

We've all seen the ads for miracle weight loss products. We're asked to buy soap that washes away fat, cream that melts fat, pills that burn fat and shoe inserts that magically make fat disappear as you walk. Yet health and fitness professionals continue to give the same advice when asked about losing weight: proper nutrition and exercise. This advice may not be new or exciting, but it is sound. Although people are often willing to make dietary changes, many simply don't want to exercise. How necessary is it to exercise in order to lose weight?

Historically, obesity has been viewed as a result of poor eating habits, but overeating may not be the problem. The general population has become more overweight since 1900, with the percentage of Americans who are obese increasing from 25% to 33% between 1980 and 1991. However, per capita caloric consumption has decreased during this century. In other words, people now eat less but weigh more. This suggests that inactivity may play a larger part than overeating in the causes of obesity.

In the U.S., the increased prevalence of obesity appears to parallel a decline in the average daily energy expenditure. Physical activity is no longer a part of our everyday lives. Technology has reduced job-related physical demands. Labor-saving devices, such as cars, elevators and remote controls, have removed substantial amounts of physical activity from our everyday lives. Reports from the Centers for Disease Control and Prevention suggest participation in vigorous activity by adults, adolescents and children has dropped substantially during the past few decades. Presently, only 15% of adults regularly engage (three times a week for at least 20 minutes) in vigorous physical activity during their leisure time, and only 22% of adults regularly engage (five times a week for 30 minutes) in sustained physical activity of any intensity during their leisure time.

Exercise and Weight Loss

Numerous studies have examined the impact of exercise training on body weight and fat. These studies demonstrate exercise favorably affects body composition by promoting fat loss. For example, William Zuti, Ph.D. and Lawrence Golding, Ph.D. examined three groups of women who maintained a caloric deficit of 500 calories per day for 16 weeks. A diet-only group decreased caloric intake by 500 calories per day, but did not alter their physical activity. The exercise-only group did not alter their diet, but burned 500 extra calories per day by increasing physical activity. The diet-exercise group reduced caloric intake by 250 calories per day and increased daily activity by 250 calories. All three groups had a similar weight loss, but the two exercise groups lost considerably more fat than the diet group, which lost a substantial amount of lean tissue.

Large population based studies consistently show a relationship between body weight and exercise. Loretta DiPietro, Ph.D. studied 19,000 men and women, and found that the prevalence of overweight was highest among sedentary people and lowest among individuals who participated in regular, intense exercise. In all age categories, people who cycled, jogged or participated in aerobics weighed less than inactive people. For people over the age of 40, walking was also associated with lower body weight.

The rate of weight loss resulting from exercise without caloric restriction is relatively slow. Experimental studies have found that exercise alone generally produces a modest loss, averaging six to seven pounds. Although some studies have reported substantial losses (13 to 26 pounds) with intensive exercise, the physical demands of these programs make them impractical for most overweight persons. Despite the seemingly discouraging nature of these findings, keep in mind that even a modest weight loss positively impacts health. In a slightly overweight person, a seven-pound loss may also be cosmetically significant.

There is some evidence that starting an exercise program will lead to changes in an exerciser's diet. The amount of physical activity in which people participate is inversely related to their fat intake; the more they exercise, the less fat they consume. This suggests that active people have a preference for carbohydrates. It may also contribute to the relative ease with which they appear to balance calories.

A combination of mild caloric restriction and regular physical activity is more effective in reducing body weight than either approach alone. Furthermore, the addition of exercise to a comprehensive weight management program has multiple health benefits, such as a reduction of the risk for developing heart disease.

Weight Loss Maintenance

Fitness professionals have been relatively successful in helping people to lose weight, but not in helping them maintain their weight loss. This is the problem on which we need to focus. According to the National Institutes of Health, most people experience significant weight regain in the first year following termination of a weight loss program with complete or almost complete weight regain in five years.

There is an impressive relationship between exercise and weight loss maintenance. Individuals who include exercise as an integral part of their weight management program are much more likely to keep weight off.

A study by K. Pavlou, Ph.D. and colleagues illustrates this point. They studied 160 overweight policemen who participated in a 12-week weight-loss program. Each policeman was assigned to either an exercise group or a non-exercise group, and then to one of four diets. Eighteen months after the program was over, the subjects were reassessed. The researchers found that regardless of diet, the non-exercise group gained back all of the weight lost in the 12-week program. In contrast, the exercise group maintained a weight loss of approximately 10 to 12 pounds.

Exercise and Fat Distribution

In addition to the effect exercise has on weight loss and fat loss, exercise favorably alters body fat distribution. Scientific evidence suggests the way some people store fat affects their health. Fat stored in the abdominal area increases the risk of coronary heart disease, Type 2 diabetes, high blood pressure and high cholesterol. A waist-to-hip ratio that exceeds .80 for women and .95 for men places them at greater risk for these diseases. Regular exercisers tend to have lower waist-to-hip ratios than sedentary individuals. This is primarily due to lower waist circumferences among the exercisers.

Higher intensity exercise (such as jogging or aerobic dance) is associated with a preferential use of abdominal fat relative to gluteal fat. During exercise, there is an increased release of epinephrine in the body; this hormone activates the breakdown of fat. Abdominal fat is more responsive to increases in epinephrine than fat stored around the hips and thighs. This explains why regular exercisers have lower waist-to-hip ratios than non-exercisers, and may help to explain why overweight men, who tend to store fat around the abdomen, lose weight more quickly and easily than overweight women who tend to deposit fat in the resistant hip and thigh region.

Exercise Intensity

Exercise is important for weight loss and critical for weight loss maintenance. It is well known that aerobic exercise is the best type of exercise for burning fat, but the question of intensity always comes up. Is high-intensity, short-duration exercise or low-intensity, long-duration exercise better for helping someone to lose weight?

From the perspective of fat loss, the answer may be "it doesn't matter." Consider the following study by Maryann Grediagan, Ph.D. She assigned overweight women to either a high intensity (80% VO_2 max) or a low intensity (50% VO_2 max) exercise group. All the women exercised four times per week for 12 weeks with a duration sufficient to expend 300 calories. The duration of the low intensity workout was considerably longer than the high intensity workout. At the end of the study, both groups had lost five pounds of fat, although the high intensity group gained more than twice as much lean tissue as the low intensity group. It can be concluded that fat loss is a function of the number of calories expended rather than exercise intensity.

There are several reasons why low intensity, long duration exercise may be more appropriate when working with an overweight population. Obese individuals are at an increased risk for injuries to their bones and joints. For this reason, it is also recommended that you select non-impact and low-impact activities. Additionally, there is an inverse relationship between exercise adherence and intensity; the harder the workouts, the more likely a person is to drop out of an exercise program.

The best way to make decisions about exercise intensity and duration is to consider the individual. Variables such as time constraints, medical problems, fitness level and personal preference should all contribute to the decision of how difficult and long to make an exercise program.

Obesity Prevention

Although fitness professionals often prescribe exercise to help people lose weight, its role in obesity prevention should not be overlooked. Physically active individuals generally weigh less, and have less body fat and fewer medical problems than their sedentary counterparts. There is a need to promote exercise to everyone, even those with ideal body weight. The adoption of even a modest exercise program helps individuals to look and feel better, and manage their weight. And they gain the many other benefits of regular physical activity.

Mechanisms Linking Exercise and Weight Control

There are several pathways by which exercise influences body weight.

- Exercise Oxygen Consumption (EPOC)—metabolism remains temporarily elevated after exercise ends. Following an exercise that burns 300 calories, the contribution of EPOC ranges from six to 42 calories. This is a small but significant contributor to energy balance.

- Prevention of the decline in metabolic rate that accompanies caloric restriction.

- The increased capacity to use fat as a fuel.

—by Deborah Riebe, Ph.D.

Deborah Riebe, Ph.D., is a professor at University of Rhode Island in Kingston.

Chapter 33

Repetitive Strain Injury and the Computer Cramp Blues

You may know all about computer virus prevention. You may even be fortified and protected against a computer crash. But what about computer encasement? No, it's not a hard drive or software problem. After sitting at your computer for hours, you suddenly realize your body is in a state of rigor mortis. Your neck feels as if it's incapable of movement and your shoulders are painfully hunched up toward your ears. At this point, you are acutely aware of every nerve ending in your spinal column. However, there is a way to untie these painful muscle cramps.

The human body is a marvelous piece of equipment capable of complex activities such as balancing, walking, stooping, reaching, twisting and lifting. In fact, the body responds favorably to being used. But when forced to remain in a static position, muscles tighten up. The legs suffer when pressed against a chair, restricting blood flow and circulation. When you limit your back movement, it becomes tight and almost locked into position. Cramped shoulders and an unnatural forward neck position only exacerbate the problem.

If you've been sitting at a desk or computer for a long time, stand up and attempt to walk slowly to encourage blood circulation. The legs will gradually loosen up. Stretch them out further by taking slightly longer steps and continue to walk until your lower body begins to relax. Once walking has increased blood circulation throughout the body, you can begin stretching out the tightness.

Reprinted with permission from the Aerobics and Fitness Association of America. *American Fitness Magazine*, © 1999, vol. 17, issue 3, p. 26, May 1999.

The following stretches can help alleviate computer encasement. These movements should be executed smoothly and accompanied by deep breaths.

Finger Flexes—These exercises can help stretch the hand and wrist and develop a stronger forearm. Starting with the little finger, curl each finger under one at a time until you make a fist. Curl the fist around in a circle, then slowly uncurl.

Shoulder Rolls—These are one of the most productive and satisfying exercises for upper body tension. Lift your shoulders as high as possible toward the ears. Then slowly and evenly roll them as far forward as possible, down and then back, attempting to press the shoulder blades together. Make these circles as complete as possible. After four rolls, reverse the direction.

Torso Twist—Turn from the waist and look over your left shoulder, then gradually rotate until you are twisted around to the right.

Pick Grapes—Stretch the right side of the body by reaching upward as high as possible, then repeat on the left side. Again, let these movements be slow and steady while breathing deeply.

Finger Stretches—One of the dreaded side effects of working long hours at a computer or engaging in other repetitive movements is carpal tunnel syndrome, which results in a loss of strength or feeling in the hands. Finger stretches can relieve stress from overuse of the hands and help prevent this condition. Hold your arms straight out in front of your body, bend the wrists down and stretch your fingers as wide as possible. Hold for 10 seconds, relax and repeat.

Neck Rotation—Once the shoulders have been loosened, the neck should be gently rotated. Imagine your head as a clock. Point your nose at 10 o'clock and slowly turn your head counterclockwise until your chin is close to your chest. Continue the rotation until your nose is pointing toward two o'clock. Reverse this partial circle while breathing deeply. Turn your head and look over your left shoulder as far as you can, then look over your right shoulder in the same manner. Swivel your head slowly from right to left four times in each direction.

Back Arch—Place your hands on your lower back and gently arch upward, lifting your chest. Release the arch and repeat four times.

By now you should feel looser and less tense. If you have time, go for a vigorous walk. Practice this routine every two hours to break the monotony and reduce tension. These movements also increase blood circulation and sharpen mental alertness. You will return to your work station more relaxed and mentally revived, no longer suffering the effects of computer encasement.

—by Lynn Difley

Lynn Difley is a freelance writer based in West Linn, Oregon

Chapter 34

Sarcopenia (Muscle Loss) and Exercise

If you're 35 to 40, although you're feeling fit as ever, you have probably begun losing skeletal muscle, the tissue that provides your strength and mobility.

Slow, inexorable muscle wasting occurs even in healthy individuals who engage in regular aerobic exercise, but it usually goes unnoticed for decades. In fact, the body hides its loss by subtly padding affected areas with extra fat. So maintaining your weight perfectly over time does not mean muscle isn't vanishing, notes Steven B. Heymsfield of St. Luke's-Roosevelt Hospital Center in New York.

This phenomenon didn't even have a name eight years ago. At that time, while speaking at a conference on aging, Irwin H. Rosenberg wondered aloud whether its anonymity accounted for the paucity of research on it—and for the medical community's apparent lack of concern over its role in crippling society's elders.

Several recent studies have indicated that while thinning bones render the elderly especially vulnerable to fractures, it's the unsteadiness caused by muscle wasting in the legs that leads to falls. To the extent that it makes walking, stair climbing, and getting in and out of chairs difficult, muscle loss can not only rob aging adults of their independence but also steer them into unhealthful, sedentary lifestyles.

"So that we could begin taking this problem seriously, I suggested, half tongue-in-cheek, that we give it a name—sarcopenia," recalls

Rosenberg, director of the Agriculture Department's Jean Mayer Human Nutrition Research Center on Aging at Tufts University in Boston. He hoped the Greek moniker's classical ring would give it the cachet to catch on. The tactic worked.

Sarcopenia, which means "vanishing flesh," has begun popping up in medical texts and gerontology papers. It even appears in a solicitation for new research proposals just issued by the National Institute on Aging (NIA) in Bethesda, Maryland. The institute convened a conference four weeks ago on techniques for studying sarcopenia, with the goal of spurring more research in the area. Next spring, NIA plans to launch an eight-year study of how this muscle loss affects activity and recovery from disease in 3,000 otherwise healthy septuagenarians.

At its annual meeting in October, the American Aging Association has scheduled a session on sarcopenia. And Miriam E. Nelson of the Tufts center has written a book for the general public, due out next year, describing exercises that her studies show can fight the ravages of muscle loss.

Sarcopenia is well on its way to becoming a household word, like osteoporosis, concludes geriatrician Tamara Harris of NIA.

Gilbert Forbes of the University of Rochester (N.Y.) School of Medicine holds the world's record for the longest chronicle of age-related muscle loss in a single individual. Since he was 44, Forbes has measured his own fat-free mass on at least 150 separate occasions spanning 37 years. He has another 27 years' worth of data on a colleague, begun when that man was 53.

Skeletal muscle comprises about half of a person's lean body weight. Because the weight of the two other major components—bone and viscera (organs)—does not drop much over time, Forbes' measurements offer an indirect gauge of vanishing muscle.

Those data, reported at the Experimental Biology '96 meeting in Washington, D.C., this past April, indicate that Forbes experienced a fairly constant one-kilogram-per-decade loss of muscle, roughly twice the rate of his heavier, more muscular colleague.

To get a speedier estimate of sarcopenia within the general population, Ronenn Roubenoff and Joseph Kehayias of the Tufts center have just finished measuring skeletal muscle in Boston area adults. By comparing people of different ages but similar builds, they're looking to identify when muscle loss begins and how quickly it proceeds.

"The data we have clearly show a decline from the thirties onward," Roubenoff told *Science News*. Though men tend to start with more muscle, they appear to lose about the same percentage as women over time. Despite large individual variability, he says, the trends indicate "that if you're a healthy elderly person in your seventies, you're down about 20 percent (in skeletal muscle) from where you were at age 25 or 30."

Moreover, there are some indications that sarcopenia's ravages accelerate with time. So far, these associations "are primarily anecdotal," Harris says. However, she adds, there haven't been many attempts to look into it.

Eric T. Poehlman of the Baltimore Veterans Affairs Medical Center and his colleagues are among the few who have tackled this question. They reported finding just such a trend in the Nov. 1, 1995 *Annals of Internal Medicine.*

For 6 years, they followed 35 healthy but sedentary women who were in their mid to late forties at the start of the study. The investigators monitored such factors as physical activity, calories burned during periods of rest, and where their bodies store fat. Over this period, half of the women entered menopause.

While all the volunteers maintained a fairly constant weight, those who became menopausal lost an average of three kg of lean tissue during the study, six times the loss seen in the women of the same age who did not enter menopause. The menopausal women also became less active over the course of the study, a factor that can itself spur muscle loss.

This study didn't continue long enough to establish whether the acceleration of sarcopenia at menopause represents a permanent change. But Poehlman says his data clearly indicate that menopause "throws you into a downward spiral of muscle loss and inactivity—two things you don't want to happen."

One hallmark of menopause is a drop in a woman's production of the sex hormone estrogen. Might such a change accelerate sarcopenia? "It's possible," says endocrinologist Clifford J. Rosen of the Maine Center for Osteoporosis Research and Education at St. Joseph Hospital in Bangor.

Estrogen helps modulate the body's production of a hormone, insulinlike growth factor 1 (IGF-1), that is important for muscle growth and development, Rosen notes. Growth hormone controls concentrations of IGF-1 even more directly. Like estrogen, growth hormone declines dramatically with age in both men and women.

Rosen therefore suspects that age-related drops in growth hormone, estrogen, and other hormones may play a driving role in sarcopenia.

To test that idea, he's conducting a year-long trial with 200 frail men and women over the age of 65. Half receive daily supplements of growth hormone, the others a placebo. If the study shows that the treatment halts muscle loss or aids an individual's ability to regain muscle strength with exercise, it may hold out the prospect of hormone therapy, he says.

Charlotte A. Peterson of the McClellan Memorial Veterans Hospital in Little Rock, Arkansas, suspects that some share of sarcopenia may also trace to problems involving satellite cells, the body's poorly understood muscle repair crews. Her data indicate that here again, IGF may play a role.

A large community of these satellite cells surrounds skeletal muscle. They do nothing until a muscle needs to grow or experiences damage—such as a bruise or those minor rips that cause aches the day after exercise. Then the satellite cells spring into action, migrating to where they're needed.

Some multiply and turn into new muscle, which eventually fuses to the old muscle. Others return to their quiet state to await the next crisis. "We're trying to figure out what signals which satellite cells to do what," Peterson explains.

What is clear, she says, is that the performance of satellite cells wanes with age. Her work with rats has shown that within just a few weeks, muscle damage in a 3- to 6-month-old young adult completely disappears. But when an elderly 24- to 28-month-old animal sustains the same damage, the satellite cells' repair proceeds much more slowly and often incompletely.

The real problem, she notes, may be not the satellite cells themselves but rather the body's difficulty in communicating with them. Other researchers have shown that when they transplant muscle and its satellite cells from an old animal into a young one, the muscle again heals rapidly.

Insulinlike growth factors "seem to be really important in controlling satellite cell function," Peterson says. Her preliminary evidence indicates "that satellite cells from older animals mount a less robust IGF response following injury." This suggests, she says, "that it's production of the growth factor that may be impaired."

Age-related neurological changes may also play a pivotal role in sarcopenia. Over decades, the body loses nerves, including those that branch out from the spinal cord into skeletal muscle throughout the body. As one of these nerves dies, a neighbor sends out branches to rescue the muscle fibers that had been abandoned. Without such a new nerve connection, that muscle would eventually shrink and die.

But there's a limit to how much a nerve can grow, according to studies by neurologist Jan Lexell of Lund University Hospital in Sweden.

"It's somewhere around two to three times its original size," he says. "So it can double the number of muscle fibers that it innervates" but probably no more. When surviving nerves are no longer numerous enough to rescue all of the abandoned muscle fibers, he says, sarcopenia becomes inevitable.

Studies that have attempted to quantify the loss of these muscle-innervating nerves find that somewhere between one-quarter and one-half of them die off between the ages of 25 and 75. Moreover, Lexell observes, because the rate of nerve loss "speeds up after age 60," persons approaching 90 are likely to have suffered dramatically more loss.

His studies indicate that the first muscle fibers to go are those used the least—rapidly contracting fibers that serve as a sort of muscular overdrive. The body calls on them to execute the most intense and rapid activities, such as heavy lifting and sprinting. The progressive loss of different types of muscle "accounts for part of the slowing of our movements with age," he says, and much of the frailty.

What all these studies confirm, Rosenberg maintains, is that although sarcopenia may represent a universal symptom of aging today, it should not be accepted as normal. Instead, he argues, it should be considered a newly recognized disease—amenable to prevention and treatment.

In fact, a series of studies at his center indicate that exercise regimen that focus on high-intensity resistance training of the arms and legs go a long way toward countering disabling frailty in the elderly. Lexell agrees, noting that this type of exercise wakes up languishing overdrive muscles by challenging them to gradually and steadily lift or move increasingly heavy weights.

"Older people who have done weight lifting over the last 15 to 20 years will have muscles the same size as someone who is 20 and sedentary," he notes.

It's never too late to start that muscle training, according to studies over the past few years led by Nelson and Maria A. Fiatarone of the Tufts center. In one 10-week study of 100 frail nursing home residents between the ages of 72 and 98, individuals more than doubled the strength of trained muscles and increased their stair-climbing power by 28 percent when they exercised their legs with resistance training three times a week.

Nelson's group then prescribed a less rigorous training regimen, with workouts only twice a week, in a year-long study with 50- to 70-year-old women. Not only did those who exercised increase their strength throughout the study, but they also gained skeletal muscle. Women who remained sedentary declined on both measures.

Moreover, this training offers payoffs that go well beyond sarcopenia, notes William J. Evans of Pennsylvania State University in University Park. A physiologist, he collaborated with the Tufts team on several of their exercise studies. While those women assigned to an exercise group in the year-long study gained a little bone over the course of their training, he notes that those who remained sedentary lost about 2 percent of their bone.

In another study, his group found that elderly men and women who performed strength training for 3 months burned 15 percent more calories over the course of a day than their sedentary counterparts. The difference was traced not so much to their increased exercise but to a boost in their metabolism, which should fight sluggishness and weight gain, he says.

In fact, he notes, those elderly adults who follow through on weight training tend to voluntarily increase their activity. In some cases, this training also enabled them to forsake wheelchairs for a walker or cane.

That's one reason the Tufts center is fighting sarcopenia so actively, Rosenberg says. Muscle loss is robbing the elderly of their freedom. "We want to give it back."

—by Janet Raloff

Part Five

Specific Activities

Chapter 35

Everday Fitness

Contents

Section 35.1

Adding More Physical Activity to Your Lifestyle

From *Tufts University Health & Nutrition Letter*, March 1999 v17 i1 p1(1). Reprinted with permission, *Tufts University Health & Nutrition Letter*, tel: 1-800-274-7581.

The researchers did not intend for Bruce MacDonald or Cynthia Gonzalez to lose any weight. Yes, they had asked the two to incorporate more physical activity into their lifestyles by walking, gardening, or engaging in other everyday activities. But, in the two-year study conducted at the Cooper Institute for Aerobics Research in Dallas, the scientists simply wanted to see if that kind of here-and-there workout was as effective as structured exercise at a health club for improving heart and lung capacity and reducing the risk for heart disease. Weight loss for the two moderately overweight subjects— along with about 120 other participants—was not a goal.

However, since the research project began (and ended) several years ago, MacDonald, a 5-foot, 10-inch tall elementary school principal now 54 years old, went from weighing "in the 190s with a paunch," as he puts it, to 170 pounds. (That's in addition to improving his heart rate and bringing his blood cholesterol from the 240s to about 200—the cutoff point for "desirable" total cholesterol.) The 5-foot, 3-inch Gonzalez, then a sales manager for AT&T, started out weighing "close to 150" and now, at age 52, gets the needle on the scale only to 135.

Edith Dersch, a participant in a similar study designed to compare the effects of structured exercise with squeezing more physical activity into the day here and there, was supposed to lose weight. Researchers at Johns Hopkins University and the University of Pennsylvania asked her and about 20 others in her group to follow a 1,200-calorie diet along with accumulating at least 30 minutes of moderate-intensity physical activity on most, if not all, days of the week.

The result: Dersch, a 5-foot, 7½-inch-tall engineering technician who weighed 188 at the start of the study, got down to 133 pounds by the time the research ended some 16 months later. She gained back 23 pounds a couple of years later, when her mother was diagnosed with a rare lymphoma and her father died of colon cancer. But now that those crises are somewhat behind her, she has since started to turn the tide by re-losing a few pounds—mostly by getting back into walking.

How could something as low-key as some casual walking or gardening contribute to such a dramatic benefit in people like MacDonald, Gonzalez, and Dersch? The answer, at least in part: it wasn't all that casual.

More Intense Than It Appears

When it comes to incorporating more physical activity into one's lifestyle, "everybody wants to make it sound like a stroll in the mall," says Andrea Dunn, PhD, study leader at the Cooper Institute for Aerobics Research. "But we're talking brisk walk," she says—"three to four miles an hour."

"One week, we took study subjects on a walk down a hallway to show them just what a brisk walk feels like," Dr. Dunn says. While it's not necessarily working up a sweat, she comments, it's also not "sauntering along." Similarly, accumulating physical activity in the back yard does not include watering the window boxes. People were "digging, relandscaping their yards," Dr. Dunn reports. They were "laying down new pathways with stones."

Ross Andersen, PhD, head researcher of the Johns Hopkins study in which Dersch participated, agrees. "If you just walk up and down the stairs a couple of times" a day, that's not going to cut it, he says. People in his program would use stairs by always going to the bathroom on another floor. Also, he remarks, they didn't "pile things on the bottom of the stairs" to carry up at the end of the day. They walked up and down the stairs every time they came across something that belonged on another floor. And when it came to chores, there was no more hiring a neighborhood kid to mow the lawn and do weeding and no more driving around the corner to the convenience store. People walked for a quart of milk; they looked for all kinds of opportunities to incorporate moving around into their days.

It wasn't always an easy shift after years of living a sedentary life. The goal was 10,000 steps a day for walkers, study participant Gonzalez explains. But a pedometer lent to her by the researchers showed her that she was doing 3,000 to 5,000 steps. And she was resistant to upping her total. She recalls complaining, "I'm too busy; I travel. It was hard at first," she says. "I made excuses—even the weather."

She also started out small and worked to a gradual buildup. "I don't have time to walk for 30 minutes," she originally told herself, "but I could walk for five. I can park my car further" away and accumulate some steps that way.

Dersch didn't have it terribly easy at first, either. "I would take a five- to eight-minute walk twice a day" at work, she says. At night, she had to make up the difference by taking a 15- or 20-minute walk. It took "a conscientious effort," she explains. "I would keep a running total every day" to be sure to accumulate 30 minutes.

Better Results Than Numbers Show

As difficult as it was to go from being sedentary to active in their daily lives, neither MacDonald, Gonzalez, nor Dersch would return to their old habits. Says MacDonald, "I felt more tired at the end of the day before I started to exercise."

He also says that having become fitter and trimmer "feels great. It feels great when I take a bath not to have a roll there. I get compliments all the time.

"I have gray hair, I'm balding," he remarks. "I look my age. But my body is trim. A guy with a flat stomach—you don't see that often at my age."

Gonzalez points out that "my stamina is longer and I can walk longer. People say I got more energized."

Dersch, who had been dealt a double blow of family illness, says, "if I hadn't gone through the program and lost the weight, it wouldn't have been as easy to handle the responsibilities." She felt she "could better handle things" as a result of "handling" her body.

Interestingly, none of the study participants had originally thought physical activity was an option. They thought exercise meant joining a health club or jogging outdoors in gym shorts, which they were all too self-conscious or too busy (or too disinterested) to do. But today, MacDonald strength-trains at a gym, while Gonzalez (who has taken early retirement) uses a health club treadmill in bad weather.

For researchers Dunn and Andersen, getting people to move from physically oriented lifestyle activities to a more structured exercise setting isn't the ultimate aim. What's important, says Dr. Dunn, is that there's "a menu of choices for people" that goes beyond what a gym or health club has to offer. "We can't expect one type of hypertension medication to work for all hypertensive people," she says. "Why should we expect all fitness programs to be the same?"

Dr. Andersen puts it this way: the lifestyle approach "affords people options. Exercise doesn't necessarily have to be incredibly vigorous or uninterrupted. But if you look at the impact of counting up at least 30 minutes of purposeful moving around most days of the week, over the course of a year it adds u to some pretty serious calories."

We're not talking about blaring Cindy Crawford tapes into the womb or anything, but evidence suggests that fitness begins just about when life does. According to a Boston University study, the more your child moves around as a preschooler, the less likely he is to become an overweight school-age child. And that could save him from becoming an overweight adult.

In this study of 103 preschoolers, those who moved around the least tended to gain body fatness, while those who moved the most tended to lose it during the 2 1/2 years of the study (*American Journal of Epidemiology*, October 15, 1993).

"Physical fitness definitely starts at a very young age," says study director Lynn L. Moore, D.Sc., M.P.H., assistant professor of medicine at Boston University School of Medicine. As Barney and Tetris become masters at keeping kids sitting still, it's increasingly up to parents to see that kids stay active. That means getting out there with the kids, says Dr. Moore. There's clear evidence that how active the parents are influences how active the children will be.

Don't let a bad back or a bum knee stop you. Lawn games like croquet or boccie keep kids running around to see where the balls land, yet can be soft on your aches until you recover. If you're totally sidelined, cheer from there—kids love to be watched and to show off what they can do.

Indoors, if possible, kids should have a place to play that's free of breakables, says Dr. Moore. In bad weather, set up an obstacle course in that space. Or hold the edges of a sheet and use it to bounce a ball into the air.

Being active as a family has benefits beyond fitness, says Dr. Moore. "Kids who learn to do physical things not only become more skilled at those activities, but also develop more self-confidence."

Section 35.2

Dynamic Gardening

Reprinted with permission from *Diabetes Forecast*, April 1995, vol. 48, no. 4, p. 26(7). © 1995 American Diabetes Association. For information on joining ADA and receiving *Diabetes Forecast*, call 1-800-806-7801.

Would you exercise if, after running for 5 miles, you were rewarded with a fresh garden salad made with just-picked lettuce, spinach, and radishes? If after a workout you returned to a bushel basket of fresh tomatoes, peppers, and zucchini? If after power walking you found a year's supply of fresh herbs for your table?

Then become a Dynamic Gardener! A Dynamic Gardener gardens while exercising. A Dynamic Gardener exercises while gardening. As a Dynamic Gardener, you don't focus on having a perfect lawn, an award-winning rose, or the largest tomato. Instead you focus on exercising while doing something meaningful and enjoyable.

Sound way out? It's not. Dynamic Gardening is full of old-fashioned family values: You can spend time with your children and grandchildren. (Not so easy on a treadmill.) You'll be caring for the environment. You'll practice the virtues of patience, perseverance, and tolerance. Dynamic Gardening is especially good for people with diabetes. You know there are three parts to diabetes management: exercise, good diet, and medication if needed. Dynamic Gardening takes care of the first two: While you exercise, you grow fresh fruits and vegetables, which are an important part of a healthy meal plan. What other exercise program does that?

No More Work

Your first step toward becoming a Dynamic Gardener is to change the way you think about yard work. If you think of raking as a chore you need to get done, you might go out on a Saturday, determined to rake the whole lawn without stopping. You'll rake with short, furious strokes without thinking about the effect on your body. Two days later, when muscle soreness is at its peak, the message is burned in your brain: Raking leaves is work.

When you embrace Dynamic Gardening, you might decide to rake for a half-hour after work on Monday and Tuesday. You work off some job-related stress, you get exercise 2 days instead of 1, and you don't overdo it. Raking becomes a feel-good activity.

Instead of saying, "I'm going to work in the yard," say, "I'm going to exercise in the yard." It's a subtle difference, yet profound. You're now doing one thing to achieve another. Think about it: Why is jumping around in leotards for 30 minutes exercise, yet digging a hole to plant an apple tree work?

Your second step is learning how to get a good, safe workout in your garden. If you have ever raked, hoed, or weeded a garden bed, you already know that gardening provides a good workout. But maybe no one has ever shown you "how" to garden: how not to strain your back, and how to avoid getting sore from repeating the same motion for hours.

Learning to use gardening as exercise is, in many ways, easiest if you have never gardened before. You won't have to unlearn old ways of gardening.

If you have gardened for years, please try to keep an open mind, allow yourself time, and use what is comfortable for you. I know I'm asking you to change habits you've developed over many years.

The core concepts of Dynamic Gardening are aerobics, resistance training, and balance. Balance means letting gardening be a part of your lifestyle. How much or how little is up to you. (Please consult with your health care team before starting this or any other exercise program. While it may appear strange to get clearance to garden, Dynamic Gardening can be every bit as strenuous as playing tennis or jogging.)

Aerobic Gardening

Plan to garden at least three times a week for a minimum of 30 minutes, and preferably for an hour. Allow yourself several weeks to build up your muscles, and start as early in the spring as possible.

If you're not in good condition, absolutely avoid marathon sessions of 4 to 8 hours of weeding, raking, or hoeing. You'll be sore all week.

Warm Up

Warm up and stretch out before you garden. Perhaps you have a favorite routine. If not, check out *Diabetes Forecast*, "Stretching," April 1994, pp. 26-31.

When it's either raining or too cold to garden outside, stretch inside your house for 5 to 15 minutes. Strive to stretch every day: Americans don't stretch enough, and it's good to keep up your routine. When the sun does come out, you'll be ready to garden.

Work Out

Plan three or more separate activities or motions for each gardening session. Each one can range from 5 minutes to an hour or more. Some examples:

- Rake, hoe, and weed—and switch your position and stance every 5 to 15 minutes.

- Exaggerate your motions. Rake and hoe with wide, sweeping motions. Keep the motions smooth and steady.

- Maintain a steady breathing rate as you rake, dig, or hoe.

Other Activities

- mow the lawn
- plant trees or bushes
- lift potted plants

- prune
- prepare flower beds
- turn the compost pile

Cool Down

Walk briskly around the garden. Plant or pick flowers or vegetables.

Resistance Gardening

Resistance training is often associated with barbells and young athletes. However, recent studies have shown that resistance training is beneficial at any age, and it's particularly good for seniors.

When you rake, hoe, or dig, you are exercising against the resistance of the weeds, grass, or soil. Therefore, resistance-training concepts can be added to gardening motions.

Repetitions and Sets

A repetition is how many times you do something. For example, raking in and out 25 times would be 25 repetitions. This can be considered one set. You might choose to rake in five sets of 25, resting after each set.

Do you need to count? Absolutely not. But thinking in terms of repetitions and sets serves to remind you that this is exercise. And that reminds you to keep your motions smooth and steady, with good extension, and to give your muscles a good workout without overdoing it.

Breathing

Breathe in and out regularly as you garden. While this might seem obvious, you'd be surprised at how often you hold your breath during strenuous activity. Breathe out as you extend your rake, breathe in as you pull it in.

Lifting

Whether you're lifting a wheelbarrow, a potted plant, or concrete blocks, the motion is the same—keep your back straight; bend from your knees, not your waist; and use your legs, not your back. Done properly and in moderation, lifting heavy objects can be beneficial to your arms, shoulders, and legs. Once again, since the focus is now on your needs and not getting the yard to look like the Smith's, avoid planting 20 bushes or moving a ton of sand in one day.

Digging

As with lifting, bend your knees as you dig. You want to let your legs do most of the work rather than your back or arms. Alternate between a right-handed and left-handed stance.

More

Want to go the extra mile? Add workout structures to your garden. I've built a pull-up/chin-up bar, a dip bar, and a sit-up board in my backyard. My "gym" is only a few steps from my back door. After planting flowers or picking vegetables, I try to get in a few sets of pull-ups, dips, and sit-ups.

Balance Gardening

Where other fitness programs focus on one diet, one exercise, or a pill, powder, or a few foods, Dynamic Gardening focuses on the whole person. It balances our relationship to our environment. Instead of a quick fix, Dynamic Gardening is a lifestyle, one that can be sustained, year after year, decade after decade. And the beauty of it is that the result of this fitness lifestyle is a cornucopia of flowers, trees, herbs, fruits, and vegetables.

Traditional Gardening

- Large garden.
- Summer garden.
- Rake with same hand all the time.
- One stance or motion.
- Grow only a few types of vegetables.
- Garden for 4,6, or 8 hours in one day.
- Use same muscles all day.
- Get the job done, whatever it takes.

Dynamic Gardening

- Small garden.
- Expand exercise time by planting a spring, summer, and fall garden.
- Alternate left-handed and right-handed raking.
- Use different stances. Vary the way you weed.
- Grow a variety of interesting fruits, vegetables, herbs, and flowers. This keeps you interested in gardening, and helps you vary your workout. If you grow just one vegetable, you might slip into working the whole garden one way. But if you have a variety of plants—some tall, some close to the ground, some that require more work in the beginning of the season, others that require work at the end of the season—you'll vary your workout. You'll avoid the one-stance, one-motion trap that leads to overuse of certain muscles.
- Garden in short sessions of 20 to 60 minutes.
- Vary garden workouts to purposely exercise your arms, legs, back, stomach, and chest.

—by Jeffrey Restuccio

Chapter 36

Aerobic Fitness: The Heartbeat of Your Fitness Program

The term aerobic means "with oxygen." During an aerobic workout, the cardiovascular system (which includes the heart, lungs, and blood vessels), responds to increased levels of physical activity by increasing the oxygen that is available to the body.

Aerobic activity involves an exercise routine that uses large muscle groups, is maintained for a sustained period of time and is rhythmic in nature. Regular aerobic exercise improves your level of fitness, as your heart becomes stronger and begins to work more efficiently. The end result is that the heart can pump more blood (thus increasing oxygen delivery to the tissues) with each heartbeat. As your aerobic fitness increases you will be able to work out longer, with greater intensity, and you will recover more quickly at the end of your workout session.

What Are Some Examples of Aerobic Exercise?

There are numerous activities that can provide an aerobic workout. Some examples include biking, jogging, running, swimming, cross-country skiing, basketball, jumping rope, roller skating, brisk walking and dancing. In addition to these activities, an aerobic workout can be achieved in a specially designed aerobic dance class or by using exercise machines (stationary bikes, treadmills, stair-steppers, rowing machines, just to name a few) that can be found at a local gym or health club. Most of these machines can also be purchased and set up for home use.

Now that you are aware of the types of activities that can provide an aerobic workout, it's easier to see how you can fit this kind of exercise activity into your routine.

Who Can Participate in Aerobic Exercise?

Most everyone can participate in some type of aerobic exercise. Since each type of aerobic exercise can be modified to varying intensity levels, people with different fitness goals, levels of physical conditioning and injury/illness history can participate.

If you are just beginning an exercise program, are over age forty, or have a known history of heart disease, high blood pressure or other cardiovascular disorder, it is advised that you consult with your physician before beginning any exercise program.

Aerobic exercise has proven beneficial for people with a variety of medical disorders like heart disease, diabetes, obesity, arthritis, anxiety, and premenstrual syndrome.

What Are the Added Benefits of Aerobic Exercise?

Studies have shown repeatedly that there are numerous health benefits to aerobic exercise. In addition to the benefits to the cardiovascular system, aerobic exercise can:

- Increase resistance to fatigue and give you more energy. Aerobic exercise can add life to your years along with years to your life.

- Improve mood, reduce depression and anxiety. Positive mood changes have been noted after as little as two to three weeks of aerobic exercise.

- Improve the quality of your sleep. Studies show that people who exercise regularly get to sleep quicker and report more restful sleep patterns. It is best to complete your aerobic exercise routine one to two hours before your regular bedtime since it takes a little time for the general emotional and physical relaxation to set in after a workout.

- Increase the good (HDL) cholesterol. This type of cholesterol is known to reduce the risk of heart disease.

- Help to control and reduce body fat. Aerobic exercise in conjunction with proper diet can decrease body fat.

- Reduce the risk of certain types of cancer. Aerobic exercise has been associated with a reduction in the incidence of colon cancer in both males and females and the incidence of breast and reproductive organ cancers in women.

What to Consider when Developing an Aerobic Workout Schedule

Three important factors affect an aerobic workout: frequency, duration, and intensity.

- Frequency refers to how often you perform aerobic activity.

- Duration refers to the amount of time spent at each aerobic session.

- Intensity refers to the percentage of your maximum heart rate that is achieved during the workout.

The American College of Sports Medicine (ACSM) recommends that aerobic activity be performed 3-5 times per week, for 20-60 minutes, at an intensity of 60-90% of maximum heart rate. (To determine your maximum heart rate subtract your age from 220, then multiply this number by .60 for the low end of your target heart range and by .90 for the higher range)

Heart Rates and Target Zones for Aerobic Exercise

For general guidelines used in determining your maximum heart rate and target heart rate ranges, refer to Table 36.1.

If you are just beginning an aerobic workout routine, it may take several months before you are able to meet these guidelines. Stick with it. It is always important to gradually increase your frequency, duration, and intensity. This is especially true if you are overweight, deconditioned, elderly, or are recovering from a recent illness or injury.

A warm up and a cool down period, both of which should incorporate stretching exercises, are essential parts of aerobic conditioning. Warm-up helps your body get ready for exercise by slowly raising your heart beat and muscle temperature. This will also decrease the likelihood of injury.

Table 36.1. Target Heart Rate Ranges.

Age	Maximum Heart Rate (beats/minute)	Target Range (beats/minute)
20-24	200	120-150
25-29	195	117-146
30-34	190	114-142
35-39	185	111-139
40-44	180	108-135
45-49	174	105-131
50-54	170	102-127
55-59	165	99-123
60-64	160	96-120
65-69	155	93-116
70 and over	150	90-113

Table 36.2. Calories burned during aerobic exercise.

Activity & cal./min.	120 lbs.	140 lbs.	160 lbs.	180 lbs.
Aerobics class	7.4	8.6	9.8	11.1
Basketball	7.5	8.8	10	11.3
Cycling (10mph)	5.5	6.4	7.3	8.2
Golf(carry clubs)	4.6	5.4	6.2	7.0
Golf (power cart)	2.1	2.5	2.8	3.2
Hiking	4.5	5.2	6.0	6.7
Jogging	9.3	10.8	12.4	13.9
Running	11.4	13.2	15.1	17.0
Skating	5.9	6.9	7.9	8.8
Skiing (cross country)	7.5	8.8	10.0	11.3
Skiing (downhill and water)	5.7	6.6	7.6	8.5
Swimming	7.8	9.0	10.3	11.6
Tennis	6.0	6.9	7.9	8.9
Walking	6.5	7.6	8.7	9.7
Weight Training	6.6	7.6	8.7	9.8

A cool down allows the heart rate to slowly return to normal and to get the blood circulating freely back to the heart. Never abruptly discontinue an aerobic activity, no matter how tired you may become, since this could result in dizziness or sudden fainting. If you are unable to maintain the pace of an aerobic workout, simply slow down, walk around for a few minutes, before discontinuing the activity.

Fluid replacement is important before, during, and after your scheduled workout.

How Many Calories Does Aerobic Exercise Burn?

The number of calories that you burn during aerobic exercise will vary with the activity and intensity of the workout. The information in Table 36.2 is taken from *ACE FitnessMatters*, Volume 1, Number 4, 1995. Calories are given for one minute of activity. To determine how many calories you would burn in 1/2 hour of aerobic activity, multiply the number shown by 30.

What Type of Equipment Do You Need for Aerobic Exercise?

The necessary equipment will vary according to your planned aerobic activity. When undergoing any type of aerobic exercise it is important to dress comfortably. Cotton clothing tends to pull moisture away from the body and will help to keep you cool. Women should wear a sports bra for support.

Select a pair of shoes designed for your particular activity. All athletic shoes are not the same. When purchasing shoes, make sure that they are well fitted and properly cushioned.

In order to determine your heart rate you will need access to a clock or watch with a sweep second hand. Devices are available that automatically calculate your heart rate and many of the newer pieces of exercise equipment are now equipped with a heart rate monitor.

What Are the Disadvantages to Aerobic Exercise?

Like any new activity, it takes time for the body to adjust to change. You may experience some soreness and stiffness as you begin a new aerobic workout. The most common injuries resulting from aerobic workouts include joint and muscle strains and sprains.

Some people with severely compromised cardiovascular systems may be advised to avoid aerobic workouts. It is best to check with your physician before engaging in any new exercise program.

In addition to cardiovascular training, experts recommend a balanced workout that includes strength and flexibility training. By adding these components to your aerobic routine, you can decrease your risk of injury.

Glossary of Terms

Aerobics: A sustained activity that relies on oxygen for energy.

Duration: The amount of time spent at each aerobic session.

Flexibility: The ability of a bone, joint, or muscle to stretch.

Frequency: How often aerobic activity is performed.

Intensity: The amount of force or energy expended during a workout.

Maximum Heart Rate (MHR): The rate at which your heart pumps blood during a very vigorous workout. Do not exceed your maximum heart rate. MHR= 220 - your age.

Stretching: Exercise which increases the ease and degree to which a muscle or joint can turn, bend or reach.

Target Heart Rate (THR): A percentage of your maximum heart rate that should be achieved during aerobic exercise. THR can be anywhere from 60 to 90% of your MHR

Workout: A planned series of exercises.

References

American College of Sports Medicine (ACSM)

American Council on Exercise (ACE)

American Heart Association

Brick, Lynne. *Fitness Aerobics*. 1996 by Human Kinetics Publishers, Inc.

President's Council on Physical Fitness and Sports: Get fit. How to Get in Shape to Meet the President's Challenge.

Disclaimer: The text presented on these pages is for your information only. It is not a substitute for professional medical advice. It may not represent your true individual medical situation. Do not use this information to diagnose or treat a health problem or disease without consulting a qualified health care provider. Please consult your health care provider if you have any questions or concerns.

Chapter 37

Test Your Walking IQ

You have probably heard about the benefits of being physically fit. You see commercials about lowering your fat and cholesterol. You hear about the latest fitness trends everywhere you go. Your friends want to lose weight or join a gym. For some, competitive sports are the answer, but you can't fit regular practices into an already busy schedule. You want an activity that's easy, doesn't take too long, but gives you the benefits of an aerobic workout. Here are some questions to test your knowledge about fitness trends in the '90s:

- You need an activity that doesn't cost much. What can you do?

- You don't have much free time, and the time you do have changes from week to week so that sticking to a routine is very difficult. How can you stay fit?

- You want to prevent the possibility of getting diabetes because people in your family have it. What can you do?

- What's the best way to lower your cholesterol level?

- You're always hungry and you want to be careful not to eat too much. What's the best way to reduce your appetite?

- What exercise is practically injury-free?

- What can you do to help increase the length of your life?

From *Current Health 2*, November 1997, vol. 24, no. 3, p. 20(2). © 1997 Weekly Reader Corporation; reprinted with permission.

- How can you become more heart healthy?

- What can you do to tone and strengthen your muscles?

- If you worry or are stressed out about something, how can you reduce that stress naturally?

- How can you lose weight and keep it off?

- If high blood pressure runs in your family, what can you do to avoid developing it?

- If your hands and feet are always cold due to poor circulation, what can help increase the blood flow?

If you answer some of these questions by saying "exercise," then you have been paying attention to the news. And if you answered each question with "walk," you are a walking genius—and you're right on track. Walking is the most popular exercise in the United States, according to *Sporting Goods Magazine*. In fact, more than 73 million people do exercise walking. It's an inexpensive, natural, and practically injury-free form of exercise. Did you know the average person will walk about 115,000 miles in a lifetime? That is more than four trips around the world.

Getting Started

You've decided to give walking a try. After all, you've been doing it since you were about a year old. You have perfected it so much by now that you don't even think about how to walk anymore. It's an easy exercise: no new rules to learn, no special equipment to buy. You don't have to gather a team together. All you have to do is get up off your couch and walk for about 20 to 30 minutes three times a week. As with all exercise programs, you will need to start with a few stretches, though. Don't forget this part because even the best walkers may get sore or injured if their muscles aren't warmed up. Spend about five minutes stretching. Include your arms, back, and sides in your stretching. When you're finished walking, spend some more time stretching your muscles. This will increase your flexibility and keep you from getting sore muscles.

You might want to plan a regular time in your schedule for walking (maybe first thing in the morning, right after school, or after dinner). This helps to ensure that you will do it and make it a habit. Find an enjoyable route to walk. Start with a 20-minute walk at a moderate pace and work up to 30 to 45 minutes at a brisk pace. Do this for at least three days a week, but no more than six days a week, using one day to rest your legs. You will be breathing harder and your heart rate will increase, but you should be able to talk to a friend while you are walking. If you find you are too out of breath to talk, you may need to slow down a little.

Walk This Way?

Believe it or not, there are different ways to walk. These include race walking, power or aerobic walking, hiking, sprint walking, and resistance walking. You have probably done most of these types of walks at one time or another, except race walking.

Race walking has a few rules. One foot must always be in contact with the ground and the leg must be straight from the time it strikes the around until it passes under the body. Power or aerobic walking refers to walking done in short spurts to build up stamina during an aerobic walk. Resistance walking is using hills to strengthen the leg muscles. Be careful while going downhill. You will want to walk slower than usual to avoid knee injury and injury to toenails by having them squeezed to the front of your shoe. Resistance walking is sometimes done by walking on level ground using ankle weights or putting on a backpack; but overall, hills are a better workout.

Shoes Made for Walking

Although walking is almost injury-free, you will want a good pair of shoes if you are going to walk regularly for fitness: sneakers that have shock absorbers in the heel and under the ball of the foot. The shoe should be lightweight, made out of canvas so it can breathe. Choose a shoe that is flexible, yet provides support and stability. Finally, make sure that your shoes fit you snugly but not tightly. This will give your feet more support and keep them from getting blisters.

Street Smarts

Yes, you say, walking is a great way to go. It will tone and develop my muscles, help me lose weight and feel great. Before you hit the streets, though, make sure you've developed your street smarts. Here are some tips to keep in mind:

- If you walk at night, always walk with a friend.
- Use reflective tape on your clothing so you will be seen.

477

- Avoid using headphones. They can put you in danger by masking sounds of traffic or someone approaching.

- Be aware of any dogs off their leashes, and cross the street, if necessary, to avoid them.

—by Tracy Early

Chapter 38

Making a Splash: Water Resistance Provides a Great Workout

Gravity got you down? Are you tired of the discomfort that accompanies pulled muscles and overworked joints? Consider taking the plunge into a less risky world of fitness. Water aerobics can provide an effective workout with the power to soothe, calm and refresh you.

The Wonder of Water Workouts

Although its popularity is at high tide, aquatic exercise has been around for years—originally used as a form of rehabilitative therapy for injured athletes. Sports medicine experts discovered water's buoyancy, resistance, and therapeutic massaging effect contributed to the healing process.

Those same characteristics proved irresistible to athletes searching for a cross-training tool and less risky exercise challenge. A water workout not only meets these needs, but provides added benefits as a bonus.

Water, acting as a giant cushion, saves wear and tear on your muscles while protecting the joints. As you work against the resistance of the water, it works with you, minimizing the sort of injuries typical of high-impact exercise. "The water pressure massages muscles, helping reduce lactic acid," says Patricia Clark, fitness and aerobics director at Hollywood-Wilshire YMCA. "Basically, the benefits of land-based aerobics are enhanced in the water."

Reprinted with permission from the Aerobics and Fitness Association of America. *American Fitness Magazine*, © 1996, vol. 14, no. 3, p. 30(5), May-June 1996.

Sports medicine specialist Daniel Kulund, M.D., of Charlottesville, Virginia uses water training to treat delicate injuries to knees and Achilles' tendons. "Water training is a good way of maintaining fitness without suffering the ravages of impact," says Kulund. In fact, when an exerciser is submerged to neck level, gravitational pull on the body is reduced by about 90%. When water workouts are employed as a cross-training device, injuries may decrease while fitness is maintained.

Water training works wonders for your overall balance and coordination, making it an ideal tool to improve your skills in other activities. "The opposition of movement between the arms and legs is the basis for all human coordination, explains Linda Huey of Huey's Athletic Network in Santa Monica, California and the creator of The Waterpower Workout®.

Building a Better Body

Increased strength is another plus. With water recruiting more muscle fibers and providing approximately 12 times the resistance of air, you can count on a heavy-duty workout. "There are benefits to water training that are simply not matched on land," says Huey, who also trains Olympic and professional athletes.

Muscle pairs (biceps/triceps, quadriceps/hamstrings and adductors/abductors) maintain a specific ratio of strength to each other. If you overtrain one of the pairs, you produce inefficiency and the potential for injury. Exercising in water forces you to work both parts of muscle pairs, according to Huey. In fact, work downward against buoyancy counterbalances the effects of gravity and strengthens the muscles that are engaged to maintain posture. "For every push against the water's resistance, you must pull backward to the starting position," she explains. "For every swing upward, you must swing downward."

To maintain flexibility and increase range of motion, stretching in water can't be beat. Your body relaxes in warm water like nowhere else, and this relaxation promotes comfortable, rhythmic breathing which enables you to further increase your limberness. Water aerobics also stimulates circulation while increasing the flow of blood to injured areas.

Unlike land-based exercise, water has its own built-in cooling system, which may keep your heart rate about 10 beats slower per minute than it would be in an aerobics class. But don't worry about lessening the intensity of your workouts. Studies have shown aqua aerobics still put sufficient demand on your heart and circulatory system to improve their efficiency. Additionally, the heart pumps 10% to 20% more blood per beat when the body is submerged in water (even in shallow depths), similar in effect to the pumping capacity of the heart of a peak-performance athlete.

In order to progress and sustain conditioning, you'll need a workout session two or three times a week, alternating water aerobics with land-based activities. A water fitness program should include the same key elements of any workout: a warm-up, 20 or 30 minutes of aerobic activity, strengthening movements, stretches to enhance flexibility and cool-down exercises. You can burn several calories, but the number varies depending on exercise design, skill, water temperature and body composition. The more muscle groups you use, the more rapidly you can achieve an aerobic effect.

Be sure to keep an eye on the water temperature. A comfortable water temperature of 84 degrees is recommended, according to fitness researchers W. McArdle, F. Katch and V. Katch.

Water at 80 degrees Fahrenheit disperses body heat about four times faster than air at the same temperature, naturally helping to maintain the core body temperature within an acceptable range and preventing the overheating common with landbased exercise.

So grab a cool drink and head for the pool or spa. Where else can you allow the day's tensions to melt away and achieve a sleek, strong body at the same time?

Gearing Up

Great strides have been achieved in the creation of water training equipment. The following items greatly amplify the natural resistance of water.

What You Need

- Aquatic dumbbells: Filled with water, they add resistance to your workout.

- Ankle weights: Usually weigh three to five pounds a pair. Add buoyancy and resistance to lower-body workouts.

- Webbed gloves: Made of lycra/nylon to enhance resistance of water.

- Flotation device: To suspend you in deep water.

- Wet vest: To keep you warm in water.

- Aquatic exercise audiotapes: To keep you moving and motivated.

Where to Buy

- Bioenergetics: (800) 433-2627
- Excel Sports Science: (800) 922-9544
- Hydro Fit, Inc.: (800) 346-7295
- Hydrophonics: (800) 794-6626
- Hydro-Tone Fitness Systems: (800) 622-8663
- Speedo Authentic Fitness Corp.: (800) 547-8770
- Sprint/Rothhammer International: (800) 235-2156
- Strom-berg Productions: (800) 82 TUNES
- WaterWear: (800) 321-7848

Aquatic Resources

Aerobics and Fitness Association of America: 15250 Ventura Blvd., Suite 200, Sherman Oaks, CA 91403; (800) 446-2322; http://www.afaa.com. Offers Aqua Fitness Home Study with Aqua Fitness video to provide instructors with valuable tools to create and teach a safe and effective class. This course brings an in-depth overview of the properties of water and how they apply to exercise science as well as the latest in research supporting the positive effects water resistance has on muscular strengthening and cardiovascular endurance. 6 AFAA CEUs.

The Aquatic Exercise Association: 3439 Technology Dr., Nokomis, FL 34275; (941) 486-8600; http://www.aeawave.com. Offers instructor training, workshops, certifications, conferences, information regarding aquatic exercise, finding a pool facility and certified aquatic instructor in your area and exercise equipment.

National Spa and Pool Institute: 2111 Eisenhower Ave. Alexandria, VA 22314-4698; (703) 838-0083; http://www.nspi.org. Publishes consumer brochures about pools, spas and water exercise.

"Aquatic Exercise" by Ruth Sova, M.S. Jones and Bartlett, $14. (508) 443-5000.

"The W.E.T. Workout" by Jane Katz, Ed.D. (Facts-on-File, $12.95) (800) 322-8755.

—by Bobbi Moreno

Chapter 39

Bicycling

Contents

Section 39.1

Ride It Off: Losing Weight through Cycling

From *Men's Health*, September 1999, vol. 14, issue 7, p. 100. © 1999 Rodale Press Inc. Reprinted with permission.

If you really want to shed your gut, pick up the first piece of fitness equipment you ever owned: your bike. Not only will cycling free you from the senses-dulling stairclimber routine, but it won't pound your joints or jiggle your gut the way running will. And done right, it can burn more calories than either.

To get fit fast, you need to ride so that you burn the maximum amount of calories and fat while steering clear of injuries. Here are nine strategies from the country's top cycling authorities.

1. **Ride at least 4 days a week**. Consistency rules when it comes to losing weight on the bike, says Edmund Burke, Ph.D., author of *Serious Cycling*. To lose a pound or two a week, aim for a minimum of three short rides of 30 to 60 minutes each during the week, and one longer trip of 1 to 2 hours on the weekend. If you haven't been on your bike for a while, stick to shorter rides until you're in good enough condition for a long one, Burke advises.

2. **Don't go too fast.** Most guys jump on their bikes and start hammering like they're Lance Armstrong, says Chris Carmichael, former head coach of the U.S. Olympic Cycling Team and currently, well, Lance Armstrong's coach. That kind of all-out riding pushes your heart rate into the anaerobic range, so your body can't send oxygen to your muscles fast enough to burn fat. A recent article in the *Journal of Strength and Conditioning Research* concluded that fat oxidation—the rate at which you burn stored fat for fuel—peaks at about 60 percent of your maximum heart rate. "I coach riders to train just above that, at 65 to 75 percent, for the best overall fitness benefits," says Carmichael. The most accurate way to tell whether you're riding in the right range is to calculate your

maximum heart rate (220 minus your age) and strap on a heart-rate monitor when you ride. But you can also judge just by the way you feel. Rate your exertion on a scale of 1 to 10, with 1 being a light spin and 10 on the verge of blowing up. Try to stay between 5 and 7.

3. **... unless you're pressed for time.** Opening up the throttle once a week can be smart, too, especially if your time is limited, says Burke. "You burn more calories per minute riding at a higher intensity; you just can't ride as long," he says. If you can ride for only 30 minutes on a particular day, take your heart rate up to between 75 percent and 85 percent of your maximum (about an 8 on the exertion scale).

4. **Stop coasting.** Cycling at 15 mph burns about 650 calories an hour. "But that's only if you're pedaling," says Burke. "Coasting doesn't burn many more calories than sitting in a recliner clicking the remote." To keep pedaling consistently, shift into a higher gear on easier terrain. "You'll burn twice as many calories as you would half-pedaling and half-coasting, and you'll lose weight faster."

5. **Use your low gears on flats and uphills.** Riding in a high gear feels more manly, but you'll save your knees and burn more calories by using a lower gear (a smaller chainring) and spinning quickly, the way the pros do, says Barney King, a U.S. Cycling Federation certified elite coach. "Spinning keeps you in that premium aerobic range. You burn fat without becoming fatigued." Aim for a cadence of 80 to 100 revolutions per minute. To determine your cadence, count the number of times your right leg hits the bottom of the pedal stroke in a 10-second period. Then multiply that number by six.

6. **Sit down when going up.** The quickest way to increase the intensity of your workout is to take it vertical, says Burke. "Hills burn a lot of calories in a short time." Adding hard hills to your itinerary will also make you stronger and faster—and therefore able to burn more calories—on the flats. "To climb most efficiently, drop into an easy low gear and keep spinning at no less than 60 to 70 rpm while seated," says Burke. "Standing drains energy."

7. **Leave the beaten path.** You don't see many fat mountain-bike riders. An hour of off-road riding burns about 600 calories and works your whole body, not just your legs. "There's more resistance on the trails, so you expend more energy," says Carmichael. You're building your upper-body muscles as you pull up over rocks and logs.

8. **Restock your cells with a sports drink.** After a hard ride, the glycogen, or stored fuel, in your muscles is low. You have about 20 minutes to replenish it or risk ravenously overeating later and jeopardizing your weight-loss goals, says Burke. Your best plan, he says, is to grab a sports drink that contains carbohydrates and protein in a 4-to-1 ratio. The protein helps repair your muscles, and the carbohydrates refuel them. "This is the step men forget," says Carmichael. "That's why they end up stuffing down $20 worth of Taco Bell in the evening and wondering why they aren't losing weight."

9. **Eat the right food at the right time.** Professional cyclists eat breakfasts that would put a lumberjack to shame. Yet they stay as skinny as their tires. "Sure, the number of hours they train helps, but the real secret is how they time their eating," says Nancy Clark, R.D., author of *Nancy Clark's Sports Nutrition Guidebook*. Most men eat a light breakfast and lunch, go out and ride hard, then eat a pound of pasta before bedtime. "That's counterproductive," says Clark. "You should eat a big meal early in the day. A large bowl of cereal, an orange, and a bagel for breakfast, along with a comfortable lunch, will let you enjoy your ride without running on empty. Then you can replenish yourself after the ride with a high-carbohydrate snack, and eat appropriately throughout the rest of the day. With the exercise and the subsequent increase in your metabolism, you'll still burn more calories than you've taken in, and you'll lose weight."

Lose the Spare Tire

Give us 4 days a week, and we'll give you a gut-busting training program. Here's what your minimum weekly workout should look like if you're riding a road bike. (You might want to get a Camelback® hydration bladder, the "look-Ma-no-hands" way to refuel with water on the road.)

- **Monday:** 45 minutes at moderate intensity (5 to 7 on an exertion scale of 10)

- **Wednesday**: 30 minutes of hills or flats at high intensity (exertion rate of 8+)

- **Friday:** 45 minutes at moderate intensity (exertion rate of 5 to 7)

- **Saturday:** 1 to 2 hours at moderate intensity (exertion rate of 5 to 7)

To build muscle while you're riding, Chris Carmichael recommends, add these drills to your workout twice a week.

- **Power starts.** Start at a very low speed (almost stopped) on a flat road. Put your bike in its biggest gear and begin hammering as hard as you can, out of the saddle, for 10 to 12 seconds or eight to 10 pedal strokes. Recover for a few minutes and repeat.

- **Stomp intervals.** On flat terrain, start rolling in your largest gear until you reach 15 to 20 mph. Then, remaining in your saddle, pedal as hard as you can for about 20 seconds. Make sure you pull through the bottom of the pedal stroke and smoothly stomp down during the downstroke. Allow at least 5 minutes of recovery time between efforts.

—by Selene Yeager

Section 39.2

Stationary Cycling: An Overview

Spinning, a type of stationary cycling, is one of the newest crazes in indoor fitness. Introduced in 1987 by super cyclist Johnny Goldberg, spinning is a non-impact indoor cycling workout that can be enjoyed by participants of all ages and fitness levels. Utilizing a specially designed stationary bike, spinning classes target both the body and mind in a unique exercise program.

What Is It?

Spinning is an exercise program that utilizes a specially designed stationary bicycle and a series of cycling movements that provide the participant with both a physical and mental workout. The spinning bike is designed to mimic an outdoor bicycle ride. The bike has fixed gear-racing handlebars, pedals equipped with clips or cages, and an adjustable bike seat. The intensity of your workout can be adjusted by manipulating the resistance knob, which is located on each spinning bicycle.

A typical spinning program lasts about 40 minutes and is often led by a spinning certified instructor. During the workout, the instructor uses a variety of visual and auditory techniques to motivate the class. Participants are often led through a simulated bike ride, where they may encounter steep hills and rolling pastures. The participants are able to make adjustments on their cycles, which correspond to the difficulty of the perceived ride. Some spinning participants wear headphones that pipe in music that simulates road conditions that may be experienced in a typical outdoor bike ride.

Heart rate monitors, often worn during the workout, allow participants to gauge how hard they are working. Once the participants get into the aerobic portion of the workout, the heart rate monitor can tell them if they are working in their target heart rate zone.

Like other well-planned aerobic workouts, spinning classes should begin with a warm-up routine and end with a cool down segment that includes stretching exercises.

Who Can Participate?

People of varying ages and fitness levels can enjoy spinning. It is considered a non-impact sport, meaning it will not place undue stress on the body's joints. Spinning is non-competitive, so people of various fitness levels can enjoy this workout together.

How Many Calories Does It Burn?

Research has shown that an average 40-minute spinning workout will burn about 500 calories. The number of calories burned by each individual will vary, depending on the intensity and duration of your workout.

Advantages

Spinning can enhance cardiovascular fitness and improve muscle tone and exercise endurance. Spinning works various muscle groups, including the quadriceps, hamstrings, calves, hips and abdominal muscles.

Participants of varying ages and fitness levels can enjoy spinning workouts. The participant determines the intensity of the workout, which fosters a non-competitive class atmosphere. For those who want to enjoy cycling year-round, spinning classes are not affected by outside weather conditions. Spinning is a great way for the outdoor cycling enthusiast to stay in shape year-round.

Spinning does not require that the participant learn any complicated dance steps, like some of the other aerobic workouts do. This eliminates the "intimidation factor" that is associated with certain aerobic workouts.

Disadvantages

The cost of a spinning program varies from one facility to another. It may be included in your overall club membership fee, or participants may be charged extra to participate. If you are interested in finding a Spinning program in your area, call 1-800-847-SPIN.

Spinning programs do require that specially designed bikes be available for use by the participant. Since spinning is still considered a relatively new form of exercise, it may not be available at many health clubs. If your fitness center does not currently provide a spinning program, express your interest to the club management.

The spinning program can be performed at home, but it requires that you purchase a specially designed bike manufactured by Schwinn, which retails for about $650.00. Experts strongly recommend that you take a few instructor-led classes before beginning this workout at home.

Many participants complain of a sore butt the first few times they take a spinning class. Bike shorts and gel seats, both of which offer special padding, can help to alleviate this discomfort.

Guidelines for Safe Spinning

The spinning program is not difficult to learn. The following guidelines are recommended for all participants.

1. Consult with your physician before beginning any new exercise program. Pre-existing health conditions, past injuries, certain medications, and other factors can all influence your ability to safely participate in a new exercise program.

2. Before beginning a spinning class, become familiar with the bicycle. Learn how to stop the pedals from moving in the event of an emergency.

3. Be sure that the bike is properly fitted and you feel comfortable before you attempt to ride it during a class.

   - **Seat height.** Your knees should be slightly bent when positioned at the bottom of the stroke pedal.

   - **Handlebar height.** Start with the handlebars at a higher level and adjust them downward as you begin to feel more comfortable riding the bike. Your elbows should be slightly bent, with your arms a comfortable distance from the handlebars.

4. Begin your ride at a comfortable pace and gradually increase it as you become more used to the bike.

5. If you should begin to feel dizzy or faint, slowly stop pedaling and inform the spinning instructor immediately.

Equipment and Gear

Cotton shirts and socks are recommended for most aerobic workouts, since this type of fiber is good at absorbing moisture. Stiffer soled shoes are recommended for spinning.

Some participants complain about soreness in the buttocks region after riding, and this can be reduced by wearing a padded cycling short or by using a gel seat. Both of these items can be found in sporting goods departments and specialty stores.

A 16-ounce sport-cap water bottle will help you to stay hydrated and can be used during the workout.

If you tend to perspire heavily during a workout, it is a good idea to bring a towel along for the ride.

Glossary of Terms

Aerobics: A sustained activity that relies on oxygen for energy.

Duration: The amount of time spent at each aerobic session.

Flexibility: The ability of a bone, joint, or muscle to stretch.

Frequency: How often aerobic activity is performed.

Hamstring: The muscle group that is located in the back of the thigh region.

Intensity: The amount of force or energy expended during a workout.

Maximum Heart Rate (MHR): The rate at which your heart pumps blood during a very vigorous workout. Do not exceed your maximum heart rate. MHR= 220 - your age.

Quadriceps: The muscle group that is located in the front of the thigh area

Spinning: A stationary bicycle exercise program aimed at achieving maximal energy expenditure utilizing a mind/body connection.

Stretching: Exercise which increases the ease and degree to which a muscle or joint can turn, bend, or reach.

Target Heart Rate (THR): A percentage of your maximum heart rate that should be achieved during aerobic exercise. THR can be anywhere from 60 to 90% of your MHR

Workout: A planned series of exercises.

491

References

- American Council on Exercise (ACE)

- E. Burke, Ph.D. and Morris, D, MS. Heart rate and caloric responses to various riding positions in well-trained individuals during a spinning class. University of Colorado, Colorado Springs, CO

- Spinning FAQs. Mad Dog Athletics, Inc.

- Schwinn Cycling and Fitness, Inc., Boulder, CO USA, 1999

Disclaimer: The text presented on these pages is for your information only. It is not a substitute for professional medical advice. It may not represent your true individual medical situation. Do not use this information to diagnose or treat a health problem or disease without consulting a qualified health care provider. Please consult your health care provider if you have any questions or concerns.

Section 39.3

Preventing Bicycle-Related Head Injuries

National Center for Injury Prevention and Control, Centers for Disease Control and Prevention. Available at www.cdc.gov/ncipc/factsheets/ bikehel.htm.

How Large a Problem Are Bicycle-Related Head Injuries in the United States?

- In 1997, 813 bicyclists were killed in crashes with motor vehicles— an increase of 7% over the previous year.[1] Of these, 31% were riders younger than 16 years old and 97% were not wearing helmets.[2]

- In 1997, an estimated 567,000 Americans sustained a bicycle-related injury that required emergency department care. Approximately two-thirds of these cyclists were children or adolescents.[3]

- An estimated 140,000 children are treated each year in emergency departments for head injuries sustained while bicycling.[4]

- In 1991, societal costs associated with bicycle-related head injury or death were estimated to exceed $3 billion.[5]

What Can Be Done?

- Riders should wear bicycle helmets every time they ride.

- In the event of a crash, wearing a bicycle helmet reduces the risk of serious head injury by as much as 85% and the risk for brain injury by as much as 88%.[6] Helmets have also been shown to reduce the risk of injury to the upper and mid-face by 65%.[7] In fact, if each rider wore a helmet, an estimated 500 bicycle-related fatalities and 151,000 nonfatal head injuries would be prevented each year—that's one death per day and one injury every four minutes.[8]

- Unfortunately, estimates on helmet usage suggest that only 25% of children ages 5-14 years wear a helmet when riding.[9] The percentage is close to zero when looking at teen riders. Children and adolescents' most common complaints are that helmets are not fashionable, or "cool," their friends don't wear them, and/or they are uncomfortable (usually too hot). Riders also convey that they do not think about the importance of bike helmets, nor about the need to protect themselves from injury, particularly if they are not riding in traffic.

- Accordingly, the national health goal for 2010 is for 50% of teenage bicyclists in 9th-12th grade to wear helmets.

What Strategies are Available to Get Bicyclists to Wear Helmets?

- The primary strategies to increase bike helmet use include education, legislation, and helmet-distribution programs. Educational programs have been conducted in different communities and schools around the nation, with generally positive results. The most successful programs are multifaceted and often multi-site campaigns that combine education with helmet giveaways or discount programs and state or local legislation requiring helmet use.

- Some evidence suggests that legislative efforts are more cost-effective than school- or community-based programs.[11]

What Is CDC Doing to Increase National Helmet Use?

- CDC developed and disseminated injury control recommendations on bicycle helmets.[12]

- CDC provides grant funding to state health departments to implement and evaluate programs that promote helmet use.

- CDC gives funds to selected injury control centers to promote helmet use.

- CDC funds research to improve helmet design.

- CDC collaborates with a host of other federal agencies and non-profit organizations to promote helmet use and bicycle safety. For more information about this collaborative effort, visit the National Bicycle Safety Network website: www.cdc.gov/ncipc/bike.

How Many States Have Bicycle Helmet Laws?

- By early 1999, 15 states and more than 65 local governments had enacted some form of bicycle helmet legislation. Most of these laws pertain to children and adolescents.[13]

What Standards Exist to Ensure that Helmets Are Truly Protective?

- The U.S. Consumer Product Safety Commission issued a new safety standard for bike helmets in 1999. The new standard ensures that bike helmets will adequately protect the head and that chin straps will be strong enough to prevent the helmet from coming off in a crash, collision, or fall. In addition, helmets intended for children up to age five must cover a larger surface of the head than before. All bike helmets made or imported into the United States must meet the CPSC standard.[14]

How Can You Help Prevent Injuries while Bicycling?

- Wear a bicycle helmet every time you ride. A bicycle helmet is a necessity, not an accessory.

- Wear your bicycle helmet correctly. A bicycle helmet should fit comfortably and snugly, but not too tightly. It should sit on top of your head in a level position, and it should not rock forward and back or from side to side. Always keep the helmet straps buckled.

- Only buy a bicycle helmet if it meets or exceeds the safety standards developed by the U.S. Consumer Product Safety Commission.

- Learn the rules of the road and obey all traffic laws. Ride with the traffic, on the right side of the road. Use appropriate hand signals. Respect traffic signals, which are meant for riders as well as drivers. Stop at all intersections; not just those intersections with pedestrian markings. Stop and look both ways before entering a street.

- Children should not ride in the street until they are 10 years old, demonstrate good riding skills, and are able to observe the basic rules of the road. And, of course, children should always wear helmets when they ride.

References

1. *NHTSA Traffic Safety Facts, 1997: Bicyclists*. Washington, D.C.: National Highway Traffic Safety Administration.

2. Insurance Institute for Highway Safety (IIHS). *1997 Fatality Facts: Bicycles*. Arlington (VA): IIHS, 1997.

3. U.S. Consumer Product Safety Commission. *National Electronic Injury Surveillance System (NEISS)*. Washington, DC: Consumer Product Safety Commission; 1997.

4. Sosin DM, Sacks JJ, Webb KW. Pediatric head injuries and deaths from bicycling in the United States. *Pediatrics* 1996;98(5):868-70.

5. U.S. Consumer Products Safety Commission (CPSC). *Bicycle-related head injury or death*. Washington (DC): CPSC, 1994.

6. Thompson RS, Rivara FP, Thompson DC. A case-control study of the effectiveness of bicycle safety helmets. *N Engl J Med*. 1989; 320:1361-7.

7. Thompson DC, Nunn ME, Thompson RS, Rivara FP. Effectiveness of bicycle safety helmets in preventing serious facial injury. *JAMA* 1996; 276:1974-1975.

8. Sacks JJ, Holmgreen P, Smith S, Sosin D. Bicycle-associated head injuries and deaths in the United States from 1984-1988. *JAMA* 1991;266:3016-8.

9.   Sacks JJ, Kresnow M, Houston B, Russell J. Bicycle helmet use among American children, 1994. *Injury Prevention* 1996; 2:258-62.

10. Public Health Service (PHS). *Healthy People 2010 Objectives: Draft for Public Comment*. Washington (DC): US Department of Health and Human Services, PHS; 1999.

11. Hatziandreu EJ, Sacks JJ, Brown R, Taylor WR, Rosenberg ML, Graham JD. The cost effectiveness of three programs to increase use of bicycle helmets among children. *Public Health Reports* 1995 May-Jun; 110(3):251-9.

12. CDC. Injury Control Recommendations: Bicycle Helmets. *MMWR* 44(RR-1)1995.

13. Bicycle Helmet Safety Institute (BHSI). *Mandatory helmet laws: summary*. Arlington (VA): BHSI, 1997.

14. *Federal Register*. U. S. Consumer Product Safety Commission. Safety standard for bicycle helmets; Final rule. FR Doc. 98-4214, February 13, 1998.

Contact Information

National Center for Injury Prevention and Control
Mailstop K65
4770 Buford Highway, NE
Atlanta, GA 30341-3724
Phone: 770-488-1506
Fax: 770-488-1667
Website: http://www.cdc.gov/ncipc
Email: OHCINFO@cdc.gov

Chapter 40

Fit to Rip:
Ski-Specific Workout

Even though it's 90 degrees out and the arrival of winter seems an ice age away, now's the time to get pumped up for ski season. So crank the AC, pour a bucket of ice cubes down your pants and imagine yourself ripping through a bump field, legs powering like jackhammers, wrists flicking poleplants, upper body perfectly poised. You can make it happen with *Skiing*'s new ski-specific workout. And when the snow does start to fly, you'll be physically amped and ready to tackle anything.

It's possible to realize huge gains in ski fitness in just 12 weeks by following a progressive, step-by-step plan. The key is periodized training in phases. Our program has four basic exercise components—call them the four food groups of ski fitness—aerobic, strength, trunk stabilization, and ski specific. In each phase, the balance of the components changes. The first four-week phase builds a foundation of overall stamina by concentrating on aerobic exercise like in-line skating and trail running. Phase two ups the strength component with a focus on weight training. And the final phase features intense, explosive ski-specific moves. Since balance is also important to skiers, the exercises we've chosen will improve that skill as well.

To develop the program, we worked with The Stone Clinic in San Francisco, one of the nation's pioneering centers for orthopedic surgery and sports-medicine research. It's where world-class athletes

From *Skiing*, September 1997, vol. 50, no. 1, p. 130(6). © 1997 Times Mirror Magazines Inc. Reprinted with permission from the publisher and the author.

turn for rehab and pre-season conditioning. Picabo Street, Megan Gerety, Julie Parisien, and other members of the U.S. Ski Team and the women's World Pro Ski Tour have made the pilgrimage to the Stone Foundation training center.

Although our program is based on the way these elite skiers train, it's geared to mere mortals. Procrastinators beware: Jumping directly into the plan's final six weeks could easily cause injury. No matter what your level of fitness now, follow the plan from the start and your body will be chiseled into a lean, mean skiing machine by the time your skis touch the snow.

Aerobic Endurance

The basic component of most fitness programs is aerobic fitness—the body's ability to suck up oxygen and put it to good use. The more efficiently your body takes in and pumps oxygen, the harder you can ski without having to stop and catch your breath and the longer you can go before skiing turns into an anaerobic sport—when you get that thigh-burning feeling, explains Michael Mullin, The Stone Clinic's head athletic-trainer. To stay aerobic, you need a powerful heart and lungs delivering the key ingredient, oxygen, to the muscles.

Although skiing doesn't require the aerobic capacity of marathon running, a solid aerobic foundation is important. The first phase of our program focuses on building an aerobic base to prepare the body for the more intense exercises of the next phases.

In a regimen that recalls the tortoise and the hare, current research suggests training at a moderate pace, 70 to 80 percent of your maximum heart rate. You'll quickly learn that 70 percent of max is quite slow and easy to maintain. As you train, you'll be able to go progressively faster without burning out, teaching your body to work at an increasingly greater intensity while maintaining a constant, fat-burning heart rate, The focus is on efficiency.

Cardio Jam

Trail running, mountain biking, and in-line skating are great ski-specific aerobic workouts. You can also get your cardio by hiking, rock climbing, rowing, kayaking, windsurfing, or playing soccer, tennis, volleyball, and racquetball. Rained in? Stair climbers, Nordic Tracks, treadmills, or rowing machines will do. Choose activities that fit into your normal lifestyle and are fun.

Strength Training

A strong heart alone won't get you through a 1,500-foot black-diamond bump run. Moreover, fighting the compressive forces of a high-speed, high-G turn takes powerful quads, poling across the flats demands strong shoulders and triceps, and staying balanced in crud necessitates a strong trunk.

In addition to the key strength exercises we've outlined here, upper-body exercises should include push-ups, dips, seated cable rows, and bench presses. Lower-body exercises should also include calf raises, hip abductions, and lunges. Vary your routine to keep things interesting, but if you're not familiar with one of these exercises, check with a trainer at your gym.

It's easy to lift too much when beginning a weight-training program. Lingering muscle soreness is a sign of damage, not of a good workout, says Emily Miller, The Stone Clinic's head strength and conditioning coach. Start with very light weight and concentrate on a smooth, full contraction and a slow, controlled recovery. For the first couple of sessions, forget about sets and reps, and focus on form.

Get Pumped

1. **Straight-arm lat pull-down:** (triceps, lats, rhomboids, deltoids) Standing with feet slightly apart for stability, grab the pull-down bar in front of and above your head, hands several inches wider than your shoulders. Keeping your arms straight, pull the bar down to about waist level. Slowly return to the start position.

2. **Overhead triceps curl:** (triceps) Sitting on a bench, grasp one end of a dumbbell with both hands and raise it above your head, straightening your arms. Lower the dumbbell behind your head, moving from the elbow. Raise it up again and repeat.

3. **Leg curl:** (hamstrings, glutes) Lie flat on your stomach, ankles under the pad. Curl your legs back smoothly, moving your feet toward your butt.

4. **Leg press:** (quads, glutes, hamstrings) Feet should be shoulder-width apart, flat on the plate, knees bent to 90 degrees. Extend your legs, pushing the weight away, but don't lock your knees. Keep your back flat on the bench throughout the movement.

5. **Squat:** (quads, glutes, hamstrings) Stand with feet shoulder-width apart, toes pointed straight ahead, with the bar centered across your shoulders, Keep your head up, eyes ahead, and heels on the floor. Lower hips until thighs are parallel to the ground. Then push up. The squat should be attempted only after you've built a strength base with the leg press and leg curl, and it's safest to learn the movement from a pro.

Trunk Stabilization

If you're weak between your hips and rib cage, "You fall over," says Aimee Mulkern, a U.S. Ski Teamer who's been to the Stone training camp. Skiing requires your legs to bob, weave, and pump underneath you while your trunk remains centered and stable. Keeping the upper body quiet while the legs move, sometimes unpredictably, requires special attention to the muscle groups connecting the upper and lower body.

A combination of abdominal and back exercises will build the muscles responsible for keeping the body poised and balanced. Just like building aerobic fitness, conditioning the muscles of the midsection takes time and repetition. For the first phase of the plan, resolve yourself to three or more days a week of doing crunches and back extensions. Your ab and back muscles recover quickly: Don't be afraid to make these exercises part of your daily routine, as long as they are low-intensity and without weight.

After the foundation phase, add the partner leg push-over, which teaches the body to perceive and react to changes in equilibrium. By resisting the unpredictable push-over attempts of a partner, you'll quickly develop a keen sense of balance, while building strength.

Trunk Tactics

1. **Back extension:** (back extensors, hamstrings, glutes) Lie flat on your stomach, feet together, arms above head (Superman position). Raise one arm and shoulder, and the opposite leg, contracting your back muscles. Hold for a few seconds, then alternate arms and legs.

2. **Crunch:** (abdominals) Lie on the ground with your legs bent and elevated on a bench. Raise your head and shoulders, keeping your lower back pressed to the ground. Think of crunching at the stomach, not bending at the waist. Start with your hands crossed on chest, progress to hands behind head, then hands holding a weight on your chest.

3. **Diagonal crunch:** (abdominals, lateral obliques) Same as crunch (including the hand progression), but move one shoulder toward the opposite knee, alternating shoulders.

4. **Leg push-over:** (trunk, legs) Lie face up on the ground. Have a partner stand straddling your head, facing toward your feet. Holding your partner's ankles, lift your legs to vertical. As your partner unpredictably shoves your legs to the ground in different directions, try to resist and then bring your legs back to vertical.

Plyometrics

You've built an aerobic base, strengthened key ski muscles, and developed intuitive sense of balance along the way. After six weeks of preparation, it's time to sculpt your athletic body into that of a skier. "If you want to get up for the ski season, plyos are the way to do it," says Mulkern.

Plyometric exercises, or plyos, convert strength and endurance into explosive power—the kind of power needed to rip a bump line, hop-turn down a narrow chute, and control your speed on steep, uneven terrain.

But if the newest research is to be believed, the benefits of plyometrics go far beyond putting a little spring in your step. A late-1996 study published by the American Orthopaedic Society for Sports Medicine found that after a six-week program of flexibility, strength, and plyometrics, female volleyball players were able to jump 10 percent higher. That's pretty good, but more impressive yet is that landing forces were reduced by 22 percent, torque on the knee was halved, and side-to-side muscle imbalances were almost totally corrected. The researchers attribute the remarkable results not only to increased muscle strength, but also to a honing of neuromuscular control. In layman's terms, plyometrics make you more coordinated.

Now the bad news: Plyometrics hearken back to the "No pain, no gain" fitness mantra of bygone eras. These are tough workouts, with lots of jumping. This is where the six weeks of aerobic and strength preparation will pay off. But it is possible to hurt yourself. If you experience pain, it's time to stop.

Start out slow and easy, learning the basic motions. Your first attempts should be low, lateral jumps. Progress to leaps over a small log, then try leaping on and off a sturdy object—a low bench, a flat rock, or a sturdy box. The taller the obstacle, the more difficult the leap. Remember to maintain good, erect posture. Just like in skiing, keep your upper body quiet, and explode from your hips and legs. Be light and quick on your feet; imagine the ground is red hot.

Table 40.1. Ski-Specific Workout (continued on next page).

Phase One (foundation)

WEEK	AEROBIC	STRENGTH	DURATION
1	Mod. intensity 2-3 days	Low intensity 2-3 days	20-36 minutes per session
2	Moderate 2-3 days	Low 3 days	30-40 min.
3	Moderate 3 days	Low 3-4 days	40-45 min.
4	Moderate 3-4 days	Low to moderate 3 days	45+ min.

Phase Two (preparation)

WEEK	AEROBIC	STRENGTH	DURATION
5	Mod. to high 3-4 days	Moderate 3-4 days	45+ min. per session
6	Same	Moderate to high	Same
7	Moderate 2-3 days	Same 2-3 days	40-45 min.
8	Same	Same	Same

Phase Three (ski specific)

WEEK	AEROBIC	STRENGTH	DURATION
9	Moderate intensity 3-4 days	Moderate to high 2-3 days	35-40 min. per session
10	Moderate 3 days	Moderate 2-3 days	35-40 min.
11	Moderate 2-3 days	Same 2-3 days	20-30 min.
12	Same	Same	Same

Table 40.1. Ski-Specific Workout (continued from previous page).

Phase One (foundation)

WEEK	TRUNK	PLYOS
1	Back extension, crunches At least 3 days	None
2	Same	None
3	Same	None
4	Same	None

Phase Two (preparation)

WEEK	TRUNK	PLYOS
5	Add partner leg push-over	None
6	Same	Low intensity, start slow
7	Same	Low
8	Same	Low to moderate

Phase Three (ski specific)

WEEK	TRUNK	PLYOS
9	Increase reps	Moderate intensity
10	Same	Moderate
11	Same	High
12	Same	High

Plyo Power

1. **Diagonal log hop:** Using a long log (or a series of boxes, cones, or small rocks), jump sideways and slightly forward, landing on the other side of the barrier. Continue jumping forward in quick progression. At the end of the series, reverse direction and repeat.

2. **Rock jumping:** Jump sideways onto a flat rock and immediately jump off to the other side, making sure to absorb the impact with, your legs. Jump back onto the surface and back to the starting position. If you can touch the rock 60 times in 60 seconds you're ready for the Olympics.

3. **Zigzag drill:** Use two parallel lines, about two to three feet apart. You can either string rope on the ground or use your imagination on a sidewalk or path. Balance on one foot on one of the lines; jump diagonally ahead to the other line, landing on the other foot. Continue bounding forward from leg to leg for about 10 meters, then rest, reverse direction, and repeat.

The Plan

Aerobic

The quick way to figure your approximate maximum heart rate is to subtract your age from 220 (226 for women). Moderate intensity is 70-80 percent of your max, high intensity is 80-90 percent.

Strength

In strength training, intensity relates to weights, repetitions, and sets, not to your heart rate, as it does in aerobic conditioning. **Low intensity:** Begin with low weight, eight to 10 reps, one set per session. During subsequent sessions, add enough weight so that you can't complete more than 15 to 20 reps. When you can easily complete 15 to 20 reps, add more weight. **Moderate intensity:** Build up to two or three sets of 10 to 15 reps each, progressively increasing the weight for each set, with two-minute rests in between. Alternate upper- and lower-body workouts each session. **High intensity:** Reduce the rest period between the three sets and push until failure in the final set.

Plyometrics

Because you will be working near your maximum heart rate, well above your aerobic rate, intensity relates to some elusive measure of desire and tolerance for pain.

Plyos are hard on the body. Do two plyo workouts each week (beginning week six) with two days' rest between workouts. Each week should systematically increase in difficulty and duration to increase coordination and power. Do three different drills during each workout. Work up to three sets of each drill with appropriate rests between each set. Continue jumping until your legs get a good burn going, then rest 1½ times as long as you jumped for.

The Stone Clinic. The Stone Clinic, supported by The Stone Foundation, specializes in orthopedic surgery, sports medicine, and rehabilitation; much of the practice is devoted to skiers. For more info, call 415-563-3110 or look at the clinic's web site: www.stoneclinic.com.

— by Steve Shimek and Jeff Stine

Chapter 41

In-Line Skating Basics

Getting Past the First Hurdles

- Fear of standing on inline skates
- Fear of falling down
- Fear of not being able to stop
- Fear of looking foolish

Most people who try inline skating for the first time expect it to be difficult to stand and keep their balance because of the in-line arrangement of the wheels. While it's true that many people need help getting to their feet the first time, it's easy to stand on inline skates, because even soft-boot skates like the K2 Flight and the Salomon TR-II have plenty of ankle support.

Inline skates are actually easier to skate on outdoors than quad (conventional) roller skates, because inline skates are more forgiving of cracks in the pavement. Quad skates are more maneuverable, which is good for roller disco and artistic skating, but inline skates are more suitable for fitness and speed skating.

The next two concerns, falling and not being able to stop, are shared by every new skater, but they can be easily overcome by a good instructor, lots of practice, and plenty of body padding—and we don't mean the natural kind!

The last item, looking foolish, should not be a concern at all. Skaters who see you learning will remember their own first attempts, and non-skaters will think you are very brave.

Starting to Skate

- Wear a helmet and protective gear

- Take lessons

- Learn to stop

Now you're almost ready to skate, but first, you need to understand how important it is to wear the proper protective gear, including a helmet, wrist guards, knee pads, and elbow pads. According to Consumer Products Safety Commission Statistics published by the International Inline Skating Association, 37% of all inline skating injuries in 1996 were injuries to the wrist or lower arm. And according to the Inline Club of Boston's Skating Safety Gear Web page, wrist guards will reduce the risk of wrist injuries by 90%, and a helmet will reduce the risk of head injuries by 85%.

Your risk of being injured on inline skates can be greatly reduced by wearing a helmet, wrist guards, knee pads and elbow pads. Protective gear is available at skate shops and sporting goods stores that sell inline skates or skateboards. A body gear 3-pack will usually cost about $40 to $60. You could easily spend more than $100 on a helmet, but you should be able to find a good one for $35 to $50.

If you are especially concerned about falling, you can practically eliminate this fear by wearing the type of padded undergarment worn by professional hockey players, and made by hockey clothing manufacturers like Crash-Pad, Austin, BiltRite, and many others. Don't worry about how you'll look in padded underwear. Why do you think aggressive skaters wear those baggy pants? It's not just to look cool!

Now that you understand the importance of wearing protective gear, you need to find a good skating instructor. Lessons are not expensive, and they will make you a much better skater. They also greatly reduce the risk of injury.

Group lessons typically cost $20, and some skate shops offer them free. Private lessons usually cost $40 to $60, but many instructors will let you share a private lesson with a friend, and reduce the per-person cost by as much as 50% The price of lessons often includes renting skates, helmet and body protection, so try to find an instructor who will include equipment rental in his or her prices.

Make sure your instructor has a current teaching certificate from the International Inline Skating Association (IISA). You can find a certified instructor by contacting your local skate shops and sporting goods stores, or you can use IISA's "Instructor Search Engine" to find an instructor in the United States and Canada and many other countries.

The first things you will learn in a class are how to put on your protective gear, how to fall safely, how to get moving, and how to STOP! Before you skate in a public place, you should be completely comfortable using your heel brake.

After you take a skating lesson, develop your stopping skills in a large, flat, empty parking lot. Practice skating and stopping, over and over, until using the brake starts to become an automatic reflex. Later you can practice in a gently sloping parking lot. Keep practicing until you are confident using your brake, and you know how far in advance you need to apply it. Using the heel brake is the one skill that will make the most difference in your confidence level and enjoyment of inline skating.

Buying Your First Skates

The best skates for you to buy will depend on the kind of skating you expect to do, and the amount of money you're willing to spend. Inline skates can be generally organized into the following categories:

- Aggressive Skates
- Artistic Skates
- Fitness and Recreational Skates
- Hockey Skates
- Speed Skates

Note that buying a particular type of skate doesn't mean you CAN'T do any other type of skating. You'll see plenty of people playing hockey in recreational skates, doing aggressive maneuvers in fitness skates and dancing in hockey skates. If you aren't sure what type of skating you'll be doing, you should probably select a comfortable, medium-priced recreational skate.

What to Spend

Plan to spend at least $200 for your first pair of skates. If you spend less, your feet will probably be so uncomfortable you won't enjoy skating at all. If you can afford to spend more than $200, your feet will definitely notice the difference. It's almost always true, that fitness and recreational skates rated highest for comfort cost between $300 and $400.

If you can't afford to buy a high-end skate, you should be quite comfortable in a mid-range skate, but there are two other options: Buy a high quality used skate, or find a discontinued high-end skate on sale. Finding good used skates may not be easy, but finding a discontinued skate on sale is very possible, especially during the winter season. We've seen top-of-the-line $350 skates on sale for under $100 after they've been replaced by a new model.

Aggressive Skates

Aggressive skates are tough, durable skates made of thick plastic. They have small wheels for maneuverability and grind plates to protect the boots when you perform aggressive stunts.

Artistic Skates

The skates most commonly used for figure skating and dancing have boots similar to ice skating boots and small wheels for maneuverability. The newest artistic skates have only three wheels, and the front and back wheels are a different hardness than the middle wheel. This allows smoother turns and spinning, and gives the skates the feel of a rockered skate or an ice skate.

Fitness and Recreational Skates

Basic recreational skates have four wheels and plenty of ankle support. They are usually made of hard plastic. If you decide to purchase one of the new soft-boot skates, make sure the one you select has a plastic cuff or some other device to provide good ankle support.

Recreational skates used for fitness and long-distance skating have larger wheels (80 mm), a slightly lower cuff, and extra comfort features. Recreational skates used for down-hill skating have a high cuff made of hard plastic, to provide the extra ankle support needed for skating down long, steep hills.

Hockey Skates

Hockey skates are made of leather and they have small wheels for maneuverability. They close with laces for a tight fit, and they are manufactured to support the agility requirements of roller hockey.

Speedskates

True speedskates are very light weight and they have a low-cut leather boot with no ankle support. They have a long wheel base and 5 large wheels for extra speed. They are not suitable for beginners because they have no brake, and the long wheel base makes it difficult to turn and do other basic maneuvers.

Skating Safety and Etiquette

Your chance of being injured on inline skates will be greatly reduced if you are aware of potential hazards and you know how to avoid them. Whenever you skate, pay attention to your surroundings and keep your eyes and ears open. Don't let yourself be surprised by changes in the terrain or the unexpected actions of other people.

Stay Alert !!!

I've never been seriously injured in a skating fall, but my three most unnerving falls were caused by surprise encounters with water on the road, sand on a bikepath, and a city sidewalk that abruptly disappeared. On those occasions, I didn't notice the danger because I allowed myself to become distracted. However, I still managed to escape injury because of...

Body Protection

Always wear your helmet, wrist guards, knee pads and elbow pads. My wrist guards are literally COVERED with scrapes and scratches and dents. I've had relatively few falls, but anyone who skates as much as I do is going to hit the ground 2 or 3 times a year. My body protection has saved me during more than one close encounter with the asphalt!

I skate about 4,000 miles a year, so I have a lot of skating experience and a lot of safety tips to share. Unfortunately I learned most of them the hard way. Here are some of the best:

Road Surfaces

• Try to skate only on smooth pavement with no surface debris.

• Be very alert for changes in the condition of the road in front of you. Don't let potholes, storm debris, rough pavement, curbs or patches of grass catch you by surprise.

- Don't skate through water, oil, mud or sand. Your wheels will have very little traction, and your feet can slide right out from under you.

- Tiny pebbles look harmless, but they can get stuck in your skate wheels and cause them to stop rolling. This one is a REAL bummer.

- Cracks in the pavement can be a serious danger, in a way that always surprises new skaters. It's not the cracks CROSSING your path that you need to worry about. Inline skates handle those cracks very well—much better than traditional quad skates. The dangerous cracks are the ones that run parallel to your skating path. If the wheels of one of your inline skates get lodged into one of those cracks, you can be thrown off balance without any warning. This typically happens when you're skating on a sidewalk with a crack down the center.

Public Paths

- Always use caution when skating in public areas with bicycles, cars, pedestrians, and other skaters.

- Learn basic skating skills before you attempt to skate in a public place. Learn how to turn, control your speed, fall safely, and most important, to stop. One of the most dangerous things on a crowded bike path is a skater who never learned how to stop!

- Always be conscious of others around you. Avoid sudden stops and last minute turns. You don't want to surprise anyone.

- When you're skating in an area with a lot of bicycle, skate or auto traffic, glance back over your shoulder every 10 or 20 seconds (remember: always be aware of your surroundings).

- Around bicycles, be very predictable. Don't make any unexpected movements. Don't swing your arms and legs wildly back and forth as you skate—many cyclists have been knocked off their bikes by careless skaters.

- Around pedestrians, always yield. Be prepared for them to run in front of you or stroll obliviously across your path.

- Around children, be prepared for ANYTHING. They will frequently run across your path when you least expect it. Children on skates or on foot usually cause me to slow down to a very cautious crawl.

- Be cautious when you approach a dog on a leash. If the dog suddenly runs run across your path, you can find yourself skating toward a leash stretched out across the path in front of you.

Street Skating

- Always be acutely aware that it is DANGEROUS to skate in the street.

- Ask your local law enforcement agency if skaters are allowed to skate in the streets, on the sidewalks, and on the bike paths in your city.

- Skate in the bicycle lane on city streets (if skaters are allowed on bike paths in your city)

- If you must skate in the street, clip two flashing bicycle lights to your helmet or your waist: one in front and one in back. I use two heavy-duty 3" by 2" flashing bicycle lights—a green one on the bow and a red one on the stern!

- Obey all traffic regulations.

- Whenever you approach a driveway, imagine a car speeding out, just as you're skating by.

- Whenever you approach a car parked on the side of the road, imagine someone flinging the door open just as you're skating by.

- Before you cross an intersection, look all around you for any car that could POSSIBLY turn in front of you. If cars drive on the right side of the road in your country, you should be especially concerned about cars making RIGHT turns in front of you. If your cars drive on the left side of the road, watch for cars making a LEFT turn in front of you. Those kinds of turns cause a lot of skating accidents because it's difficult for drivers to see you in time to stop.

Equipment

- Wear good-quality, well-fitting skates that provide adequate ankle support.

- Check your skates regularly to make sure they're in good condition.

- Rotate your wheels when they wear unevenly.

- Replace worn-out wheels and bearings.

- Replace your brake BEFORE it wears out.

- Make sure your wheels are securely tightened

- Make sure your wheels are never blocked by debris or grass.

- Always have an all-purpose skate tool with you when you skate.

Other Safety Tips

- Never skate at night. When it's dark, you can't see hazards in the road and you can't be seen by others. If you ever DO have to skate in the dark, clip two flashing bicycle lights to your helmet or your waist (one in front and one in back).

- Wear protective gear every time you skate. Long-sleeved shirts and long trousers will give you additional protection from scrapes and cuts.

- Always skate under control and within your abilities. Avoid hills until you are ready for them. Remember that you will gain speed quickly on even a very small hill.

- Many people recommend against skating with headphones, because they block out sounds that can alert you to approaching danger. If you must skate with headphones, keep the volume low, and use headphones that don't block out surrounding noise.

- When you can't avoid falling, try to fall in sand or grass, and fall forward onto your wrist guards and knee pads.

Skating Etiquette and Courtesy

The best thing you can do to prevent skating bans in your area, is to demonstrate that skaters are an asset to your community rather than a nuisance and a hazard. Give skating a good name!

- Be courteous, friendly, and helpful to those around you.

- Be tolerant of the shortcomings of others.

- Do your most weird and dangerous tricks out of eye-sight and out of camera-sight. This tip is from Dave Cooper, Government Relations Chair for the International Inline Skating Association.

- Don't swing legs and arms wildly to the left and right.

- Always skate single file, even when you skate with friends.

- Skate on the FAR right side of sidewalks, bike paths and trails.

- Pass pedestrians, cyclists and other skaters on the left (skate on the right, pass on the left)

- Don't pass without warning and pass only when it's safe, and you know there's enough room.

- Warn others before passing. Say "Passing on your left." Say it loudly, but don't bark it out angrily. If you say it with a smile, the smile will be reflected in your voice. (I usually smile and wave to the person I'm passing.)

All this passing etiquette might seem like overkill, but for some reason, people often become annoyed when someone skates up behind them shrieking, "ON YOUR LEEEEEEEEFT!!!!"

To avoid being the victim of someone's bike-path road rage, AND to prevent skating bans in your area, always be a courteous, friendly, helpful, polite, and civic-minded skater.

Practice Tips for Beginners

Take a Lesson First!

Before you start practicing on inline skates, you should take a skating lesson from an IISA-certified skating instructor. You will be a much better skater, and much less likely to injure yourself, if you take at least one lesson before you try skating on your own. You can use the IISA Instructor Search Engine to find a class in the USA or almost anywhere in the world. Please take a lesson before you try skating on your own. Attempting to skate without taking lessons is scary and dangerous to yourself and others!

Things to Bring when You Skate

- Skates and socks

- Helmet, wrist guards, knee pads, elbow pads

- All-purpose skate tool

- Water or money for drinks

- Money for phone calls, taxi, snacks

- Phone numbers you might need

- Pencil and paper for new phone numbers

- Band-Aids, moleskin, blister kit, athletic tape

- Sunglasses

- Sunscreen lotion

- Elastic bands for tying back your hair

- Bike lights if you might be out after dark

- MP3 player or tape player if you skate to music

Your Very First Practice Sessions

Rollerblade's *Tips for Beginning Skaters* suggests that first-time skaters walk around on a flat, grassy surface before they try skating on pavement. It's a good way for new skaters to get the feel of their skates, and to practice standing and balancing. You might want to start several of your first sessions this way.

When you feel you're ready, carefully move to the pavement and just BALANCE on your skates, without trying more. Position your feet a few inches apart, bend your knees, and balance your weight on the balls of your feet.

When you're ready to roll, begin to skate gradually. Practice moving forward but don't get going too fast. You should ease into your first practice sessions. Don't push yourself too hard and don't try to skate beyond your abilities. There's plenty of time!

Warm Up before You Skate

Warm up before each practice session. You will be less likely to injure yourself if you begin each skating session with a few stretching exercises and a slow five-minute warm-up skate.

When I first started skating, I always felt very unsteady when I first put on my skates. It felt like I had never been on skates before! After about 10 or 20 minutes, I always got my "skating legs" back. It still happens to me, to a lesser extent, so don't get discouraged if you experience the same thing.

Where and What to Practice

Find a large, flat, empty parking lot for your first practice sessions. When I say flat, I mean VERY flat. The slightest grade will make you gain speed faster than you expect, and you will quickly find yourself skating out of control.

Practice the striding and stopping skills you learned in your skating lesson. Skate and stop, over and over, until stopping starts to become an automatic reflex. Later you should practice skating and stopping in a gently sloping parking lot.

Bend Your Knees

It's very important to bend your knees when you skate. It keeps your center of gravity low so you will be more stable and less likely to fall. Bending your knees also adds power to your stride. If you stand up straight, your stride is only about 1 foot wide on each side, but if you bend your knees deeply, your stride is more like 3 feet wide on each side. This longer stride adds power to your skating, and your stride will be more productive with less effort. (I learned this tip from Jay Etheredge, winner of many U.S. speedskating competitions.)

Bending the knees is difficult for most beginners. Actually, it's not really difficult for them to DO, it's just difficult for them to KNOW whether or not they're doing it. They think they're bending their knees, but they're really bending at the waist. To overcome this very common problem, try bending your knees until you can feel the cuff of your skates pressing against the front of your shins. If you can't feel your skates pressing hard against your shins, you aren't bending your knees deeply enough.

Learn to Fall

Keep your weight forward on the balls of your feet when you're skating. Always remember that you don't want to fall backwards onto your unprotected back or tailbone. Of course, most of us don't want to fall at ALL, but when you can't avoid it, you should make sure you fall forward onto your wrist guards and knee pads.

Skate Every Day

Try to skate every day, even if it's only once around the block. Your skating skills will develop quickly if you make time for frequent practice sessions. Even 15 or 20 minutes a day will make a big difference.

Go Back to School

After you are comfortable with basic skating skills like stopping and striding, take an intermediate class to learn T-stops, slalom (turning) techniques, skating backwards, and other more advanced maneuvers.

Chapter 42

How to Use a Jog Stroller

Three years ago, the sight of a "super mom," half-dazed and painting behind a jogging stroller containing a 20-plus pound bundle of joy, would have left me in awe. Two children later, I consider pushing just one child in a jogging stroller light training. Having graduated to the "deluxe playground on wheels" (double stroller) to accommodate an infant and a toddler, I know the secrets to making a stroller run an experience everyone can enjoy.

Most parents break into a cold sweat just thinking about taking a jogging stroller around the block. Where does a novice runner begin? How do you run without using your arms? If you think that a jogging stroller is beyond your parenting, running and aerobic skills, you may be pleasantly surprised.

The jogging stroller can be intimidating, especially if you have little to no hands-on experience with this rugged, all-terrain contraption that looks more like a high-tech moon buggy than a stroller. Fortunately, however, a jogging stroller may actually be more user-friendly than a standard stroller—even on roads, sidewalks and gravel—thanks to three 14-inch to 20-inch tires. Additionally, the large tires make pushing 45 pounds surprisingly easy (unless you happen to be running up a hill). Don't be surprised if, after doing a few trial runs, you find you never want to use a standard stroller again.

Reprinted with permission from the Aerobics and Fitness Association of America. *American Fitness Magazine*, © 1997, vol. 15, no. 4, p. 46(20), July-August 1997.

There are two types of jogging strollers: the single and double passenger. While the single typically comes with more perks (it's lighter, has hand brakes, larger tires, it's easier to maneuver, folds for an easy fit into most car trunks and sports a more comfortable seat), it only holds one child. The double passenger stroller, often already equipped with a windscreen/rain tarp and removable front wheel to adapt to a pull-cart for bicycles, is slightly more cumbersome—especially to the novice jogging stroller operator. However, it's ideal if you have two children and are interested in packing lots of weight training into your running routine.

Both types of strollers cost between $150 and $300. If you want to purchase a used jogging stroller, be prepared to buy at a moment's notice. It's a hot item, especially during the spring and summer months. One of the greatest advantages of the used stroller is that it is already assembled. However, if you can put together a crib, you can easily master the stroller.

If you purchase a two-passenger jogging stroller with a hard plastic shell and no padding on the seats, you can make it more comfortable for your children with a standard outdoor chair cushion with ties ($10 to $20). Cut holes or slits in the cushion for the shoulder straps and lap belts to pull through, and tie to the frame of the stroller. In less than five minutes, you have a comfortable stroller ready for an all-terrain ride.

Once your stroller is ready for its first run, help yourself and your passenger(s) prepare for a successful run with the following guidelines.

For Parents

- Make sure you spend at least five to 10 minutes stretching.

- Start out slowly. Runners who typically travel five to seven miles may want to consider starting off with one to two miles. Beginners may want to experiment with one to two miles of speed walking mixed with five to 10 minute intervals of jogging. It will be hard to motivate yourself for a second day of running if you are an aching mass of raw muscle.

- Drink lots of fluids.

- Invest in sports bras that provide adequate support. Although an underwire push-up bra may give you some impressive cleavage, it may not give you the support and comfort you need. Nursing moms might try wearing two sports bras, or a combination of a sports and full-support bra to minimize or alleviate breast discomfort. Also, they should empty breasts, especially if running first thing in the morning. Breasts tend to become engorged after a full night's sleep.

- Invest in a good pair of running shoes ($45 to $100). Many running enthusiasts recommend buying a new pair of shoes every 300 miles. If you are prone to impact injuries (ankles, shins, knees and hips), you may want to switch your shoes more often. (Helpful hint: When trying on new shoes, if the shoe is uncomfortable or falls into that "all it needs is a little breaking in" category, don't buy them. Your feet and body will thank you later.)

For Passengers

- Feed your kids, change wet pants, and take toddlers on a last visit to the bathroom prior to venturing down the road. You may want to pack along a spare water or juice bottle, or spill-proof sip cup—especially for longer runs or hot weather.

- Dress your passengers appropriately for the weather. Keep in mind they are passive participants in your exercise plans, and the elements will affect them differently. Don't forget the sunscreen, hats and sunglasses.

- Avoid running close to nap times. Exercising first thing in the morning can be a great way to start the day and take advantage of cooler temperatures—especially during the hot summer months.

- If the scenery doesn't appear to hold your children's attention long, try throwing in a couple of their favorite toys. Be sure to avoid anything with small or moving parts that can easily break off and be swallowed.

- If you find yourself stopping and starting because your passengers are fighting over toys or can't seem to keep their hands to themselves, place a piece of foam, pillow or board between them to create a safe barrier.

- Always remember to properly strap in your precious cargo with the appropriate safety belts. Also, you may want to post lists of emergency phone numbers on the inside and outside of the stroller in lieu of advertising any personal identification information.

Running Forms

Before you even reach the end of your driveway, you will notice there is nothing natural about running behind a jogging stroller. In fact, the more experienced you are at running, the harder it will be to break old habits like running with a long stride or using your freely swinging arms to help keep your pace. However, you'll soon adapt to a new running form.

You can use one hand or two to push the stroller. If you are running with a single passenger stroller, it may be easier to travel with one hand on the stroller handle and allow the other arm to swing freely at your side. If you are using a two passenger stroller, however, most runners recommend using both hands to compensate for the additional awkwardness of the larger stroller and extra weight. Allowing your shoulders to swing slightly, in lieu of your arms, will help alleviate some of the initial awkwardness. Avoid the temptation to run along beside the stroller since your ability to steer in a straight line will be impaired. Additionally, you may want to decrease the length of your stride to avoid hitting or tripping over the stroller. Remember to allow your hands to comfortably rest on the stroller handle and bend your arms slightly at the elbows.

If you want to add an additional challenge to your run, try experimenting with hills of varying grades and lengths. Leaning into the hill and flattening out your body will help make ascension easier. Contrary to any thoughts you may have on your way up a hill while staring at the rear tires of the stroller, no one has ever been severely maimed, injured or died from being backed over by a jogging stroller. While descending, lean back away from the stroller and try to resist running full-force down the hill in order to avoid a runaway stroller.

With a little practice, running behind a jogging stroller will not only be second nature, but it will be a great way to spend some special time with your children and work off those last few pregnancy pounds. While you may be a super parent for exercising with your children, it doesn't take a super hero to master the jogging stroller.

— by Suzanne P. Lamp

Suzanne P. Lamp is a freelance writer, long distance runner and mother of two, who resides in Bloomington, Illinois.

Part Six

Additional Help and Information

Chapter 43

Glossary

A

abduction: To draw away from or deviate from the midline of the body; opposite of adduction; side movement away from the midline of the body. Example: a side leg raise moving the leg away from the body's center.

abrasion: A scraping away of skin or mucous membrane as the result of an injury or by other mechanical means.

abs: Slang for rectus abdominus muscle.

accommodative resistance: The application of a resistive force that controls the speed with which an individual is able to move, thereby allowing him to work at maximal resistance throughout the complete range of motion; this is very useful during rehabilitation, when injuries are present, and also in sports training for speed-strength; also referred to as isokinetic resistance; see also isokinetic resistance.

Achilles tendinitis: Inflammation of the Achilles tendon (tendon found at the back of the heel); rest and ice are the two recommended treatments for Achilles tendinitis.

acid-base balance: The mechanisms by which the pH of the body fluids are kept in a state of balance so that arterial blood is kept at a constant pH level of 7.35 to 7.45. The pH of blood is kept from becoming too acidic or alkaline through respiration, buffers, and work done by the kidneys.

active (dynamic) stretching: A technique in stretching muscle and tissue that requires muscle contraction through a range of motion; no outside force is involved.

active recovery: Performing light aerobic exercise, stretching exercises, or working other body parts to facilitate recovery after intense exercise to allow for more productive use of exercise time and to encourage blood flow to the muscles.

acute: Having a rapid onset; sharp, severe; opposite of chronic.

adduction: To bring toward the midline of the body; opposite of abduction. Example: bringing the elbows together in front of the body like a chest press working the pectoralis muscle.

adenosine triphosphate (ATP): A high-energy molecule from which the body derives its energy; produced aerobically and anaerobically, and stored in the body.

adipose tissue: Fatty tissue; connective tissue made up of fat cells.

ADP: Adenosine di-phosphate, a high energy phosphate molecule involved in the production and storage of energy; the end product of the mono-phosphate reduction of ATP.

aerobic: With, or in the presence of, oxygen; aerobic metabolism most efficiently produces the basic energy source, adenosine triphosphate (ATP). Walking, jogging, biking, an aerobic exercise class and any activity which maintains the heart rate in the THR zone for a minimum of 20 minutes is aerobic activity. Tennis and basketball are not considered aerobic activities.

aerobic exercise: Aerobic exercise refers sustained exercise that uses large muscle groups and places demands on the cardiovascular system.

aerobic exercise (training): Exercise with the purpose of developing aerobic or cardiovascular conditioning; activities in which oxygen from the blood is required to fuel the energy-producing mechanisms of muscle fibers. Examples: running, cycling, rowing, cross-country skiing.

aerobic interval training: Training method characterized by intervals of high and low intensity of pre-determined duration; heart rate typically remains at 60-80% of MHR, with 2- to 15-minute intervals; used to develop the aerobic energy system.

aerobic threshold intervals: Used to develop ability to use oxygen while performing at a higher intensity; exercise is performed for a pre-determined time at anaerobic threshold, combined with a period of active recovery; This training can be modified in terms of intensity and duration of the exercise interval and the number of work intervals per workout.

afterburn: Calories used due to an increase in metabolic rate following exercise activities.

agonist (muscle): Muscle that is directly involved in contraction; primarily responsible for movement; opposes the action of an antagonist (opposite) muscle. During a bicep curl, the bicep is the active muscle or agonist; compare antagonist.

all-or-none principle: The principle of muscle contraction that states that when a motor unit is activated, all of the muscle fibers in that given motor unit will maximally contract or not contract at all.

amenorrhea: The absence of menstruation; somewhat more common in women engaging in excessive exercise; thorough medical exam is required to determine the exact cause.

amino acids: Amino acids function as the building blocks of proteins. Chemically, amino acids are organic compounds containing an amino (NH2) group and a carboxyl (COOH) group. Amino acids are classified as essential, nonessential and conditionally essential. If body synthesis is inadequate to meet metabolic need, an amino acid is classified as essential and must be supplied as part of the diet. Essential amino acids include leucine, isoleucine, valine, tryptophan, phenylalanine, methionine, threonine, lysine, histidine and possibly arginine (conditionally essential). Nonessential amino acids can be synthesized by the body in adequate amounts, and include alanine, aspartic acid, asparagine, glutamic acid, glutamine, glycine, proline and serine. Conditionally essential amino acids become essential under certain clinical conditions.

AMP: Adenosine mono-phosphate, a phosphate molecule involved in the production of energy in the body. The end product of the monophosphate reduction of ADP or the di-phosphate reduction of ATP. Used to regenerate ATP levels.

anabolic androgenic steroids: A general class of hormones (or synthetic derivatives) of the male sex hormone testosterone which simulates testosterone's tissue building and masculinizing properties.

anabolism: The metabolic processes which build up body tissue. Example: muscle-building; anabolism is the opposite of catabolism.

anaerobic: Outside the presence of oxygen; not requiring oxygen; anaerobic activities produce higher levels of lactic acids and carbon dioxide than aerobic activities. Short duration activities, requiring bursts of energy, are usually anaerobic.

anaerobic exercise: Short-term, highly intense activities in which muscle fibers derive energy for contraction from stored internal energy sources without the use of oxygen from the blood; stored energy sources include ATP, CP, and glycogen. Example: short burst, intense efforts, such as in sprinting or weightlifting.

anaerobic glycolysis: The metabolic pathway that uses glucose or stored glycogen for energy production without requiring oxygen; sometimes referred to as the lactic acid system or anaerobic glucose system, it produces lactic acid as a by-product.

anaerobic interval training: Training designed to teach the body to derive energy from the anaerobic system to improve muscular strength and speed and develop the athlete's ability to remove lactate from the muscles; characterized by intervals of higher and lower intensity; aerobic interval training typically exceeds 85% of MHR with 30-second to 4-minute intervals.

anaerobic threshold: The point during high intensity activity when the body can no longer meet its demand for oxygen and anaerobic metabolism predominates; also called lactate threshold.

anatomical planes: Three planes of the human body in the anatomical position: sagittal, frontal, and transverse.

anatomical position: Description of human body when body is erect, arms are down at sides, and palms are forward; used for describing positions on the body or directions of movement of the body.

anatomy: The study of the structure of an organism or its elements; human anatomy refers to the study of the human body.

anemia: Anemia is a condition in which a deficiency in the size or number of erythrocytes (red blood cells) or the amount of hemoglobin they contain limits the exchange of oxygen and carbon dioxide between the blood and the tissue cells. Most anemias are caused by a lack of nutrients required for normal erythrocyte synthesis, principally iron, vitamin B_{12}, and folic acid. Others result from a variety of conditions, such as hemorrhage, genetic abnormalities, chronic disease states or drug toxicity.

anemic: Condition characterized by a reduction below normal of the number of red blood cells or hemoglobin in the blood, often displaying symptoms of fatigue.

angina pectoris: Pain in the chest due to insufficient blood supply and oxygen to the heart; can be characterized as a crushing pain or by a substantial "pressure" sensation within the chest, commonly radiating down the arm, up into the jaw, or to another site; angina pectoris is caused by an obstructed coronary artery and insufficient oxygen to the heart muscle.

anorexia nervosa: A psychological eating disorder characterized by refusal to maintain a minimally normal weight for height and age. This condition includes weight loss leading to maintenance of body weight 15 percent below normal; an intense fear of weight gain or becoming fat despite the individual's underweight status; a disturbance in the self-awareness of one's own body weight or shape; and in females, the absence of at least three consecutive menstrual cycles that would otherwise be expected to occur. Metabolic abnormalities are commonly associated with this disorder and can sometimes be fatal.

antagonist: Muscle that works against or in opposition to an agonist muscle; while one muscle group flexes, another extends; during a biceps curl, the biceps is the agonist and the triceps is the antagonist; see also agonist.

anterior: Toward the front; frontal segment. Example: the quadriceps are anterior to the hamstring.

anthropometric measurements: Measurement and analysis of parts of the human body. Examples, skinfold, girth, and body weight.

antibody: Protein produced by the immune system of humans and higher animals in response to the presence of a specific antigen.

antigen: A foreign substance (almost always a protein) that, when introduced into the body, stimulates an immune response.

antioxidant: Antioxidants protect key cell components by neutralizing the damaging effects of "free radicals," natural byproducts of cell metabolism. Free radicals form when oxygen is metabolized, or burned by the body. They travel through cells, disrupting the structure of other molecules, causing cellular damage. Such cell damage is believed to contribute to aging and various health problems. Antioxidants include vitamins A, C, E, and selenium. Other potential antioxidants include pycnogenol, nordihydroguairetic acid (NDGA), glutathione, superoxide dismutase, and others. Antioxidants are also referred to as free-radical "scavengers."

aorta: The main arterial vessel; arises from the left ventricle of the heart and carries blood to all parts of the body; The aorta is the largest artery in the body.

arrhythmia: Abnormal heart rhythm or beat.

arteries: Vessels that carry oxygenated blood away from the heart; the carotid artery is commonly used to monitor the heart rate.

arterioles: Smaller divisions of the arteries as they get farther away from the heart and lead to capillaries.

arteriosclerosis: The hardening, thickening or loss of elasticity of the wall of an artery; precedes cardiovascular disease such as stroke and coronary artery disease; arteriosclerosis is sometimes referred to as "hardening of the arteries."

arthritis: Inflammation of one or more joints; a potentially painful disorder that limits comfortable range of motion; The exercise prescription for arthritis should include slow, controlled exercises that work the full range of motion; see also osteoarthritis and rheumatoid arthritis.

articulation: Place of union or junction between two or more bones; joint.

asthma: An intermittent obstruction of the tubes that carry air to and from the lungs characterized by episodes of difficulty breathing; for some, asthma is brought on only by exercise. Symptoms of exercise-induced asthma are coughing and shortness of breath after only 8-12 minutes of exercise. Participants should consult a doctor and obtain an exercise prescription.

atherosclerosis: The most common and serious form of arteriosclerosis; fatty substances and other debris collect in the inner lining of the arteries, forming plaques that encroach upon the passageway and gradually obstruct the flow of blood. Atherosclerosis is associated with a high-fat diet.

athlete's heart: An enlarged heart muscle found in endurance athletes; athlete's heart is the result of large, strong muscle fibers in the heart's left ventricle, which are well-conditioned by pushing out a great volume of blood.

atom: The smallest divisible unit of an element in nature in which that element still holds its natural properties as that element.

ATPase: Enzyme which acts to split the ATP molecule.

ATP: Adenosine triphosphate, a high-energy molecule from which the body derives its energy.

ATP-CP system: Energy system that utilizes ATP and creatine phosphate; see also adenosine triphosphate and creatine phosphate.

atrium: One of the two (left and right) upper chambers of the heart (Pl. atria); acts as a collection chamber for the heart prior to entering the ventricles to leave the heart.

atrophy: Decrease in the cross-sectional size of a muscle due to lack of use or disease. Example: the arm, after it has been in a cast for a period of time, is usually smaller than before it was broken.

avascular: Lacking in blood vessels or having a poor blood supply; not vascular; said of tissues such as cartilage and ligaments.

avulsion: The forcible separation or tearing of tissue from the body.

axis of rotation: The imaginary line or point about which an object, such as a body or a lever, rotates.

B

ball and socket joints: Triaxial joints constructed as they sound: a rounded or ball-shaped surface which fits into a concave hole or socket; the hip joint and shoulder joint are examples of ball and socket joints.

ballistic: A bouncing movement relying on gravity; ballistic stretching was once thought to be the best way to improve flexibility. It has since been found that ballistic stretching can potentially tear muscles resulting in scar tissue that is inflexible.

basal metabolic rate (BMR): The lowest rate of energy metabolism of a person at rest, 12-18 hours after eating; the lowest rate of metabolism compatible with life; physical exertion speeds up the basal metabolic rate.

beta-carotene: A carotenoid (pigment) found in yellow, orange, and deep green vegetables which provides a source of vitamin A when ingested; this substance has been found to have antioxidant properties.

beta-oxidation: The process by which fats, in the form of Acyl-CoA molecules, are broken down in the mitochondria to generate Acetyl-CoA, the entry molecule for Kreb's Cycle.

bi-axial joint: Joint that allows motion in two planes of motion. Example: condyloid joint such as the wrist.

bilateral: Affecting two sides.

biochemistry: The study of the chemistry within biological organisms.

biomechanics: The study of the internal and external forces acting on the body and the effects produced by these forces; the study of the mechanical aspects of physical movement, such as torque, drag, and posture, that is used to enhance athletic technique.

blind (single or double) experiment: In a single blind experiment, the subjects do not know whether they are receiving an experimental treatment or a placebo. In a double blind experiment, neither the researchers nor the participants are aware of which subjects receive the treatment until after the study is completed.

blood doping: A technique that consists of giving a blood transfusion to add red blood cells to increase the oxygen-carrying ability of the blood. An athlete using this technique will usually have blood drawn and stored. Once the athlete's blood levels have returned to normal, adding back in the removed red blood cells gives the athlete an increased number of red blood cells. It is illegal in most competitions. Risks include blood coagulation in the arteries, presenting a risk of death. Blood doping has been suggested in the deaths of some elite endurance athletes.

blood glucose: Blood glucose (blood sugar) refers to sugar in the form of glucose. The blood sugar level in humans is normally 60 to 100 milligrams per 100 milliliters of blood; it rises after a meal to as much as 150 milligrams per 100 milliliter of blood, but this may vary.

blood pressure: The force exerted against heart and blood vessel walls by passing blood. When a blood pressure reading is taken, the systolic over diastolic value is determined. Systolic pressure is primarily caused by the heartbeat or contraction. The diastolic pressure is taken when the heart is filling with blood between beats. Blood pressure values vary appreciably depending on age, sex, and ethnicity. A typical adult reading may be 120mm Hg over 80mm Hg, stated "120 over 80." Blood pressures above 140 over 90 at rest are considered high; see diastolic and systolic.

BMR (basal metabolic rate): See basal metabolic rate.

body composition test: A test or tests used to determine percentage of body fat. Examples: underwater or hydrostatic, skinfold, anthropometric, or electrical impedance.

body composition: The proportion of body fat to fat free mass.

body mass index (BMI): A relative measure of body weight (in kg) to body height (in meters squared) for determining degree of obesity; BMIs over 30 are considered obese according to U.S. standards.

bodybuilding: Training with the specific goal to enhance musculature and physical appearance.

body fat: Term often used to describe the percentage of fat in the body.

bone: Dense connective tissue that composes the skeleton. Bones may be strengthened through proper exercise — typically through exercise that requires weight bearing on the bone.

Borg's scale (of perceived exertion): A scale using perceived exertion with a numerical code to determine the level of exertion. The scale helps participants tune into their bodies since metabolism and functions can vary from day to day. There are two versions of the Borg scale: classical, based upon a scale of zero to 20 and the modified Borg scale, which is more common, based upon a scale of zero to 10.

brachial artery: The main artery of the arm, located in the upper inside of the arm.

bradycardia: Slower than average resting heart rate, due to the increased efficiency of the heart through aerobic conditioning in an athlete. A heart rate of less than 60 beats per minute is typical of bradycardia. Slow HR is considered to mean poor health for a non-athlete, but a sign of cardiac fitness for an athlete.

branched chain amino acids (BCAA): The essential amino acids valine, leucine, and isoleucine. The "branched chain" refers to the chemical structure of these amino acids. Thought to be important because they can be used to generate glucose for use as energy.

bronchioles: The smallest tubes that supply air to the alveoli (air sacs) of the lungs.

bronchitis: Acute or chronic inflammation of the mucous membranes of the bronchial tubes; see chronic obstructive pulmonary disease.

bronchodilators: Drugs that are designed to expand the bronchial tubes by relaxing the constricted bronchial smooth muscle, used by asthmatics. Example: Proventil.

bulimia nervosa: An eating disorder also known as "binge and purge." A bulimic person often overeats then induces vomiting and/or the use of diuretics or laxatives. Bulimia is a disorder that can become life threatening. This condition requires medical intervention; treatment involves psychotherapy.

bursa: A lubricating and protective sac located between certain connective tissue, i.e., between tendon and bone, tendon and ligament, or other structures, usually in the vicinity of joints; (Pl. bursae).

bursitis: The inflammation of a bursa; occurs most often in the knees, hips, shoulders, and elbows.

C

caffeine: Caffeine is a naturally occurring substance found in the leaves, seeds or fruits of over 63 plant species worldwide and is part of a group of compounds known as methylxanthines. The most commonly known sources of caffeine are coffee and cocoa beans, cola nuts and tea leaves. Caffeine is a pharmacologically active substance and, depending on the dose, can be a mild central nervous system stimulant. Caffeine does not accumulate in the body and is normally excreted within several hours of consumption.

calorie: A calorie is the amount of energy required to raise the temperature of one milliliter (ml) of water at a standard initial temperature by one Celsius degree, specifically between 14.5 and 15.5 degrees Celsius at 1 atmosphere of pressure (sea level). Use of a capital "C" for Calorie indicates 1,000 calories, or one kilocalorie. Calorie is the standard unit for energy measurement in nutrition.

capillaries: Tiny blood channels that are the point of nutrient exchange. Capillaries deliver oxygen to the tissues and withdraw carbon dioxide to be carried through the veins to the heart and lungs. They connect the arterial and venous systems.

carbohydrate (CHO): An essential nutrient that provides energy to the body; CHOs are also the most efficient fuel for other body functions. Sources of CHO include vegetables, fruit, rice, bread, pasta and whole grains. 1 gm CHO yields 4 kilocalories of energy.

carbohydrate loading: Sequence of up to a week-long regimen of manipulating intensity of training and carbohydrate intake to achieve maximum glycogen storage for an endurance event; primarily benefits athletes participating in events over 60 minutes long, where glycogen can become depleted to inhibit work capacity.

cardiac cycle: The period from the beginning of one heart beat to the beginning of the next; the systolic and diastolic movement, and the interval in between.

cardiac muscle: One of the body's 3 types of muscle, found only in the heart.

cardiac output: The volume of blood expelled by the ventricles of the heart each minute; equal to the amount of blood ejected at each beat multiplied by the number of beats per minute; usually expressed in liters of blood per minute. The cardiac output can increase with regular aerobic exercise.

cardiopulmonary: Pertaining to the heart and lungs.

cardiorespiratory endurance: The ability to perform large muscle movement over a sustained period; the capacity of the heart-lung system to deliver oxygen for sustained energy production; also called cardiovascular endurance.

cardiorespiratory: Referring to the heart, lungs, and blood vessels working together to deliver oxygen to the body and to remove unwanted waste products such as carbon dioxide.

cardiovascular disease (CVD): General term for any disease of the heart and blood vessels; includes coronary artery disease, hypertension, stroke, congestive heart failure, peripheral vascular disease and valvular heart disease.

cardiovascular endurance: See cardiorespiratory endurance.

cardiovascular: Referring to the heart (cardio), blood, and blood vessels (vascular).

carnitine (L-carnitine): Carrier protein that assists in the transportation of fats, in the form of Acyl-CoA, across the mitochondrial membrane so they may be oxidized to generate energy. L-carnitine is available as a dietary supplement. Formed from the essential amino acids lysine and methionine.

carotid artery: This artery is located in the neck. It is commonly used for palpating the pulse rate. *Note*: it is generally considered safest to monitor the pulse at the radial artery when monitoring the pulse of someone other than one's self.

cartilage: The dense connective tissue that covers the joint surfaces of the bones. The area where bones meet this smooth, semi-opaque material provides a "frictionless" surface for the joint.

catabolism: The breaking down of body tissue, including all processes in which complex substances are progressively broken down into simpler ones. Example: the catabolism of protein in muscle tissue into component amino acids, which occurs in intense training. Both anabolism and catabolism usually involve the release of energy, and together constitute metabolism.

cell membrane: The enveloping capsule of a cell, composed primarily of a lipid bilayer, but including carbohydrates and proteins in addition to the fats and cholesterol that make up the lipid bilayer.

cellulite: Subcutaneous fat (fat stored beneath the skin); although no different from other fat, it has a dimpled appearance caused by the structure of skin fibers covering it.

Centers for Disease Control and Prevention (CDC): The CDC, composed of 11 Centers, Institutes and Offices, aims to promote health and quality of life by preventing and controlling disease, injury and disability.

cervical curve: Curve in the rear neck formed by the seven vertebrae found between the base of the skull to the base of the neck. The cervical curve is slightly concave.

cervical vertebra: One of seven vertebrae found between the base of the skull and the base of the neck.

cholesterol (dietary): Cholesterol is not a fat, but rather a lipid, which is a classification of molecules that include fats. Cholesterol is vital to life and is found in all cell membranes. It is necessary for the production of bile acids and steroid hormones. Dietary cholesterol is found only in animal foods. Abundant in organ meats and egg yolks, cholesterol is also contained in meats and poultry. Vegetable oils and shortenings are cholesterol-free.

cholesterol (serum, or blood): High blood cholesterol is a risk factor in the development of coronary heart disease. Most of the cholesterol that is found in the blood is manufactured by the body, in the liver, at a rate of about 800 to 1,500 milligrams a day. By comparison, the average American consumes 300 to 450 milligrams daily in foods. Cholesterol is carried by proteins in the body in the form of lipoproteins. The most abundant lipoproteins include low-density (LDL), high-density (HDL), and very-low density lipoproteins (VLDL). LDL seems to be the culprit in coronary heart disease and is popularly known as the "bad cholesterol." By contrast, HDL is increasingly considered desirable and known as the "good cholesterol."

chondromalacia: The wearing away or softening of articular cartilage, usually occurring in the back of the kneecap; A cracking sound in the knee or grating feeling is typical of chondromalacia.

chromosome: Thread-like components in the cell that contain DNA. They make proteins. Genes are carried on the chromosomes.

chronic disuse: Any disease state that persists over a long period of time.

circuit training: A form of training that takes the participant through a series of exercise stations, sometimes with brief rest intervals in between; can emphasize muscular endurance, aerobic conditioning, muscular strength, or a combination of all three.

circumduction: The circular movement of a limb; a combination of flexion, abduction, extension and adduction movements.

clinical trials: Clinical trials undertake experimental study of human subjects. Trials may attempt to determine whether the finds of basic research are applicable to humans, or to confirm the results of epidemiological research. Studies may be small, with a limited number of participants, or they may be large intervention trials that seek to discover the outcome of treatments on entire populations. The "gold standard" clinical trials are double-blind, placebo-controlled studies which employ random assignment of subjects to experimental and control groups unknown to the subject or the researcher.

collagen: The main constituent of connective tissue, such as ligaments, tendons and muscles.

complete proteins: Foods that contain all essential amino acids; Most meats and dairy products are considered complete protein foods.

concentric (contraction/action): A muscle develops enough force to overcome a resistance, thus shortening the muscle and creating a movement in the direction of the pull; a shortening of the muscle due to a contraction.

conduction: Means of heat transfer through direct contact. Heat transfers from the body to another object through physical contact.

condyloid joint: Bi-axial joint with movement ability that includes flexion, extension, abduction, adduction and circumduction; considered a partial ball-and-socket joint; also referred to as an ellipsoid joint; This joint appears similar to the ball and socket joint except it is smaller and more oval shaped. Example: the wrist joint.

confounding variable or confounding factor: A "hidden" variable that may cause an association which the researcher attributes to other variables.

connective tissue: The tissue that binds together and supports various structures of the body. Examples: ligaments, tendons, and fascia.

continuous training: Conditioning exercise, such as walking, jogging, cycling or aerobic dancing, in which the prescribed intensity is maintained continuously between 50 and 85 percent of maximal oxygen consumption (functional capacity) and for a prolonged period of time.

contraction: The shortening or tightening of a muscle. The two phases of contraction include the concentric (shortening) phase and the eccentric (lengthening) phase.

contra-indicated (movements): Movements that present a very high risk of injury and that should normally be avoided.

control group: The group of subjects in a study to whom a comparison is made in order to determine whether an observation or treatment has an effect. In an experimental study it is the group that does not receive a treatment. Subjects are as similar as possible to those in the test or treatment group.

controlled experiment: In this type of research, study subjects (whether animal or human) are selected according to relevant characteristics, and then randomly assigned to either an experimental group, or a control group. Random assignment ensures that factors known as variables, which may affect the outcome of the study, are distributed equally among the groups and therefore could not lead to differences in the effect of the treatment under study. The experimental group is then given a treatment (sometimes called an intervention), and the results are compared to the control group, which does not receive treatment. A placebo, or false treatment, may be administered to the control group. With all other variables controlled, differences between the experimental and control groups may be attributed to the treatment under study.

convection: Means of heat transfer through the movement of air or other particles in a medium; similar to the effect of a fan blowing on body; a means of eliminating heat.

cool-down: The tapering-off period of very light activity at the end of a vigorous workout; this slowly cools the body down to a nearly normal core temperature.

core temperature: The temperature of vital internal organs.

coronary artery disease (CAD): The major form of cardiovascular disease; almost always the result of atherosclerosis; also called coronary heart disease (CHD).

coronary heart disease (CHD): See coronary artery disease (CAD).

coronary: Of, or relating to, the heart. Coronary arrest is a term for a heart attack; see myocardial infarction.

correlation: An association, or when one phenomenon is found to be accompanied by another. A correlation does not prove cause and effect. Correlation may also be defined statistically.

creatine monohydrate: Supplement that is composed of creatine bound to one molecule of water; thought to increase recovery during intense training by providing a somewhat elevated level of creatine phosphate stores in muscles; see also creatine phosphate or CP.

creatine phosphate (CP): A high-energy phosphate molecule that is stored in cells and can be used to immediately resynthesize ATP; one of the phosphagens.

creatine phosphate system: System of transfer of chemical energy for resynthesis of ATP supplied rapidly and without oxygen from the breakdown of creatine phosphate (CP); also called ATP-CP system.

cross-bridges: Projections of myosin molecules that link with actin filaments to create a grabbing, pulling effect, resulting in contraction.

cross-bridging: Term used to refer to the process of the myosin head attaching to the actin filament during muscular contraction.

cross-training: The incorporation of various modalities of exercise. Cross training reduces stress on any one structure, provides variety and can increase exercise adherence.

crunch(-es): Abdominal exercise used to isolate the abdominals while, at the same time, eliminates unwanted action from the iliopsoas muscles (hip flexors) and reduces the risk of stress on the lower back; preferred method of abdominal training over sit-ups.

cryotherapy: The use of cold therapy for treatment of injury; sprains, tears, twists, bruises and bleeding under the skin respond favorably to cryotherapy; suggested use: repeated applications for 24-48 hours or until external swelling is gone.

D

defibrillation: Stopping of atrial or ventricular fibrillation (rapid, randomized contractions of the myocardium), by the use of drugs or mechanical means, often by electroshock.

dehydration: Condition of having a less than optimal level of body water.

delayed onset muscle soreness (DOMS): Muscle soreness that occurs 24 to 48 hours after intense exercise; typically associated with eccentric muscle contractions, and thought to be the result of microscopic tears in muscle or connective tissue.

delts: Slang term referring to the deltoid muscles.

dextrose: A monosaccharide, which is a major part of corn syrup and honey.

diabetes: Diabetes is the name for a group of medical disorders characterized by high blood sugar levels. Normally when people eat, food is digested and much of it is converted to glucose—a simple sugar—which the body uses for energy. The blood carries the glucose to cells where it is absorbed with the help of the hormone insulin. For those with diabetes, however, the body does not make enough insulin, or cannot properly use the insulin it does make. Without insulin, glucose accumulates in the blood rather than moving into the cells. High blood sugar levels result.

diabetes mellitus: A disease of carbohydrate metabolism in which an absolute or relative deficiency of insulin results in an inability to metabolize carbohydrates normally; may require insulin injections. Exercise may influence a diabetic's need to inject insulin.

diastolic blood pressure: The amount of pressure maintained in the arteries between heart beats, as the heart relaxes and fills. The National High Blood Pressure Education Program recommends that anyone with a diastolic pressure of 105 or greater should be treated with drug therapy. Persons with readings of 90-104 should be individually treated as needed by a physician.

distal: Anatomical term meaning farthest away from the point of attachment or body's midline. Example: the foot is distal to the knee.

diuretic: Medication that produces an increase in the volume of urine and sodium (salt) that is excreted; sometimes used to reduce water weight and volume in the body. Use of diuretics by athletes can be very unsafe and is not recommended.

DNA: Deoxyribonucleic acid. This is the molecule that carries the genetic information for most living systems. The DNA molecule consists of four bases (adenine, cytosine, guanine and thymine) and a sugar-phosphate backbone, arranged in two connected strands to form its characteristic double-helix.

dorsal: The backside.

dorsiflexion: Bending backward of the hand or foot; opposite of plantarflexion.

duration: Length of time one works or exercises. Duration is one way of increasing resistance to a muscle or system to improve its function.

dynamic constant-resistance: Strength training exercises and/or equipment that provide a constant resistance throughout the movement range.

dynamic flexibility: The range of motion about a joint when speed is involved during physical performance; strength, power, neuromuscular coordination and tissue resistance are all factors.

dynamic variable-resistance (isokinetic): Strength training exercises and/or equipment that automatically vary the resistance throughout the movement range; see also accommodative resistance.

dyspnea index: An index which measures shortness of breath for calculating exertion levels; The dyspnea index is useful for people with lung disorders and those on heart-rate depressant drugs.

dyspnea: Shortness of breath or difficult breathing; the subjective feeling of being out of breath; caused by heart or lung disorders, strenuous activity, high anxiety or stress.

E

ectomorph: A thin body type; low fat content.

edema: Swelling due to abnormal accumulation of fluid in tissues or cavities.

elasticity: The ability of a tissue or other material to return to its original size or shape after stretching or elongation.

electrolytes: The minerals sodium, potassium and chlorine, which are present in the body as electrically charged particles called ions. Electrolytes are molecules that dissociate into cations or anions when fused or in solution, thus capable of conducting electricity; see ion.

emphysema: Chronic lung disease characterized by loss of air sacs resulting in a decreased ability to exchange gases; carbon dioxide levels are increased and oxygen levels are decreased, causing rapid breathing and dyspnea.

empty calories: Calories obtained from foods high in sugar and fat without significant nutritional value (vitamins and minerals).

endocrine: Pertaining to a gland that secretes directly into the bloodstream; the opposite of exocrine.

endocrine glands: Organs which secrete hormones into the blood or lymph systems to regulate or influence general chemical changes in the body or the activities of other organs. Major endocrine glands are the thyroid, adrenal, pituitary, parathyroid, pancreas, ovaries and testicles.

endomorph: A person whose body build is soft and round, with fat throughout the body; compare ectomorph and mesomorph.

endorphins: A natural chemical released by the body during exercise. Endorphins help relieve pain and leave the participant with a "natural high."

energy balance: The balance between energy taken in and energy used.

energy balance theory: The theory that body weight will stay the same when caloric intake equals caloric expenditure, and that a positive or negative energy balance will cause weight gain or weight loss.

enzymes: Proteins that speed specific chemical reactions.

epidemiology: The study of distribution and determinants of diseases or other health outcomes in human populations. It seeks to expose potential associations between aspects of health (such as cancer, heart disease, etc.) and diet, lifestyle, habits or other factors within populations. Epidemiological studies may suggest relationships between two factors, but do not provide the basis for conclusions about cause and effect. Possible associations inferred from epidemiological research can turn out to be coincidental.

essential amino acids: Eight of the 23 different amino acids needed to make proteins in adults; called essential because they must be obtained from the diet, since they cannot be manufactured by the body.

essential fatty acid: Fatty acid that can not be generated by other fatty acids in the body. The essential fatty acids include linoleic, linolenic, and arachadonic acids.

etiology: The study of the causes of disease.

essential nutrient: A nutrient that must be supplied by the diet because it cannot be produced in sufficient quantities by the body.

eversion: Turning outward.

exercise physiologist: A scientist who conducts controlled investigations of responses and adaptations to muscular activity utilizing human subjects or animals within a clinical, research, or academic setting. Exercise physiologists are degreed and certified in exercise physiology or a related field.

exercise physiology: The study of life processes as they relate to exercise.

exercise prescription: A physician's recommendations or referral for exercise; the recommended volume of exercise including frequency, intensity, duration, and type of exercise.

exercise-induced asthma: Intermittent labored breathing precipitated by exertion during exercise; see also asthma.

exertional headaches: Pain triggered by a variety of exercise activities ranging from weightlifting to jogging, and including sexual intercourse.

experimental group: The group of subjects in an experimental study which receives a treatment.

extension: To straighten; movement of a body part away from the body; to increase the angle at a joint. Example: triceps extension.

external rotation: Rotary motion away from the midline of the body.

F

fartlek training: Training method that alternates fast and slow activity over varied terrain, utilizing perceived exertion.

fascia: Sheet or band of fibrous tissue that lies deep to the skin or forms an attachment for muscles and organs and covering individual muscles.

fast-twitch (Type II) fiber: Large muscle fiber characterized by its fast speed of contraction; utilized in high intensity, short duration activities.

fat soluble vitamins: Vitamins soluble in fat, not water. Fat soluble vitamins can be stored in the fat within the body. Therefore, fat soluble vitamins pose the greatest threat of reaching toxic levels from Megadosing. Each of the fat-soluble vitamins A, D, E and K has a distinct and separate physiologic role. Vitamins A and E have antioxidant properties to depress the effects of metabolic byproducts called free radicals, which are thought to cause degenerative changes related to aging.

fat soluble: Able to be dissolved in fat; relating to vitamins, those that are stored in the body fat, principally in the liver: vitamins A, D, E and K.

fat-free mass: That part of the body composition that represents everything but fat: blood, bones, connective tissue, organs and muscle; the same as lean body mass; also called fat-free weight.

fatigue: State of decreased capacity for work due to previous workload; working a muscle to fatigue refers to working to "failure"; the inability to perform another repetition in good form.

fats (dietary fats): Fats are referred to in the plural because there is no one type of fat. Fats are composed of the same three elements as carbohydrates—carbon, hydrogen and oxygen, However, fats have relatively more carbon and hydrogen and less oxygen, thus supplying a higher fuel value of nine calories per gram (versus four calories per gram from carbohydrates and protein). One molecule of fat can be broken down into three molecules of fatty acids and one molecule of glycerol. Thus, stored fats are known chemically as triglycerides. Fats are a vital nutrient in a healthy diet. Fats supply essential fatty acids, such as linoleic acid, which is especially important to childhood growth. Fat helps maintain healthy skin, regulate cholesterol metabolism and is a precursor of prostaglandins, hormone-like substances that regulate some body processes. Dietary fat is needed to carry fat-soluble vitamins A, D, E and K and to aid in their absorption from the intestine.

fatty acid: Fatty acids are generally classified as saturated, monounsaturated or polyunsaturated. These terms refer to the number of hydrogen atoms attached to the carbon atoms of the fat molecule.

fiber: Dietary fiber generally refers to parts of fruits, vegetables, grains, nuts and legumes that can't be digested by humans. Meats and dairy products do not contain fiber. Studies indicate that high-fiber diets can reduce the risks of heart disease and certain types of cancer. There are two basic types of fiber—insoluble and soluble. Soluble fiber in cereals, oatmeal, beans and other foods has been found to lower blood cholesterol. Insoluble fiber in cauliflower, cabbage and other vegetables and fruits helps move foods through the stomach and intestine, thereby decreasing the risk of cancers of the colon and rectum.

flex: Contracting or tightening a muscle (or muscles) isometrically; also refers to joint movement; see flexion.

flexibility: The range of movement in a joint and corresponding muscle groups. Flexibility training increases the length and elasticity of the muscles.

flexion: Bending of a limb at a joint; decreasing the angle of the joint.

flush: Cleansing a muscle of metabolic toxins by increasing the blood supply to it through exertion.

Food and Drug Administration (FDA): The Food and Drug Administration is part of the Public Health Service of the U.S. Department of Health and Human Services. It is the regulatory agency responsible for ensuring the safety and wholesomeness of all foods sold in interstate commerce except meat, poultry and eggs (which are under the jurisdiction of the U.S. Department of Agriculture). FDA develops standards for the composition, quality, nutrition, safety and labeling of foods including food and color additives. It conducts research to improve detection and prevention of contamination. It collects and interprets data on nutrition, food additives and pesticide residues. The agency also inspects food plants, imported food products and feed mills that make feeds containing medications or nutritional supplements that are destined for human consumption. And it regulates radiation-emitting products such as microwave ovens. FDA also enforces pesticide tolerances established by the Environmental Protection Agency for all domestically produced and imported foods, except for foods under USDA jurisdiction.

Food Guide Pyramid: a graphic design used to communicate the recommended daily food choices contained in the Dietary Guidelines for Americans. The information presented in the Food Guide Pyramid was developed and promoted by the U.S. Department of Agriculture and the U.S. Department of Health and Human Services. It was published in 1992 by the U.S. Dept. of Agriculture and the U.S. Dept. of Health & Human Services.

forced repetitions or reps: A weight training system where assistance is given by a spotter to perform additional repetitions of an exercise when muscles can no longer complete the positive contraction on their own.

form: Manner in which a particular exercise is performed.

free radicals: Free radicals are highly reactive molecules which contain an odd number of electrons and target the body's tissues; thought to be involved in generation of some cancers.

frequency: How often a person exercises.

frontal plane: An imaginary longitudinal section that divides the body into anterior and posterior halves; lies at a right angle to the sagittal plane.

fulcrum: The support on which a lever rotates when moving or lifting something.

functional capacity: The maximum physical performance represented by maximal oxygen consumption.

functional foods: Foods that may provide health benefits beyond basic nutrition. Examples include tomatoes with lycopene, thought to help prevent the incidence of prostate and cervical cancers; fiber in wheat bran and sulfur compounds in garlic also believed to prevent cancer.

G

glucagon: Hormone responsible for increasing the rate of gluconeogenesis when blood sugar becomes low. Glucagon regulates blood sugar levels with insulin which inhibits glucagon and helps store sugar when blood sugar becomes too high.

glucose: A sugar, most commonly in the form of dextroglucose, that occurs naturally, has about half the sweetening power of regular sugar and does not crystallize easily. Glucose comes from grape juice, honey and certain vegetables, among other things. Glucose is the simple sugar utilized in the body for energy and storage of energy in the form of carbohydrates.

gluteals: Abbreviation for gluteus maximus, medius and minimus; the hip extensor muscles; also called buttocks or glutes.

glycemic index: A rating scale which measures the increase in blood sugar and the rise in insulin levels following the consumption of a given food.

glycogen: The storage form of carbohydrate in the muscles and the blood, composed of chains of glucose molecules.

gram (g): Approximately 1/5 of a level teaspoon.

grand mal seizure: Major motor seizure characterized by violent and uncontrollable muscle contractions.

growth hormone (GH): A hormone that regulates cell division and protein synthesis necessary for normal growth. The growth hormone exerts a direct effect on protein, carbohydrate and lipid metabolism, and controls the rate of skeletal, connective (collagenous) tissue and visceral growth.

H

hams: Slang for hamstring muscles.

health-related physical fitness: Components of physical fitness that are associated with some aspect of health; these important factors include cardiorespiratory endurance, muscular endurance, muscular strength, body composition, and joint flexibility.

health: The absence of disease or injury along with physical, mental, and social well-being.

heart attack: See myocardial infarction.

heart rate (HR): Number of times the heart beats in one minute.

heart rate reserve (HRR): The result of subtracting the resting heart rate from the maximal heart rate; represents the working heart-rate range between rest and maximal heart rate within which all activity occurs; used in the Karvonen method of calculating target heart rates.

heat cramps: Painful cramps occurring in muscles caused from laboring in hot conditions in which excessive amounts of electrolytes are lost in the sweat.

heat exhaustion: The most common heat-related illness; usually the result of intense exercise in a hot, humid environment and characterized by profuse sweating, which results in fluid and electrolyte loss, a drop in blood pressure, light-headedness, nausea, vomiting, decreased coordination and often syncope (fainting).

heat stroke: Exertional heat stroke is caused when the body generates more heat through muscle activity than it can dissipate, which can lead to permanent damage or death. Symptoms of heat stroke include red dry skin, cessation of perspiration, fast strong pulse, dizziness or fainting. A true medical emergency, heat stroke can be prevented by working out at a cooler time, dressing lightly and drinking plenty of water before, during and after exercising.

hemoglobin: Protein that holds and transports oxygen within the blood consisting of an iron-containing pigment called heme and a simple protein, globin.

hernia: Protrusion or projection of part of an organ through the wall of the cavity that normally contains it. Example: protrusion of the abdominal contents into the groin (inguinal hernia) or through the abdominal wall (abdominal hernia).

high energy phosphates: Molecules within the body that provide the energy to drive chemical reactions within the body. Example: ATP.

high-density lipoprotein (HDL): A type of cholesterol that has scavenger characteristics in removing some fats, making it beneficial. Exercise can increase the production of HDL.

homeostasis: The tendency toward stability and balance in normal body states.

hormones: Chemical substances which originate in an organ, gland, or body part, and are conveyed by the blood to affect functions in other parts of the body.

human growth hormone (HGH): Hormone secreted by the anterior pituitary gland in response to various stressful stimuli such as heat, starvation and intense physical stress (e.g., exercise). The principle functions of HGH are to stimulate anabolism and to mobilize stored fat (triglycerides) for energy, thus sparing muscle glycogen.

hypercholesterolemia: A condition characterized by having elevated cholesterol in the blood.

hyperextension: Extreme or excessive extension of a joint beyond the normal range of motion.

hyperglycemia: A condition characterized by an abnormally high content of glucose in the blood.

hyperlipidemia: A condition characterized by an excess of lipids in the blood.

hyperplasia: An increase in cell growth through splitting of cells.

hypertension: Hypertension is the persistently elevated arterial blood pressure. It is the most common public health problem in developed countries. Emphasis on lifestyle modifications has given diet a prominent role for both the primary prevention and management of hypertension. Hypertension is considered as resting blood pressure levels over 140/90.

hypertension: A condition characterized by high blood pressure, or the elevation of blood pressure above 140/90 mmHg.

hyperthermia: A condition characterized by abnormally high body temperature.

hypertrophy: An increase in the cross-sectional size of a muscle in response to progressive resistance (strength) training.

hyperventilation: A condition characterized by a greater-than-normal rate of breathing that results in an abnormal loss of carbon dioxide from the blood; dizziness may occur.

hypoglycemia: A condition characterized by a deficiency of sugar in the blood commonly caused by too much insulin, too little glucose, or too much exercise in the insulin-dependent diabetic.

hypokalemia: A condition characterized by a deficiency of potassium in the blood.

hypokinesis: A condition characterized by a lack of activity or energy.

hypothermia: A condition characterized by an abnormally low body temperature.

I

inferior: Anatomical term meaning situated below or nearer the soles of the feet in relation to a specific reference point; opposite of superior.

innervation: Nerve root extended from a particular vertebrae to attach to a given muscle or part of the body.

insertion: Attachment point of a muscle that is more distal or inferior; attachment point of a muscle onto the more moveable structure.

insulin-dependent diabetes mellitus (IDDM): A form of diabetes caused by the destruction of the insulin-producing beta cells in the pancreas, which leads to little or no insulin secretion; generally develops in childhood and requires regular insulin injections.

intensity: The physiological stress on the body during exercise; indicates how hard the body should be working to achieve a training effect; workload.

internal rotation: Rotary motion toward the midline of the body. Example: internally rotating the hip to point the knees and toes inward.

interval training: Exercise performed in an intermittent manner using a pre-established spacing of work and rest intervals. By changing the duration of work and rest intervals, a specific energy transfer system can be emphasized and overloaded; see aerobic intervals, aerobic threshold intervals and anaerobic intervals.

inversion: Turning inward.

ischemia: Insufficient blood flow to some part of the body, resulting in decreased oxygen availability.

isokinetic: Refers to a type of contraction where the speed of movement is fixed and the resistance varies in accordance with the muscular force exerted; see accommodative resistance.

isometric: Working a muscle against an immovable object; tension is developed but no mechanical work is performed; contraction of a muscle in which shortening or lengthening is prevented; involves muscular force equal to, but not greater than the resistance.

isotonic: Refers to a type of muscle contraction performed while equal tension is maintained on the muscle, and the length of the muscle is decreased or lengthened.

J

jerk: The part of the Olympic lift known as the "clean and jerk," where the lifter drives the barbell from his or her shoulders overhead to a locked position.

joint: Point where two bones come together; articulation.

K

Karvonen formula: A mathematical calculation for determining target heart rates: [(220 - age) - (RHR) x (50-85%)] + RHR - THR.

Kegel exercises: Exercises for strengthening the pubococcygeus muscles. Kegel exercises can be especially beneficial for women in the childbearing years.

ketogenic diet: Low-carbohydrate diet designed to generate a state of ketosis.

ketosis: A condition characterized by an abnormal increase of ketone bodies in the body; usually the result of a low-carbohydrate diet, fasting or starvation; see ketone bodies.

Kilocalorie: 1,000 calories or a "Calorie" which is used as the standard for energy measurement in nutrition.

kinesiology: The study of human movement.

kinesthetic awareness: The ability of individuals to feel where their bodies are in relation to space; a body awareness.

Krebs cycle: Cycle by which high energy intermediates are formed prior to generating ATP through the Electron Transport System.

kyphosis: Abnormal outward curvature of the upper back; Examples, hunchback or dowager's hump.

kyphosis-lordosis: An increase in the normal inward curve of the low back, combined with an increased outward curve of the thoracic spine.

L

lactate: The anaerobic product of glycolysis in animals. Formed under conditions that do not favor aerobic breakdown of pyruvate, the end product of glycolysis.

lactic acid (lactate): A bi-product of anaerobic energy production known to cause localized muscle fatigue when it accumulates during short-term, high intensity exercise. It is associated with fatigue.

lactic acid system: See anaerobic glycolysis.

lactose: A sugar naturally occurring in milk, also known as "milk sugar," that is the least sweet of all natural sugars and used in baby formulas and candies.

lactose intolerance: Lactose intolerance is an inherited inability to properly digest dairy products, due to a deficiency in the amount of the enzyme, lactase in the small intestine. This enzyme is necessary for the hydrolysis of lactose (a disaccharide) into its constituent monosaccharides, glucose and galactose. Symptoms of lactose intolerance, including abdominal cramps, flatulence and frothy diarrhea, can increase with age.

lateral: Anatomical term meaning away from the midline of the body, toward the side.

lats: Slang referring to the latissimus dorsi, the large muscles of the back that are the prime movers for adduction, extension and hyper-extension of the shoulder joints.

law of acceleration: Force (F) acting on a body in a given direction is equal to the body's mass (m) multiplied by the body's acceleration (a) in that direction; F = ma, or a = F/m.

law of inertia: The tendency of all objects and matter to remain at rest, or, if moving, to continue moving in the same straight line unless acted on by an outside force; proportional to body mass.

lean body mass: See fat-free mass.

ligament: A band of non-elastic tough connective tissue connecting the articular ends of the bones; frequently the stabilizing element of a joint.

lipids: Fats or fat-like substances.

lipolysis: The splitting of a fat molecule.

lipoprotein: Vehicle that transports fat throughout the body; made up of protein, fat, and cholesterol.

locomotion: Movement from one place to another.

longevity: Length of life.

lordosis: A normal curvature of the lower back; this can also refer to an excessive inward curvature (hyperlordosis) or lack of curvature in the lumbar area (hypolordosis). Hyperlordosis predisposes the participant to a higher risk of injury.

low-density lipoproteins (LDLs): Plasma complex of lipids and proteins that contains relatively more cholesterol and triglycerides and less protein. High LDL levels are associated with an increased risk of coronary heart disease.

lumbar curve: Curve which is formed from the 5 vertebrae found in the lower back; this curve is slightly concave; see lordosis.

lycopene: Lycopene is a carotenoid related to the better known beta-carotene. Lycopene gives tomatoes and some other fruits and vegetables their distinctive red color. Nutritionally, it functions as an antioxidant. Research shows lycopene is best absorbed by the body when consumed as tomatoes that have been heat-processed using a small amount of oil. This includes products such as tomato sauce and tomato paste. Also, see *functional foods*.

M

macronutrient: Substance required in large amounts to sustain life (Carbohydrate, protein, fat, and water).

maximal heart rate (HRmax or MHR): Maximal number of times an individual's heart beats within one minute; HRmax is determined in part by age and genetics; also referred to as maximum heart rate.

maximal oxygen consumption (VO2max): The highest volume of oxygen a person can consume during exercise; maximum-aerobic capacity; VO2max is a measure of maximal cardiovascular performance.

maximal oxygen uptake: See maximal oxygen consumption (VO2 max).

max: Maximum effort for one repetition of a weight training exercise; also expressed as one's "1-RM" or "one rep max."

medial: Anatomical term meaning situated or occurring in the middle of the body; toward the midline.

mega-dose (Mega-dosing): A dose of a nutrient that is 10 times or more than the RDA for that nutrient.

meniscal tear: A tear in the meniscal cartilage (found in the knee). Torn meniscus, a common and painful injury, plagues many athletes and dancers.

menopause: Cessation of menstruation in the human female, usually occurring between the ages of 48 and 50.

mesomorph: A person whose body shape consists mostly of muscle, bone and connective tissue, with a predisposition to muscular development; compare ectomorph and endomorph.

meta-analysis: A quantitative technique in which the results of several individual studies are pooled to yield overall conclusions.

metabolic equivalents (METS): A simplified system for classifying physical activities where one MET is equal to the resting oxygen consumption, which is approximately 3.5 milliliters of oxygen per kilogram of body weight per minute (3.5 ml/kg/min).

metabolic pathways: A series of consecutive enzymatic reactions that produce specific products; pathways involved in metabolic processes. Example: the breakdown of glucose, the storing of glycogen, the breakdown of fats, etc.

metabolic rate: The rate at which the body utilizes energy. Exercise raises the metabolic rate.

metabolism: The sum total of all chemical reactions taking place in a living organism; typically broken down into the energy-producing and absorbing processes that are occurring in the body. Metabolism describes the energy utilized by the body.

MET: See metabolic equivalents (METs).

micronutrient: Substance required in small amounts to sustain life (vitamins and minerals).

mitochondria: Specialized subcellular structures located within body cells that contain oxidative enzymes needed by the cells to metabolize foodstuffs into energy sources. They are the source of energy in the cell and are involved in protein synthesis and lipid metabolism.

monounsaturated fats: A type of unsaturated fat (liquid at room temperature) that has one spot available on the fatty acid for the addition of a hydrogen atom; moderate intake is associated with a lower risk for cardiovascular disease. Example: oleic acid in olive oil; generally considered to be a "healthy" fat.

morbid obesity: This is a state of adiposity or overweight, in which body weight is 100 percent above the ideal and a body mass index of 45 or greater.

morbidity: The disease rate; the ratio of sick to well persons in a community.

mortality: The death rate, or ratio of deaths that take place to expected deaths.

motive force: The force that starts or causes a movement.

motor learning effect: Improvement in performance during the initial weeks of strength training due to more efficient motor unit utilization.

motor unit: A motor nerve and all the muscle fibers it stimulates. In the quadriceps muscle, one neuron can activate as many as 1,000 fibers. In the eye, where great precision is required, one nerve cell may control only 3 fibers.

muscle cramp: Painful involuntary contraction due to overexertion and imbalance of oxygen, minerals and carbon dioxide. Stretch the cramped muscle with one hand and squeeze and release the body of the muscle rhythmically with the other hand. Deep breathing helps to release cramps since it increases oxygen availability.

muscle fiber: A muscle cell.

muscle spindle: The sensory organ within a muscle that is sensitive to stretch and thus protects the muscle from being stretched too far; Muscle spindles cause the muscle to contract instead of allowing it to stretch during rapid stretching.

muscle tear: The tearing of a muscle bundle caused by severe stretching accompanied by acute pain and spasm. A muscle tear is called a strain.

muscle tone: The degree of tension and vigor in a gross muscle. Muscle tone is increased through weight training, which results in a greater number of muscle fibers "firing" while at rest.

muscular endurance: The ability to sustain a sub-maximal contraction (isometric) over time, or the ability to perform a maximum number of sub-maximal repetitions (isotonic).

muscular strength: The ability of the muscle to exert force; usually measured with one maximal repetition or with a hand dynamometer.

myocardial infarction (MI): An interruption of blood supply to the heart; may be caused by blockage of a heart artery caused by atherosclerosis or a blood clot; MI causes tissue damage to the heart muscle. It may begin with a crushing chest pain that moves to the left arm, neck or upper abdomen, and it may seem like indigestion. Signs of MI are rapid, irregular heart rate, low blood pressure and fever. Emergency treatment may require CPR; commonly called a heart attack.

myofibril: The functional units within muscle fibers that cause contractions. The more myofibrilla (plural) a person has, the greater his or her strength.

myoglobin: Protein that holds and stores oxygen within the muscles and tissues.

myosin: Thick contractile protein in a myofibril which overlaps with actin to produce contractions.

myotatic stretch reflex: Muscular reflex created by excessive muscle spindle stimulation; prevents potential tissue damage during periods of rapid muscle stretching.

N

National Health and Nutrition Examination Survey (NHANES): A series of surveys that include information from medical history, physical measurements, biochemical evaluation, physical examination and dietary intake of population groups within the United States. The NHANES is conducted by the U.S. Department of Health and Human Services approximately every five years.

Nationwide Food Consumption Survey (NFCS): A survey conducted by the USDA roughly every ten years that monitors the nutrient intake of a cross-section of the U.S. public.

negatives: Weight training technique in which the exerciser must obtain assistance to perform a concentric contraction to raise the weight; assistance may be through a spotter(s) as in forced reps or through the breaking of proper training form, as in cheat sets; This type of exercise is extremely damaging to connective tissue and often leads to DOMS.

non-insulin-dependent diabetes mellitus (NIDDM): Most common form of diabetes; typically develops in adulthood; is characterized by a reduced sensitivity of the insulin target cells to available insulin and is usually associated with obesity.

nutraceuticals: One term used to describe substances in or parts of a food that may be considered to provide medical or health benefits beyond basic nutrition, including disease prevention. Also, see functional foods.

nutrient: Something that nourishes, especially as found in food.

nutrient density: Quantitative analysis of the amount of nutrients versus the amount of calories in a given food. Nutrient-dense foods provide more nutrients than calories.

nutrition: Process by which a living organism takes in and uses food for the purpose of growth and tissue replacement.

O

obesity: Definitions vary, but are typically based upon calculations of body mass index (weight in kilograms divided by height in meters squared) over 30, or percent body fat over 30.

obliques: Short for external and/or internal obliques; the muscles to either side of the abdominals that rotate and flex the trunk.

one repetition maximum (1-RM): The amount of resistance that can be moved through the range of motion one time before the muscle is temporarily fatigued and the motion cannot be performed with good form again.

onset of blood lactate (OBLA): Point at which lactate begins to accumulate faster in the blood than it can be removed. This point is often referred to as a "lactate" or "anaerobic" threshold and is often considered the point where the body begins to get a high percentage of its energy from sugars as opposed to fats. The point just before the OBLA is often considered a "fat utilization" zone.

opposing muscle group: See antagonist muscle.

origin: Attachment of a muscle that is more superior or proximal.

orthostatic hypotension: Drop in blood pressure associated with rising to an erect position.

orthotics: Shoe inserts; can be helpful for persons who pronate (foot rotating inward) or supinate (foot rolling out).

osteoarthritis: Degenerative joint disease occurring chiefly in older persons; characterized by degeneration of the articular cartilage, hypertrophy of the bones, and changes in the synovial membrane.

osteoporosis: Thinning of the bones; density diminishes as calcium absorption is reduced; Exercised bones become denser and stronger, as long as dietary calcium is adequate.

outcomes research: A type of research increasingly used by the health industry which provides information about how a specific procedure or treatment regimen results: the subject (clinical safety and efficacy), the subject's physical functioning and lifestyle, and economic considerations such as saving/prolonging life and avoiding costly complications.

overfat: Typically defined as a BMI in excess of 25.

overload: To work intensely and vigorously beyond what you are used to; resistance, intensity, duration or frequency can be increased by increments of up to 10% in a workout to achieve overload in a progressive manner (followed by 48 hours for recovery); see progressive overload.

overload principle: One of the principles of human performance that states that beneficial adaptations occur in response to demands applied to the body at levels beyond a certain threshold (overload), but within the limits of tolerance and safety.

overtraining: Excessive hard training day-after-day without proper rest to ensure recovery.

overuse: Doing too much, too intensely, too frequently, or for too long; many injuries are caused by overuse.

overuse injury: An injury caused by activity that places too much stress on one area of the body over an extended period.

overweight: More than "normal" body weight based on standard charts, after adjustment for height, body build and age; overweight is not the same as overfat.

oxidation: The process of combining with oxygen, often associated in nutrition with the breakdown of a nutrient.

oxidation: Use of oxygen to split or breakdown molecules. Example: When oxygen is available, fat can be broken down (oxidized) by the oxygen molecule.

oxygen consumption: The amount of oxygen the body can take in and utilize.

oxygen debt: The extra oxygen (above normal resting levels) needed to recover from physical activity.

oxygen deficit: A temporary shortage of oxygen due to exercise.

P

palpation: Use of hands and/or fingers to detect anatomical structures or an arterial pulse (e.g., carotid pulse).

palpitation: A pounding or racing of the heart; associated with emotional responses or with certain heart disorders.

patella: Kneecap.

pecs: Slang for pectoral muscles of the chest.

perceived exertion: The subjective perception of exercise effort; see Borg's scale (of perceived exertion).

percent body fat: Refers to the ratio of fat to lean tissue and muscle mass.

periodization: The alternating of training intensities over periods of days, weeks, months, or years.

peripheral vascular resistance: Impedance of blood flow in the peripheral (farthest from the center) blood vessels.

phosphagens: High-energy phosphate molecules that can be broken down for immediate use by the cells; adenosine triphosphate (ATP) and creatine phosphate (CP).

physical fitness: A set of attributes that relates to the ability to perform physical activity.

physiological adaptations: Changes that occur as a result of stimuli to the various systems involved in life functions (muscular, cardiovascular, skeletal, etc.).

physiology: The study of essential life processes, functions, and activities.

placebo: Sometimes casually referred to as a "sugar pill," a placebo is a "fake" treatment which seems identical to the real treatment. Placebo treatments are used to eliminate bias that may arise from the expectation that a treatment should produce an effect.

plantar flexion: Ankle movement pointing toes toward ground, or away from body.

plantar: Of or pertaining to the sole of the foot.

plateau: A point in training at which one no longer sees improvements from one's current exercise routine; maintaining one's muscular size, strength, and/or athletic performance in spite of increased training efforts.

plyometric exercises: The sudden eccentric loading and stretching of muscles followed by their forceful concentric contraction; the sudden stretch causes a forceful contraction; i.e., jumping from a bench to the ground, then jumping back onto the bench.

polypeptide: Chain of amino acids.

polyunsaturated fats: A bond of at least 3 fatty acids with two or more points of unsaturation; polyunsaturated fats are found in raw nuts, some vegetables and grains; preferable to saturated fats.

posterior: Back portion or toward the back. Example: a tendon located behind the inner ankle is the posterior tibialis tendon.

post-menopausal: Pertaining to the period of time after menopause.

power: The speed at which one can apply a force over a given distance. Power = Force x Distance/Time.

premenopausal: Pertaining to the time before menopause.

prime mover: A muscle or set of muscles that acts directly to bring about a specific movement; most body movements are a combined action of many muscles.

progressive overload: Incremental increases of the workload, frequency, intensity, duration, load prescription, interval time, number of repetitions, or number of sets.

pronation: Rotation of a limb toward the midline of the body; turning the palm downward or flattening the arch of the foot. Pronation is a common foot problem which could predispose an athlete to injury; see orthotics.

prospective study: Epidemiological research that follows a group of people over a period of time to observe the potential effects of diet, behavior and other factors on health or the incidence of disease. In general, this is considered a more valid research design than retrospective research.

protagonists: Muscles working together to create a certain movement.

protein: Chemically, a protein is a complex nitrogenous compound made up of amino acids in peptide linkages. Dietary proteins are involved in the synthesis of tissue protein and other special metabolic functions. In anabolic processes they furnish the amino acids required to build and maintain body tissues. As an energy source, proteins are equivalent to carbohydrates in providing 4 calories per gram. Proteins perform a major structural role in all body tissues and in the formation of enzymes, hormones and various body fluids and secretions. Proteins participate in the transport of some lipids, vitamins and minerals and help maintain the body's homeostasis.

protraction: Scapular abduction.

proximal: Anatomical term meaning closer to the trunk of the body; nearest the point of attachment or nearest the center of the body.

pulmonary: Affecting the lungs or lung tissue.

pyruvic acid/pyruvate: End product of the glycolytic pathway; three-carbon metabolite that in aerobic conditions becomes acetyl Co-A and enters the Kreb's cycle, or, under anaerobic conditions will become lactic acid.

Q

quads: Slang for quadriceps; the four thigh muscles that extend the knee.

R

'roids: Slang for anabolic steroid.

R.I.C.E.: Rest, Ice, Compression, Elevation; the immediate treatment for most sudden athletic injuries.

radial artery: The artery in the wrist commonly used to take the pulse; The radial artery is located above the wrist, directly below the base of the thumb; generally considered the safest site for pulse monitoring.

random sample: A random sample is a procedure to select subjects for a study in which all individuals in a population being studied have an equal chance of being selected. Using a random sample allows the results of the study to be generalized to the entire population. The term random also applies to assignments within controlled studies, or the division of subjects into groups. Random assignment ensures that all subjects have an equal chance of being in the experimental and control groups, and increases the probability that any unidentified variable will systematically occur in both groups with the same frequency. Randomization is crucial to control for variables that researchers may not be aware of or cannot adequately control, but which could affect the outcome of an experimental study.

randomization, or random assignment: A process of assigning subjects to experimental or control groups in which the subjects have an equal chance of being assigned to each group. Randomization is used to control for known, unknown and difficult-to-control-for variables.

range of motion (ROM): The maximum motion allowed by muscles, joints, ligaments, tendons, and the structure of the bones.

rating of perceived exertion (RPE): Developed by Borg, this scale provides a standard means for evaluating a participant's perception of their physical exertion; the original scale was 6-20; the revised scale is 0-10; see also Borg's scale (of perceived exertion).

RDA: The Recommended Dietary Allowance (RDA) is the dietary intake level that is sufficient to meet the nutrient requirements of nearly all individuals in a specific age and gender group.

RDI: The values listed on the food labels for nutrients reflect average allowances based on the RDA. These values are referred to as Reference Daily Intakes (RDIs).

reciprocal innervation: Reflex utilized with stretch reflex to inhibit activity of an opposing muscle group.

recombinant DNA (rDNA): The DNA formed by combining segments of DNA from different organisms.

recruitment: Activation of motor units; the greater the resistance encountered, the greater will be the recruitment necessary to overcome its inertia.

repetition maximum (RM): Maximal number of repetitions one can perform a given exercise at a given weight and intensity while using proper exercise form.

repetitions (reps): Number of times a particular movement is performed.

research design: How a study is set up to collect information, or data. For valid results, the design must be appropriate to answer the question or hypothesis being studied.

residual volume: The air that stays in the lungs after breathing out as much as possible; the portion of the lungs which is not ventilated.

resistance: The amount of weight used in each set of an exercise.

respiratory or pulmonary: Referring to the lungs.

resting heart rate (RHR): The heart rate upon awakening from sleep before sitting up, averaged over a three-day period; normally, the lower the heart rate at rest, the better aerobic condition the person is in.

resting metabolic rate (RMR): Rate of body metabolism while conscious, but inactive.

retraction: Scapular adduction.

retrospective study: Research that relies on recall of past data, or on previously recorded information. Often this type of research is considered to have limitations, because the number of variables that cannot be controlled, and because memory is not infallible.

rheumatoid arthritis: Autoimmune disease that causes inflammation of connective tissues and joints.

RM: Acronym for "repetitions maximum." Example: 5RM stands for the maximum amount of weight you can perform for five repetitions.

RNA: Also known as ribonucleic acid. RNA is a molecule similar to DNA that functions primarily to decode the instructions carried by genes for protein synthesis.

ROM: See range of motion.

rotator cuff: Four intrinsic muscles of the shoulder that help to rotate the arm and keep the humerus in the glenoid fossa during activity.

S

sacral curve: Curve which is formed from the sacrum and coccyx in the area of the lower back and buttocks.

saddle joint: Joint in which the concave surfaces of two bones articulate with one another; movement is possible in two planes; a biaxial joint; resembles a saddle; capable of flexion, extension, abduction, adduction and circumduction. Example: the thumb is a saddle joint.

sagittal plane: Anatomical term referring to the imaginary longitudinal line that divides the body or any of its parts into right and left sections; the mid-sagittal line divides both halves equally. Motions within the sagittal plane include flexion and extension.

SAID principle: Acronym for the exercise training principle "specific adaptations to imposed demands"; training must be relative to the sport or activity for physiological change to take place and is specific to the action, energy systems, and muscle fibers.

sarcomere: Repeating base unit that composes a muscle fiber.

saturated fats: Fatty acids that have the maximum number of hydrogen atoms they can accommodate; found primarily in animal sources and a few plant fats; may lead to high cholesterol and heart disease; these fats are solid at room temperature.

scoliosis: Lateral curvature of the spine; usually evident in the upper or lower back.

secondary assessment: Assessment performed on an injured person after immediate life or limb-threatening injuries and illnesses have been identified; this more thorough evaluation is performed to identify more subtle, yet still important, injuries such as broken bones, sprains, strains, cuts, and other injuries.

sedentary: Not active.

seizure: A disorder originating from the brain in which there is a disturbance of movement, behavior, sensation, or consciousness.

set: A grouping of repetitions performed without rest. Example: an exerciser may perform 8 repetitions in a set of leg extensions.

set-point theory: A weight-control theory that states that each person has an established normal body weight, deviation from this set point will lead to changes in body metabolism to return to established 'normal weight' of that individual's body.

shin splints: An overuse syndrome including pain in the anterior lower leg; recommended treatment: R.I.C.E., wrap the shin, and support the plantar arch if necessary; see R.I.C.E.

side stitch (ache): A pain in the side usually caused by insufficient oxygen to the diaphragm, improper breathing, or intestinal gas.

sliding filament theory: An accepted theory explaining the interaction between actin and myosin proteins and ATP to cause muscle contraction.

slow-twitch (type I fiber): Muscle fiber characterized by its slow speed of contraction and a high capacity for aerobic glycolysis; also referred to as "red muscle fibers."

smooth muscle: Involuntary muscle tissue found in the walls of almost every organ of the body.

somatotype: Body type; see endomorph, ectomorph, and mesomorph.

spasm: See muscle cramp.

specificity of training: Principle of exercise training which refers to the fact that training the muscles in a specific way for a specific sport does not condition the body for different sports or exercises. Example: a marathon runner trains for distance running, but may not be able to do intense weight lifting. Only the systems we overload become stronger. See also SAID principle.

sphygmomanometer: An instrument used for measuring blood pressure in the arteries, usually at the brachial artery.

spondylolisthesis: Forward displacement of one vertebra over another; usually occurs at the 4th or 5th lumbar vertebrae.

spondylolysis: The breaking down (dissolving into another) of a vertebra; usually beginning with a stress fracture.

sport performance: The ability to achieve a high level of physical function within a given sport.

spot reducing: A myth suggesting that a high number of exercise repetitions in a particular area can significantly reduce the fat content in that area.

sprain: Stretching or tearing of ligaments of a joint, following a sudden twisting, wrenching or external force.

stabilizer muscle: Muscle that stabilizes (or fixes) one joint so a desired movement can be performed in another joint.

static: Position held without noticeable movement. Static stretching involves a slow, deliberate stretch until you feel a tightness in the muscle, but before you feel pain. Hold the stretch for 15-60 seconds.

statistical power: A mathematical quantity that indicates the probability a study has of obtaining a statistically significant effect. A high power of 80 percent, or 0.8, indicates that the study—if conducted repeatedly—would produce a statistically significant effect 80 percent of the time. On the other hand, a power of only 0.1 means there would be a 90 percent chance that the research missed the effect—if one exists at all.

statistical significance: The probability of obtaining an effect or association in a study sample as or more extreme than the one observed if there was actually no effect in the population. Based on the hypothesis that if there truly is no effect, the results of a study are unlikely to have occurred. A P value of less than five percent (P<0.05) means the result would occur less than five percent of the time if there were no effect, and is generally considered evidence of a true treatment effect or a true relationship.

steroids: Naturally occurring and synthetic chemicals that include some hormones, bile acids, and other substances; see anabolic androgenic steroids and 'roids.

strain: An injury of muscles or tendons or adjacent tissue such as the fascia as a result of over stretching or overexertion; see muscle tear.

strength: The ability to apply a force for a given distance; the ability to move a given amount of weight for a given distance; Strength = Force x Distance.

stress fracture: Fine, hairline fracture of the bone usually from repetitive stress; it may not show in an X-ray for several weeks; characterized by sharp persistent pain. Stress fractures are commonly caused by overuse, hard surfaces, or improper footwear.

stretch reflex: The body's automatic defensive action that stops the stretch action and protects against severe injury or abuse during stretching; see proprioceptive neuromuscular facilitation, Golgi tendon organ (GTO), and muscle spindle.

stroke volume: Amount of blood pumped per beat by the left ventricle; increases with regular aerobic exercise.

stroke: A sudden and often severe attack due to blockage of an artery into the brain; see cerebrovascular accident.

subluxation: A partial dislocation of a joint that usually reduces itself.

submaximal aerobic exercise test: A cardiorespiratory fitness test designed so that the intensity does not exceed 85 percent of heart-rate reserve or maximal oxygen uptake; this provides an estimation of maximal oxygen uptake without the risks associated with maximal exercise testing.

sucrose: Sucrose, a type of sugar, is a disaccharide composed of glucose and fructose. Also, see "carbohydrates."

sugar: Although the consumer is confronted by a wide variety of sugars—sucrose, raw sugar, turbinado sugar, brown sugar, honey, corn syrup—there is no significant difference in the nutritional content or energy each provides, and therefore no advantage of one nutritionally over another. There also is no evidence that the body can distinguish between naturally occurring or added sugars in food products.

superficial: External; located close to or on the body surface.

superior: Anatomical term meaning located closer to the head; opposite of inferior.

superset: Alternating between two exercises until the prescribed number of sets is completed; the two exercises generally involve a protagonist and antagonist (e.g., the pectoralis major and latissimus dorsi), but common usage of the term can mean any two exercises alternated with one another.

supination: Upward rotation of a limb, usually the hand or forearm, in an opened position.

supine: Horizontal position of the body, lying with the face upwards.

sympathetic nervous system: A division of the autonomic nervous system that activates the body to cope with some stressor (i.e., fight or flight response).

syncope: Fainting; a transient state of unconsciousness resulting from a lack of oxygen to the brain.

synergistic: Working together in a coordinated fashion; a synergistic muscle assists another muscle in its function.

synovial fluid: Transparent, viscous lubricating fluid found in the joints, bursae, and tendon sheaths; a proper warm-up stimulates its secretion.

systole: The contraction phase of the cardiac cycle during which blood leaves the ventricles.

systolic blood pressure: The pressure exerted by the blood on the blood vessel walls during ventricular contractions.

T

talk test: Subjective test for measuring exercise intensity by observing respiration effort and the ability to talk while exercising.

target heart rate (THR): The number of heartbeats per minute at which one should exercise for a desired result; 60-85% of the maximum heart rate is recommended for most people.

tendinitis: The inflammation or swelling of a tendon as a result of injury or overuse.

tendon: A tough cord or band of dense, white, fibrous connective tissue connecting a muscle to a bone; a tendon transmits the force exerted by a muscle.

testosterone: Testosterone is an androgen, a sex hormone produced by all humans. It is important in the development of male gonads and sex characteristics and it stimulates growth in tissues on which it acts.

thoracic curve: Outward curve formed by the thoracic vertebrae in the area of the upper back between the cervical and lumbar areas.

thrombosis: The formation, development or presence of a blood clot (thrombus).

torque: Moment of force causing rotation about a fixed axis of rotation; the act or process of turning around on an axis.

total lung capacity: The volume of gas in the lungs at the end of a maximum inhalation.

training effect: Change in functional capacity of muscles and other bodily tissues as a result of overload placed upon them during training.

training heart rate: Heart rate range at which an individual exercises to elicit a specific response. Example: the fat utilization training zone.

training to failure: Performing a set in weight training until inability to complete another repetition without assistance or breaking proper form.

training zone: Training heart rate range; see also target heart rate.

trans fats: Trans fats occur naturally in beef, butter, milk and lamb fats and in commercially prepared, partially hydrogenated margarines and solid cooking fats. The main sources of trans fats in the American diet today are margarine, shortening, commercial frying fats and high-fat baked goods. Partially hydrogenated vegetable oils were developed in part to help displace highly saturated animal and vegetable fats used in frying, baking and spreads. However, trans fats, like saturated fats, may raise blood LDL cholesterol levels (the so-called "bad" cholesterol). At high consumption, levels may also reduce the HDL or "good" cholesterol levels.

transient ischemic attack (TIA): Momentary dizziness, loss of consciousness or forgetfulness caused by a short-lived lack of oxygen (blood) to the brain; usually due to a partial blockage of an artery, it is a warning sign for a stroke.

transverse plane: Dissection of the body (or body part) into a top and a bottom portion; motions within this plane include rotation of the particular body part.

traps: Slang for trapezius muscles; the largest muscles of the back and neck that elevate the shoulder girdle and draw the scapulae medially.

tri's: Slang for triceps brachii muscle, located at the back of the arm.

triathlon: Race with three parts: a swim, a bicycle ride, and a run.

triglyceride: The storage form of fat consisting of three free fatty acids and glycerol.

troponin: A contractile protein that reacts with calcium to set the contractile mechanism into action within muscle fibers.

U

U.S. Department of Agriculture (USDA): The United States Department of Agriculture is comprised of many agencies charged with different tasks related to agriculture and our food supply. Among these is ensuring a safe, affordable, nutritious and accessible food supply. The USDA also enhances the quality of life for the American population by supporting production of agricultural products; caring for agricultural, forest and range lands; supporting sound development of our rural communities; providing economic opportunities for farm and rural residents; expanding global markets for agricultural and forest products and services; and working to reduce hunger in America and throughout the world.

unilateral: Affecting only one side.

V

validity: The extent to which a study or study instrument measures what it is intended to measure. Refers to accuracy or truthfulness in regard to a study's conclusion.

valsalva maneuver: To force the breath against a closed throat, i.e., holding the breath, tightening the muscles, and making a strong effort to lift a weight. The valsalva maneuver is especially dangerous to clients with high blood pressure or heart disease.

variability: The training technique of changing (varying) exercise sessions to prevent overuse, to prevent injuries, and to increase interest and adherence while minimizing staleness in a training program.

variable resistance equipment: Strength training equipment which can, through the use of elliptical cams and other such technology, vary the amount of weight being lifted to match the strength curve for a particular exercise. Example: Nautilus machines.

vascularity: The degree to which veins are observable.

vasoconstriction: Decrease in diameter of a blood vessel.

vasodilation: Increase in the diameter of a blood vessel.

vasodilator: An agent (motor nerve or drug) that acts to relax (dilate) a blood vessel.

ventricle: One of the two (left and right) lower chambers of the heart. The muscular left ventricle pumps blood to the body and is the portion of the heart in which adaptation to exercise is usually most visible. The smaller right ventricle pumps blood to the lungs.

vitamins: Vitamins are organic compounds that are nutritionally essential in small amounts to control metabolic processes and cannot be synthesized by the body. Vitamins are usually classified by their solubility, which to some degree determines their stability, occurrence in foodstuffs, distribution in body fluids, and tissue storage capacity. Each of the fat-soluble vitamins A, D, E and K has a distinct and separate physiologic role. Several have antioxidant properties that depress the effects of metabolic byproducts called free radicals, which are thought to cause degenerative changes related to aging. Most of the water-soluble vitamins are components of essential enzyme systems; many are involved in the reactions supporting energy metabolism. These vitamins are not normally stored in the body in appreciable amounts and are normally excreted in the urine. Thus, a daily supply is desirable to avoid depletion and interruption of normal physiologic functions.

VO2 max: See maximal oxygen consumption.

W

waist-to-hip circumference ratio (WTH): Measure for determining health risk due to the site of fat storage; taken by dividing the abdominal girth (waist measurement) by the hip measurement to form a ratio.

warm-up: A pre-workout routine that prepares the body for strenuous exercise. Warming up generally consists of light, progressive movements that stimulate heart, lungs, and muscles. The goal of the warm-up is to increase nutrient flow and heat of the muscles through increased blood flow throughout the body. Stretching is not advised as a warm-up strategy because of the damage that is easily caused to cold muscles.

water: Although deficiencies of energy or nutrients can be sustained for months or even years, a person can survive only a few days without water. Experts rank water second only to oxygen as essential for life. In addition to offering true refreshment for the thirsty, water plays a vital role in all bodily processes. It supplies the medium in which various chemical changes of the body occur, aiding in digestion, absorption, circulation and lubrication of body joints. For example, as a major component of blood, water helps deliver nutrients to body cells and removes waste to the kidneys for excretion.

water soluble vitamins: Vitamins that are soluble in water, not fat. Most of the water-soluble vitamins are components of essential enzyme systems. Many are involved in the reactions supporting energy metabolism. These vitamins are not normally stored in the body in appreciable amounts and are normally excreted in the urine. Thus, a daily supply is desirable to avoid depletion and interruption of normal physiologic functions.

water soluble: Able to dissolve in water.

work load: Amount of physical effort required for a specified task (often referred to in watts).

work: Physical effort required to accomplish a task.

X

xenobiotics: Synthetic chemicals believed to be resistant to environmental degradation. A branch of biotechnology called bioremediation is seeking to develop biological methods to degrade such compounds.

Chapter 44

Resources

Contents

Section 44.1

Resources in the Federal Government

Contact information was updated in December 2000.
Inclusion does not constitute endorsement.

Centers for Disease Control and Prevention

The Centers for Disease Control and Prevention (CDC), located in Atlanta, Georgia, USA, is an agency of the Department of Health and Human Services. The Centers for Disease Control and Prevention (CDC) performs many of the administrative functions for the Agency for Toxic Substances and Disease Registry (ATSDR), a sister agency of CDC, and one of eight federal public health agencies within the Department of Health and Human Services. The Director of CDC also serves as the Administrator of ATSDR: Agency for Toxic Substances and Disease Registry.

CDC Mission: To promote health and quality of life by preventing and controlling disease, injury, and disability.

CDC Pledge: CDC pledges to the American people:

- To be a diligent steward of the funds entrusted to it.

- To provide an environment for intellectual and personal growth and integrity.

- To base all public health decisions on the highest quality scientific data, openly and objectively derived.

- To place the benefits to society above the benefits to the institution.

- To treat all persons with dignity, honesty, and respect.

CDC's Physical Activity Efforts

- Provides state and national estimates of the prevalence of physical activity.

- Investigates the association of physical inactivity with cardio-vascular disease and other chronic conditions.

- Provides technical assistance to state risk-reduction programs to increase physical activity.

- Conducts annual research and practice seminars for public health professionals in collaboration with the University of South Carolina.

- Conducts regional seminars on physical activity training to increase the capacity of state health departments to promote physical activity.

- Convenes national physical activity meetings such as the May 1999 Expert Panel Meeting on School Physical Education Programs.

- As a World Health Organization (WHO) Collaborating Center for Physical Activity and Health Promotion, convenes international physical activity meetings such as the July 1999 WHO Workshop on the Economic Benefits of Physical Activity/Burdens of Inactivity.

- Produces physical activity resource materials for national and international distribution (e.g., Promoting Physical Activity: A Guide for Community Action).

CDC Contact Information: For information on any of the various topics with which CDC is involved, call 1-800-311-3435 or visit http://www.cdc.gov

Morbidity and Mortality Weekly Report: The data in the weekly *MMWR* are provisional, based on weekly reports to CDC by state health departments. The reporting week concludes at close of business on Friday; compiled data on a national basis are officially released to the public on the succeeding Friday. Inquiries about the *MMWR* Series should be directed to: Editor, *MMWR* Series, Mailstop C-08, Centers for Disease Control and Prevention, Atlanta, GA 30333 http://www.cdc.gov/epo/mmwr

Other CDC Resources

http://www.cdc.gov: The website for the Centers for Disease Control and Prevention. This site includes information on health issues in the news, data and statistics on health ad health-related issues, health-related topics "from A to Z" and information on how to order CDC publications, software and products.

http://www.cdc.gov/nchs/hphome.htm:

Click on *Healthy People 2000:* This is the CDC's National Center for Health Statistics' homepage for the Healthy People 2000 initiative. In September 1990, the Department of Health and Human Services released *Healthy People 2000: National Health Promotion and Disease Prevention Objectives,* a strategy for improving the health of Americans by the end of the century. Healthy People 2000 contains 319 unduplicated main objectives grouped into 22 priority areas. Because some priority areas share identical objectives, there are a total of 376 objectives including duplicates.

Click on *Healthy People 2010:* This is the CDC's National Center for Health Statistics' homepage for the Healthy People 2010 initiative. In January 2000, the Department of Health and Human Services launched Healthy People 2010, a comprehensive, nationwide health promotion and disease prevention agenda. Healthy People 2010 contains 467 objectives designed to serve as a road map for improving the health of all people in the United States during the first decade of the 21st century. Healthy People 2010 builds on similar initiatives pursued over the past two decades. Two overarching goals—increase quality and years of healthy life, and eliminate health disparities—served as a guide for developing objectives that will actually measure progress. The objectives are organized in 28 focus areas, each representing an important public health area.

For more information on Healthy People 2010 objectives or on physical activity and fitness, visit www.health.gov/healthypeople or call 1-800-336-4797.

http://www.cdc.gov/nchs/data/statnt18.pdf: This is the CDC's website for the statistical notes on the Healthy People 2000 initiative. To order a copy of the publication, call 301-458-4636 or email nchsquery@cdc.gov.

http://www.cdc.gov/nccdphp/dnpa: In CDC's National Center for Chronic Disease Prevention and Health Promotion, the Division of Nutrition and Physical Activity provides science-based activities for children and adults that address the role of nutrition and physical activity in health promotion and the prevention and control of chronic diseases. The scope of DNPA programs includes epidemiology, applied research, public health policy, surveillance, community interventions, evaluation, and communications. Find consumer information on various nutrition and fitness-related topics. Send requests for information to Division of Nutrition and Physical Activity, National Center for Chronic Disease Prevention and Health Promotion, Centers for Disease Control and Prevention, 4770 Buford Highway, NE, MS/K-24, Atlanta, GA 30341-3717, Phone (770) 488-5820, Fax (770) 488-5473

http://www.cdc.gov/nccdphp/sgr/sgr.htm: These pages contain the contents of the *Surgeon General's Report on Physical Activity and Health*. The entire report can be viewed and downloaded or it can be obtained by requesting a copy. Fax request to: (202)512-2250. Phone orders to: 202-512-1800 (7:30 a.m. - 4:30 p.m. ET). Mail request to: Superintendent of Documents, P.O. Box 371954, Pittsburgh, PA 15250-7954.

Department of Health and Human Services

The Department of Health and Human Services is the United States government's principal agency for protecting the health of all Americans and providing essential human services, especially for those who are least able to help themselves.

More information at The U.S. Department of Health and Human Services, 200 Independence Avenue, S.W., Washington, D.C. 20201. Phone: (202) 619-0257; toll-free: 1-877-696-6775, http://www.os.dhhs.gov

Consumer Health Information: healthfinder® is a free gateway to reliable consumer health and human services information developed by the U.S. Department of Health and Human Services. healthfinder® can lead you to selected online publications, clearinghouses, databases, web sites, and support and self-help groups, as well as the government agencies and not-for-profit organizations that produce reliable information for the public: http://www.healthfinder.gov

HS Partner Gateway: Together with many partner organizations, the Department works on a broad array of health and human services. This Gateway for Partner Organizations provides an easily navigable roadmap to HHS resources on the Web and points of contact off the Web that are of special interest to our partners. As such, the Gateway may not offer a comprehensive search of all the services and resources offered by the U.S. Department of Health and Human Services. Go to: http://www.hhs.gov/partner

Office of Disease Prevention and Health Promotion: The Office of Disease Prevention and Health Promotion, Office of Public Health and Science, Office of the Secretary, U.S. Department of Health and Human Services, works to strengthen the disease prevention and health promotion priorities of the Department within the collaborative framework of the HHS agencies.

To receive a list of ODPHP publications, call the ODPHP fax-back system at (301) 468-3028, or visit http://www.odphp.osophs.dhhs.gov

Administration on Aging: http://www.aoa.dhhs.gov is the website for the Department of Health and Human Services Administration on Aging. It includes information on fitness and exercise for the elderly. To contact the AoA, E-mail AoAInfo@aoa.gov, write to Administration on Aging, 330 Independence Avenue, SW, Washington, DC 20201, or call any of these numbers: (800) 677-1116 (Eldercare Locator—to find services for an older person in his or her locality); (202) 619-7501 (AoA's National Aging Information Center—for technical information and public inquiries); (202) 401-4541 (Office of the Assistant Secretary for Aging) (Congressional and media inquiries) Fax: (202) 260-1012.

The President's Council on Physical Fitness and Sports. *Provides "Pep Up Your Life," a free exercise booklet for older adults, in partnership with the American Association of Retired Persons. For more information:* DHHS/OS/OPHS, 200 Independence Ave., SW, HHH Bldg. Room 738 H, Washington, DC 20201. Phone: (202) 690-9000. Website: http://www.os.dhhs.gov

Federal Trade Commission

The FTC publishes free brochures on many consumer issues. For a complete list of publications, write for Best Sellers, Consumer Response Center, Federal Trade Commission, Room H-130, 600 Pennsylvania Ave, NW, Washington, DC 20580; or call toll-free 1-877-FTC-HELP (382-4357); TDD: (202) 326-2502. Website: http://www.ftc.gov

Food and Drug Administration

FDA is one of our nation's oldest consumer protection agencies. Its approximately 9,000 employees monitor the manufacture, import, transport, storage and sale of about $1 trillion worth of products each year. It does that at a cost to the taxpayer of about $3 per person.

First and foremost, FDA is a public health agency, charged with protecting American consumers by enforcing the Federal Food, Drug, and Cosmetic Act and several related public health laws. To carry out this mandate of consumer protection, FDA has some 1,100 investigators and inspectors who cover the country's almost 95,000 FDA-regulated businesses. These employees are located in district and local offices in 157 cities across the country.

For more information, call toll-free 1-888-INFO-FDA (1-888-463-6332), or visit the agency's website at http://www.fda.gov.

National Institutes of Health

The NIH mission is to uncover new knowledge that will lead to better health for everyone. NIH works toward that mission by: conducting research in its own laboratories; supporting the research of non-Federal scientists in universities, medical schools, hospitals, and research institutions throughout the country and abroad; helping in the training of research investigators; and fostering communication of medical information.

The NIH is one of eight health agencies of the Public Health Services which, in turn, is part of the U.S. Department of Health and Human Services. Comprised of 25 separate Institutes and Centers, NIH has 75 buildings on more than 300 acres in Bethesda, MD. From a total of about $300 in 1887, the NIH budget has grown to more than $15.6 billion in 1999. Write to: National Institutes of Health (NIH), Bethesda, Maryland 20892, or visit http://www.nih.gov

National Library of Medicine

Under the umbrella of the National Institutes of Health, the National Library of Medicine provides a wealth of reference information on hundreds of health topics, including MedlinePlus, a reference site for health topics, drug information, dictionaries, and other resources. Phone Numbers: (888) FIND-NLM, (888) 346-3656, (301) 594-5983 (local and international calls); http://www.nlm.nih.gov

Other NIH Resources

http://www.niddk.nih.gov/health/nutrit/win.htm: The website for The Weight-control Information Network (WIN), a national information service of the National Institute of Diabetes and Digestive and Kidney Diseases (NIDDK), National Institutes of Health (NIH). WIN was established in 1994 to provide health professionals and consumers with science-based information on obesity, weight control, and nutrition. For more information, contact: The Weight-control Information Network, 1 WIN Way, Bethesda, MD 20892-3665, Tel: (202) 828-1025 or 1-877-946-4627, Fax: (202) 828-1028, E-mail: win@info.niddk. nih.gov

http://www.nhlbi.nih.gov/health/public/heart/obesity/ lose_wt/patmats.htm: The website for The National Heart, Lung, and Blood Institute's (part of the National Institutes of Health) Obesity Education Intitiative. Information on Obesity and Physical Activity. Available NHLBI published pamphlets include: Aim for a Healthy Weight, Energize Yourself! Stay Physically Active, Embrace Your Health! Lose Weight if You are Overweight, Check Your Physical Activity and Heart Disease I.Q., Cut Down on Fat—Not on Taste, Facts About Heart Disease and Women: Be Physically Active, Stay Active and Feel Better, Watch Your Weight, Stay Young at Heart Recipes.

Weight-Control Information Network: The Weight-control Information Network (WIN) is a service of the National Institute of Diabetes and Digestive and Kidney Diseases, part of the National Institutes of Health, under the U.S. Public Health Service. Authorized by Congress (Public Law 103-43), WIN assembles and disseminates to health professionals and the general public information on weight control, obesity, and nutritional disorders. WIN responds to requests for information; develops, reviews, and distributes publications; and develops communication strategies to encourage individuals to achieve and maintain a healthy weight.

Publications produced by WIN are reviewed for scientific accuracy, content, and readability. Materials produced by other sources are also reviewed for scientific accuracy and are distributed, along with WIN publications, to answer requests. For more information: 1 WIN Way, Bethesda, MD 20892-3665, Tel: (202) 828-1025 or 1-877-946-4627, Fax: (202) 828-1028, E-mail: WIN@ info.niddk.nih.gov. Website: http://www.niddk.nih.gov/health/nutrit/win.htm.

National Heart, Lung and Blood Institute: Part of the National Institutes of Health. Offers free publications, on exercise, diet, and cholesterol. For more information: NHLBI Information Center, P.O. Box 30105, Bethesda, MD 20824-0105, phone: (301) 592-8573. Internet: http://www.nhlbi.nih.gov, or E-mail at nhlbinfo@rover.nhlbi.nih.gov

National Institute of Arthritis and Musculoskeletal and Skin Diseases: Part of the National Institutes of Health. Provides free information about exercise and arthritis; large print copies available on request. For more information: National Arthritis and Musculoskeletal and Skin Diseases Information Clearinghouse/NIAMS National Institutes of Health, 1 AMS Circle, Bethesda, MD 20892-3675. Phone: (301) 495-4484 Fax copies on request (301) 881-2731 (follow instructions and enter "10301" for the publication number). Website: http://www.nih.gov/niams/healthinfo

National Institute on Aging: Part of the National Institutes of Health. Call or write to receive free publications about health and fitness for older adults. For more information: Bldg. 31, Rm. 5C27 31, Center Drive, MSC 2292, Bethesda, MD 20892-2292. Information Center toll free phone: 800-222-2225. Toll Free TTY: 800-222-4225. Website: http://www.nih.gov/nia

The Osteoporosis and Related Bone Diseases National Resource Center, funded by the National Institutes of Health, offers free information for consumers and healthcare providers. Call 800-624-BONE (2663). Website: http://www.osteo.org

National Kidney and Urologic Diseases Information Clearinghouse: The National Kidney and Urologic Diseases Information Clearinghouse is a service of the National Institute of Diabetes and Digestive and Kidney Diseases, of the National Institutes of Health, under the U.S. Public Health Service. Established in 1987, the clearinghouse provides information about diseases of the kidneys and urologic system to people with these disorders and to their families, health care professionals, and the public. The clearinghouse answers inquiries; develops, reviews, and distributes publications; and works closely with professional and patient organizations and government agencies to coordinate resources about kidney and urologic diseases. Publications produced by the clearinghouse are reviewed carefully for scientific accuracy, content, and readability.

Let's Talk about Bladder Control for Women is a public health awareness campaign conducted by the National Kidney and Urologic Diseases Information Clearinghouse (NKUDIC), an information dissemination service of the National Institute of Diabetes and Digestive and Kidney Diseases (NIDDK), National Institutes of Health. Toll-Free 1-800-891-5388.

For more information: 3 Information Way, Bethesda, MD 20892 3580. Website: http://www.niddk.nih.gov/health/kidney/nkudic.htm

The National Heart, Lung, and Blood Institute: NHLBI provides leadership for a national program in diseases of the heart, blood vessels, lung, and blood; blood resources; and sleep disorders. For more information: NHLBI Information Center, PO Box 30105, Bethesda, MD 20824-0105. 301-592-8573; Fax 301-592-8563. Website: http://www.nhlbi.nih.gov. E-mail: NHLBIinfo@rover.nhlbi.nih.gov

Presidential Sports Award/Amateur Athletic Union

Call or write to receive a log on which to record your physical activities or sports activities. When you accomplish your goals, return the log with $8 to cover materials and shipping. You will receive a personalized certificate of achievement from the President of the United States, a congratulatory letter from the co-chairpersons of the President's Council on Physical Fitness and Sports, and an embroidered emblem that can be sewn onto a blazer or sweater. (All sales support the Amateur Athletic Union/Presidential Sports Award.) Walt Disney World Resort, P.O. Box 10000, Lake Buena Vista, FL 32830-1000. Phone: (407) 828-3711. Internet: http://www.aausports.org

United States Department of Agriculture

USDA's Center for Nutrition Policy and Promotion: To see an explanation of the food guide pyramid on the Internet, visit http://www.usda.gov/cnpp and choose "food guide pyramid," then choose "interactive food guide pyramid."

Section 44.2

Private Sector Resources

This list was compiled from several sources deemed accurate; inclusion does not constitute endorsement. Contact information was updated in December 2000.

Aerobics and Fitness Association of America
15250 Ventura Blvd., Suite 200
Sherman Oaks, CA 91403
Toll-Free: 800-446-2322
Toll-Free: 877-YOUR BODY
Fax: 818-788-6301
Website: http://www.afaa.com

Amateur Athletic Union/ Presidential Sports Award
Walt Disney World Resort
P.O. Box 10000
Lake Buena Vista, FL 32830-1000
Phone: 407-934-7200
Website: http://
www.aausports.org

American Academy of Orthopedic Surgeons
6300 North River Road
Des Plaines, IL 60018-4262
Toll-Free: 1-800-824-BONES
(2663)
Phone: 847-823-7186
Fax: 847-823-8125
E-Mail: custserv@aaos.org
Website: http://www.aaos.org

American Academy of Pediatrics
141 Northwest Point Boulevard
Elk Grove Village, IL 60007-1089
Phone: 847-434-4000
Fax: 847-434-8000
E-Mail: kidsdocs@aap.org
Website: http://www.aap.org

American Association of Diabetes Educators
100 West Monroe St., Suite 400
Chicago, IL 60603-1901
Toll-Free: 800-338-3633
Phone: 312-424-2426
Fax: 312-424-2427
Website: http://www.aadenet.org

American College of Rheumatology/Association of Rheumatology Health Professionals
1800 Century Place, Suite 250
Atlanta, GA 30345
Phone: 404-633-3777
Fax: 404-633-1870
Website: http://
www.rheumatology.org
E-Mail: acr@rheumatology

American College of Sports Medicine
401 W. Michigan St.
Indianapolis, IN 46202-3233
Phone: 317-637-9200
Fax: 317-634-7817
Website: http://www.acsm.org

American Diabetes Association
1701 North Beauregard Street
Alexandria, VA 22311
Toll-Free: 800-232-3472
Phone: 703-549-1500
Website: http://www.diabetes.org

The American Dietetic Association
216 West Jackson Boulevard
Chicago, IL 60606-6995
Phone: 312-899-0040
Nutrition Information Line:
800-366-1655
Website: http://www.eatright.org

American Heart Association National Center
7272 Greenville Ave.
Dallas, TX 75231-4596
Toll-Free: 1-800-AHA-USA1
Website: http://
www.americanheart.org

American Physical Therapy Association
1111 North Fairfax St.
Alexandria, VA 22314-1488
Phone: 1-800-999-2782
Website: http://www.apta.org

American Red Cross
430 17th Street, NW
Washington, DC 20006
Phone: 202-639-3520
Website: http://www.redcross.org

American Running and Fitness Association
4405 East West Highway
Suite 405
Bethesda, MD 20814
Toll Free: 800-776-2732
Phone: 301-913-9517
Fax: 301-913-9520
Website: http://
www.americanrunning.org
E-Mail:
run@americanrunning.org

The Aquatic Exercise Association
3439 Technology Dr.
Nokomis, FL 34275
Phone: 941-486-8600
Fax: 941-486-8820
Website: http://
www.aeawave.com

Arthritis Foundation
1330 West Peachtree Street
Atlanta, GA 30309
Phone: 1-800-283-7800
Website: http://
www.arthritis.org
E-Mail: help@arthritis.org

The Cooper Institute for Aerobics Research
12330 Preston Road
Dallas, TX 75230
Toll Free: 800-635-7050, ext. 3230
Fax: 972-341-3225
Website: http://www.cooperinst.org
E-Mail: products@cooperinst.org

Diabetes Exercise and Sports
1647 West Bethany Home Rd. #B
Phoenix, AZ 85015
Toll Free: 800-898-IDAA
Phone: 602-433-2113
Fax: 602-433-9331
Website: http://www.diabetes-exercise.org
E-Mail: idaa@diabetes-exercise.org

50-Plus Fitness Association
P.O. Box 20230
Stanford, CA 94309
Phone: 650-323-6160
Website: http://www.50plus.org

Juvenile Diabetes Foundation International
120 Wall Street, 19th Floor
New York, NY 10005
Toll-Free: 800-533-CURE
Phone: 212-785-9500
Fax: 212-785-9595
Website: http://www.jdfcure.org
E-Mail: info@idf.org

Mature Fitness Awards USA
1850 W. Winchester Rd.
Suite 213
Libertyville, IL 60048
Phone: 847-816-8660
Fax: 847-816-8662
Website: http://www.acpinc.com/seniors/mfausa
E-Mail: seniorprograms@aol.com

National Association for Health and Fitness/Network of State and Governor's Councils
Pan American Plaza
201 S. Capitol Avenue
Suite 560
Indianapolis, IN 46225
Phone: 317-237-5630
Fax: 317-237-5632
Website: http://www.physicalfitness.org

National Osteoporosis Foundation
1232 22nd Street, NW
Washington, DC 20037
Phone: 202-223-2226
Fax: 202-223-2237
Website: http://www.nof.org

National Spa and Pool Institute
2111 Eisenhower Ave.
Alexandria, VA 22314-4698
Phone: 703-838-0083
Fax: 703-549-0493
Website: http://www.nspi.org

Spondylitis Association of America (SAA)
14827 Ventura Blvd., Suite 222
Sherman Oaks, CA 91403
Toll-Free: 800-777-8189
Phone: 818-981-1616
Fax: 818-981-9826
Website: http://
www.spondylitis.org

Chapter 45

Further Reading

Benefits of Physical Activity

A Report of the Surgeon General: Physical Activity and Health. 1996. Produced by the Centers for Disease Control and Prevention, this report compiles decades of research concerning physical activity and health. It addresses the nationwide health problems associated with physical inactivity and outlines the benefits of becoming more physically active. Available for $19.00 from the U.S. Government Printing Office, Superintendent o f Documents, Washington, DC 20402; (202) 512-1800. Stock Number 017-023-00196-5.

Fitness: A Way of Life, free with stamped, self-addressed, business-size envelope. American Physical Therapy Association, 111 North Fairfax St., Alexandria, VA 22314-1488.

Better Health and Fitness Through Physical Activity, free with stamped, self-addressed business-size envelope. American Academy of Pediatrics Department C, Better Health and Fitness Through Physical Activity, 141 Northwest Point Blvd., Elk Grove Village, IL 60007-1089.

Fitness Fundamentals, single copy free. President's Council on Physical Fitness and Sports, Room 738-H, 200 Independence Avenue SW, Washington, DC 20201.

Exercise Lite, single copy free with self-addressed, stamped business-size envelope. American College of Sports Medicine, 401 W. Michigan St., Indianapolis, IN 46202-3233.

More Reading

- American Heart Association. *Strategic plan for promoting physical activity*. Dallas, TX: American Heart Association, 1995.

- Bouchard, C., Shephard, R. J., & Stephens, T. (Eds.). (1994). *Physical activity, fitness, and health*. Champaign, IL: Human Kinetics.

- Fletcher GF, Blair SN, Blumenthal J, et al. Statement on exercise. Benefits and recommendations for physical activity programs for all Americans. *Circulation* 1992;86(1):340-4.

- Ibrahim MA, Yankauer A. The promotion of exercise. *Am J Public Health* 1988;78(11):1413-4.

- McGinnis JM. The public health burden of a sedentary lifestyle. *Med Sci Sports Exercise* 1992;24(6 suppl):S196-S200.

- Paffenbarger RS Jr, Hyde RT, Wing AL, Lee I-M, Kampert JB. Some interrelations of physical activity, physiological fitness, health, and longevity. In: Bouchard C, Shephard RJ, Stephens T, eds. *Physical activity, fitness, and health: international proceedings and consensus statement*. Champaign, IL: Human Kinetics, 1994:119-33.

- Pate RR, Pratt M, Blair SN, et al. Physical activity and public health: a recommendation from the Centers for Disease Control and Prevention and the American College of Sports Medicine. *JAMA* 1995;273(5):402-7.

- Powell KE, Blair SN. The public health burdens of sedentary living habits: theoretical but realistic estimates. *Med Sci Sports Exercise* 1994;26(7):851-6.

- Shephard, R. J. (1986). *Economic benefits of enhanced physical activity*. Champaign, IL: Human Kinetics.

- Telama, R. (1991). Nature as motivation for physical activity. In P. Oja & R. Telama (Eds.), *Sport for all* (pp. 607-616). Amsterdam: Elsevier.

- Verschuur, R. (1987). *Daily physical activity and health*. Haarlem, The Netherlands: Uitgeverij de Vrieseborch.

- Vuori, I. (1995a). Exercise and physical health: Musculoskeletal health and functional capabilities. *Research Quarterly for Exercise and Sport*, 66, 276-285.

Fitness at Work

- Kannel WB, Belanger A, D'Agostino R, Israel I. Physical activity and physical demand on the job and risk of cardiovascular disease and death: the Framingham Study. *Am Heart J* 1986; 112(4):820-5.

- Shephard, R. J. (1995). Worksite health promotion and productivity. In R. Kaman (Ed.), *Worksite health promotion economics* (pp. 147-173). Champaign, IL: Human Kinetics.

Leisure Time Physical Activity

- Dannenberg AL, Keller JB, Wilson PWF, Castelli WP. Leisure time physical activity in the Framingham Offspring Study. *Am J Epidemiol* 1989;129(1):76-88.

- Godin, G., Valois, P., Shephard, R. J., & Desharnais, R. (1987). Prediction of leisure-time exercise behavior: A path analysis (LISREL V model). *Journal of Behavioral Medicine*, 10, 145-158.

- Leon AS, Connett J, Jacobs DR Jr, Rauramaa R. Leisure-time physical activity levels and risk of coronary heart disease and death: the Multiple Risk Factor Intervention Trial. *JAMA* 1987; 258(17):2388-95.

- Salonen JT, Slater JS, Tuomilehto J, Rauramaa R. Leisure time and occupational physical activity: risk of death from ischemic heart disease. *Am J Epidemiol* 1988;127(1):87-94.

Miscellaneous

- Calfas KJ, Sallis JF, Lovato CY, Campbell J. Physical activity and its determinants before and after college graduation. *Med Exercise Nutr Health* 1994;3:323-34.

- Marcus BH, Eaton CA, Ross JS, Harlow LL. Self-efficacy, decision-making, and stages of change: an integrative model of physical exercise. *J Appl Soc Psychol* 1994;24(6):489-508.

- McGinnis JM, Foege WH. Actual causes of death in the United States. *JAMA* 1993; 270(18):2207-12.

- Perusse L, Tremblay A, LeBlanc C, Bouchard C. Genetic and environmental influences on level of habitual physical activity and exercise participation. *Am J Epidemiol* 1989;129(5):1012-22.

- Robinson TN, Killen JD. Ethnic and gender differences in the relationships between television viewing and obesity, physical activity, and dietary fat intake. *J Health Educ* 1995;26(2 suppl):S91-S98.

Physical Fitness and Children, Adolescents

- Bailey, D. A. (1974). Exercise, fitness, and physical education for the growing child. In W. A. R. Orban (Ed.), *Proceedings of the National Conference on Fitness and Health* (pp. 13-22). Ottawa, Ontario, Canada: Health & Welfare, Canada.

- Bailey D.A., Martin AD. Physical activity and skeletal health in adolescents. *Pediatr Exercise Sci* 1994;6:330-47.

- Borra ST, Schwartz NE, Spain CG, Natchipolsky MM. Food, physical activity, and fun: inspiring America's kids to more healthful lifestyles. *J Am Diet Assoc* 1995;95(7):816-8.

- Brownell KD, Kaye FS. A school-based behavior modification, nutrition education, and physical activity program for obese children. *Am J Clin Nutr* 1982;35:277-83.

- Calfas KJ, Taylor WC. Effects of physical activity on psychological variables in adolescents. *Pediatr Exercise Sci* 1994;6:406-23.

- Epstein LH, Valoski A, Wing RR, McCurley J. Ten-year follow-up of behavioral, family-based treatment for obese children. *JAMA* 1990;264(19):2519-23.

- Epstein LH, Valoski AM, Vara LS, et al. Effects of decreasing sedentary behavior and increasing activity on weight change in obese children. *Health Psychol* 1995;14(2):109-15.

- Kemper, H., Storm-van Essen, L., & Verschuur, R. (1989). Tracking of risk indicators for coronary heart disease from teenager to adult: The Amsterdam growth and health study. In S. Oseid & H. -K. Carlsen (Eds.), *Children and exercise XIII* (pp. 235-245). Champaign, IL: Human Kinetics.

- Luepker RV, Perry CL, McKinlay SM, et al. Outcomes of a field trial to improve children's dietary patterns and physical activity: the Child and Adolescent Trial for Cardiovascular Health (CATCH). *JAMA* 1996;275(10):768-76.

- McCullagh P, Matzkanin KT, Shaw SD, Maldonado M. Motivation for participation in physical activity: a comparison of parent-child perceived competencies and participation motives. *Pediatr Exercise Sci* 1993;5:224-33.

- Pate RR, Long BJ, Heath G. Descriptive epidemiology of physical activity in adolescents. *Pediatr Exercise Sci* 1994;6:434-47.

- Reynolds KD, Killen JD, Bryson SW, et al. Psychosocial predictors of physical activity in adolescents. *Prev Med* 1990;19:541-51.

- Rubin K, Schirduan V, Gendreau P, Sarfarazi M, Mendola R, Dalsky G. Predictors of axial and peripheral bone mineral density in healthy children and adolescents, with special attention to the role of puberty. *J Pediatr* 1993;123:863-70.

- Tappe MK, Duda JL, Menges-Ehrnwald P. Personal investment predictors of adolescent motivational orientation toward exercise. *Can J Sport Sci* 1990;15(3):185-92.

- Tinsley BJ, Holtgrave DR, Reise SP, Erdley C, Cupp RG. Developmental status, gender, age, and self-reported decision-making influences on students' risky and preventive health behaviors. *Health Educ Q* 1995;22(2):244-59.

- Tappe MK, Duda JL, Ehrnwald PM. Perceived barriers to exercise among adolescents. *J Sch Health* 1989;59(4):153-5.

Physical Activity and Communities

- Blair SN, Booth M, Gyarfas I, et al. Development of public policy and physical activity initiatives internationally. *Sports Med* 1996;21(3):157-63.

- CDC. *Promoting physical activity: a guide for community action*. Atlanta: U.S. Department of Health and Human Services, Public Health Service, CDC (in press).

- Iverson DC, Fielding JE, Crow RS, Christenson GM. The promotion of physical activity in the United States population: the status of programs in medical, worksite, community, and school settings. *Public Health Rep* 1985;100(2):212-23.

- King AC. Community and public health approaches to the promotion of physical activity. *Med Sci Sports Exercise* 1994;26(11): 1405-12.

- King AC, Jeffery RW, Fridinger FW, et al. Environmental and policy approaches to cardiovascular disease prevention through physical activity: issues and opportunities. *Health Educ Q* 1995;22(44):499-511.

- Owen N, Lee C. Development of behaviorally-based policy guidelines for the promotion of exercise. *J Public Health Policy* 1989;10(1):43-61.

- McGinnis JM, Kanner L, DeGraw C. Physical education's role in achieving national health objectives. *Res Q Exercise Sport* 1991;62(2):138-42.

- Schmid TL, Pratt M, Howze E. Policy as intervention: environmental and policy approaches to the prevention of cardiovascular disease. *Am J Public Health* 1995;85(9):1207-11.

- U.S. Consumer Product Safety Commission. *Handbook for public playground safety*. Washington, DC: U.S. Government Printing Office, 1991. Publication no. 305-724.

- Winkleby MA. The future of community-based cardiovascular disease intervention studies. *Am J Public Health* 1994;84(9):1369-72.

Physical Activity and Diet/Weight Control

Binge-Eating Disorder. NIH Publication No. 94-3589. This fact sheet describes the symptoms, causes, complications, and treatment of binge-eating disorder, along with a profile of those at risk for the disorder. 1993. Write to National Institutes of Health (NIH), Bethesda, Maryland 20892.

Nutrition and Your Health: Dietary Guidelines for Americans, Fourth Edition. Home and Garden Bulletin No. 232. 1995. This booklet answers some of the basic questions about healthy eating and the link between poor nutrition and disease. It stresses the importance of a balanced diet and a healthy lifestyle. Write to National Institutes of Health (NIH), Bethesda, Maryland 20892.

Physical Activity and Weight Control. NIH Publication No. 964031. This fact sheet explains how physical activity helps promote weight control and other ways it benefits one's health. It also describes the different types of physical activity and provides tips on how to become more physically active. 1996. Write to National Institutes of Health (NIH), Bethesda, Maryland 20892.

The Facts About Weight-Loss Products and Programs. DHHS Publication No. (FDA) 92-1189. This pamphlet provides basic facts about the weight-loss industry and what the consumer should expect from a diet program and/or product. Available from the Food and Drug Administration, Office of Consumer Affairs, HFE-88, Rockville, MD 20857.

Weight Cycling. NIH Publication No. 95-3901. Based on research, this fact sheet describes the health effects of weight cycling, also known as "yo-yo" dieting, and how it affects obese individuals' future weight-loss efforts. 1995. Available from WIN.

Are You Eating Right? *Consumer Reports*. October 1992, pp. 644-55. This article summarizes advice from 68 nutrition experts, including a discussion on weight control and health risks of obesity. Available in public libraries.

Losing Weight: What Works. What Doesn't and **Rating the Diets.** *Consumer Reports*. June 1993, pp. 347-57. These articles report on a survey of readers' experiences with weight-loss diets, discuss research related to weight control, and outline pros and cons of different diet programs. Available in public libraries.

More Reading

- Chang-Claude J, Frentzel-Beyme R. Dietary and lifestyle determinants of mortality among German vegetarians. *Int J Epidemiol* 1993;22(2):228-36.

- Ching PLYH, Willett WC, Rimm EB, Colditz GA, Gortmaker SL, Stampfer MJ. Activity level and risk of overweight in male health professionals. *Am J Public Health* 1996;86(1):25-30.

- French SA, Jeffery RW, Forster JL, McGovern PG, Kelder SH, Baxter JE. Predictors of weight change over two years among a population of working adults: the Healthy Worker Project. *Int J Obes* 1994;18:145-54.

- Lampman RM, Schteingart DE, Foss ML. Exercise as a partial therapy for the extremely obese. *Med Sci Sports Exerc* 1986; 18:19-24.

- Slattery ML, McDonald A, Bild DE, et al. Associations of body fat and its distribution with dietary intake, physical activity, alcohol, and smoking in blacks and whites. *Am J Clin Nutr* 1992;55:943-9.

- Williamson DF, Madans J, Anda RF, Kleinman JC, Kahn HS, Byers T. Recreational physical activity and ten-year weight change in a US national cohort. *Int J Obes* 1993;17:279-86.

Physical Activity and Different Groups of People

- Cardinal BJ. The stages of exercise scale and stages of exercise behavior in female adults. *J Sports Med Physical Fitness* 1995;35(2):87-92.

- Ettinger B, Friedman GD, Bush T, et al: Reduced mortality associated with long-term postmenopausal estrogen therapy. *Obstet Gynecol* 1996;87(1):6-12.

- Fiatarone MA, O'Neill EF, Ryan ND, Clements KM, Solares GR, Nelson ME, et al. Exercise training and nutritional supplementation for physical frailty in very elderly people. *N Engl J Med* 1994;330:1769-75.

- Hammar M, Berg G, Lindgren R: Does physical exercise influence the frequency of postmenopausal hot flushes? Acta *Obstet Gynecol* Scand 1990;69(5):409-412.

- Kaplan GA, Seeman TE, Cohen RD, Knudsen LP, Guralnik J. Mortality among the elderly in the Alameda County Study: behavioral and demographic risk factors. *Am J Public Health* 1987;77(3):307-12.

- Kritz-Silverstein D, Barrett-Connor E: Long-term postmenopausal hormone use, obesity, and fat distribution in older women. *JAMA* 1996;275(1):46-49.

- Lee I-M, Hsieh C-C, Paffenbarger RS Jr. Exercise intensity and longevity in men: the Harvard Alumni Health Study. *JAMA* 1995;273(15):1179-84.

- MacArthur RD, Levine SD, Birk TJ. Supervised exercise training improves cardiopulmonary fitness in HIV-infected persons. *Med Sci Sports Exerc* 1993;25:684-8.

- Notelovitz M, Martin D, Tesar R, et al: Estrogen therapy and variable-resistance weight training increase bone mineral in surgically menopausal women. *J BoneMiner Res* 1991;6(6):583-590.

- Paffenbarger RS Jr, Hyde RT, Wing AL, Lee I-M, Jung DL, Kampert JB. The association of changes in physical-activity level and other lifestyle characteristics with mortality among men. *N Engl J Med* 1993;328:538-45.

- Paffenbarger RS Jr, Kampert JB, Lee I-M, Hyde RT, Leung RW, Wing AL. Changes in physical activity and other lifeway patterns influencing longevity. *Med Sci Sports Exercise* 1994; 26(7):857-65.

- Rode, A., & Shephard, R. J. (1995). *"Modernization" and the health of the circumpolar peoples*. London: Cambridge University Press.

- Sallis JF, Patterson TL, Buono MJ, Atkins CJ, Nader PR. Aggregation of physical activity habits in Mexican-American and Anglo families. *J Behav Med* 1988;11(1):31-41.

- Shangold M, Mirkin G: *Women and Exercise: Physiology and Sports Medicine, ed 2*. Philadelphia, FA Davis, 1994.

- Shephard, R. J. (1987). *Physical activity and aging (2nd ed.)*. London: Croom Helm.

- Shephard, R. J. (1989). Exercise and lifestyle change. *British Journal of Sports Medicine*, 23, 11-22.

- Shephard, R. J. (1991). Fitness and aging. In C. Blais (Ed.), *Aging into the twenty first century* (pp. 22-35). North York, Ontario, Canada: Captus Publications.

- Donahue RP, Abbott RD, Reed DM, Yano K. Physical activity and coronary heart disease in middle-aged and elderly men: the Honolulu Heart Program. *Am J Public Health* 1988;78(6):683-5.

- Taylor PA, Ward A: Women, high-density lipoprotein cholesterol, and exercise. *Arch Intern Med* 1993;153(10):1178-1184.

- Wells TJ, Brink CA, Diokno AC, Wolfe R, Gillis GL. Pelvic muscle exercise for stress urinary incontinence in elderly women. *J Am Geriatr Soc* 1991;39:785-91.

Physical Activity and Medical Conditions

Blood Diseases

- Alcorn R, Bowser B, Henley EJ, Holloway V. Fluidotherapy and exercise in the management of sickle cell anemia. A clinical report. *Phys Ther* 1984;64:1520-2.

- Greene WB, Strickler EM. A modified isokinetic strengthening program for patients with severe hemophilia. *Dev Med Child Neurol* 1983;25:189-96.

- Sopko G, Jacobs DR Jr, Jeffery R, Mittelmark M, Lenz K, Hedding E, et al. Effects on blood lipids and body weight in high risk men of a practical exercise program. *Atherosclerosis* 1983;49:219-29.

Cancer

- Bernstein L, Henderson BE, Hanisch R, Sullivan-Halley J, Ross RK. Physical exercise and reduced risk of breast cancer in young women. *J Natl Cancer Inst* 1994;86:1403-8.

- Gerhardsson M, Floderus B, Norell SE. Physical activity and colon cancer risk. *Int J Epidemiol* 1988;17(4):743-6.

- Gerhardsson de Verdier M, Steineck G, Hagman U, Rieger ·, Norell SE. Physical activity and colon cancer: a case-referent study in Stockholm. *Int J Cancer* 1990;46:985-9.

- Giovannucci E, Ascherio A, Rimm EB, Colditz GA, Stampfer MJ, Willet WC. Physical activity, obesity, and risk for colon cancer and adenoma in men. *Ann Intern Med* 1995;122:327-34.

- Lee, I.-M. (1995). Exercise and physical health: Cancer and immune function. *Research Quarterly for Exercise and Sport*, 66, 286-291.

- Lee I-M, Paffenbarger RS Jr, Hsieh C-C. Physical activity and risk of developing colorectal cancer among college alumni. *J Natl Cancer Inst* 1991;83:1324-9.

- Longnecker MP, Gerhardsson de Verdier M, Frumkin H, Carpenter C. A case-control study of physical activity in relation to risk of cancer of the right colon and rectum in men. *Int J Epidemiol* 1995;24(1):42-50.

- Markowitz S, Morabia A, Garibaldi K, Wynder E. Effect of occupational and recreational activity on the risk of colorectal cancer among males: a case-control study. *Int J Epidemiol* 1992; 21(6):1057-62.

- Shephard, R. J. (1993). Exercise in the prevention and treatment of cancer: An update. *Sports Medicine*, 15, 258-280.

- Slattery ML, Schumacher MC, Smith KR, West DW, Abd-Elghany N. Physical activity, diet, and risk of colon cancer in Utah. *Am J Epidemiol* 1988;128(5):989-99.

- Whittemore AS, Wu-Williams AH, Lee M, et al. Diet, physical activity, and colorectal cancer among Chinese in North American and China. *J Natl Cancer Inst* 1990;82(11):915-26.

- Yoshioka H. Rehabilitation for the terminal cancer patient. *Am J Phys Med Rehabil* 1994;73:199-206.

Chronic Fatigue Syndrome/Chronic Pain

- Darling M. The use of exercise as a method of aborting migraine. *Headache* 1991;31:616-8.

- Davis VP, Fillingim RB, Doleys DM, Davis MP. Assessment of aerobic power in chronic pain patients before and after a multidisciplinary treatment program. *Arch Phys Med Rehabil* 1992; 73:726-9.

- Johannsen F, Remvig L, Kryger P, Beck P, Warming S, Lybeck K, et al. Exercises for chronic low back pain: a clinical trial. *J Orthop Sports Phys Ther* 1995;22:52-9.

- McCully KK, Sisto SA, Natelson BH. Use of exercise for treatment of chronic fatigue syndrome. *Sports Med* 1996;21:35-48.

Diabetes

- Burchfiel CM, Sharp DS, Curb JD, et al. Physical activity and incidence of diabetes: the Honolulu Heart Program. *Am J Epidemiol* 1995;141(4):360-8.

- Campaigne BN, Gilliam TB, Spencer ML, Lampman RM, Schork MA. Effects of a physical activity program on metabolic control and cardiovascular fitness in children with insulin-dependent diabetes mellitus. *Diabetes Care* 1984;7:57-62.

- *Diabetes Self-Management*, published by R.A. Rapaport Publishing Company P.O. Box 52890, Boulder, CO 80322, 1-800-234-0923.

- *Diabetes Interview*, published by Diabetes Interview, 3715 Balboa Street, San Francisco, CA 94121, 1-800-473-4636.

- Gudat, U., Berger, M., & Lefebvre, P. (1994). Physical activity, fitness, and non-insulin dependent (Type II) diabetes mellitus. In C. Bouchard, R. J. Shephard, & T. Stephens (Eds.), *Physical activity, fitness, and health* (pp. 669-683). Champaign, IL: Human Kinetics.

- Helmrich SP, Ragland DR, Leung RW, Paffenbarger RS Jr. Physical activity and reduced occurrence of non-insulin-dependent diabetes mellitus. *N Engl J Med* 1991;325(3):147-52.

- Helmrich SP, Ragland DR, Paffenbarger RS Jr. Prevention of non-insulin-dependent diabetes mellitus with physical activity. *Med Sci Sports Exercise* 1994;26(7):824-30.

- Lehmann R, Vokac A, Niedermann K, Agosti K, Spinas GA. Loss of abdominal fat and improvement of the cardiovascular risk profile by regular moderate exercise training in patients with NIDDM. *Diabetologia* 1995;38:1313-9.

- Manson JE, Nathan DM, Krolewski AS, Stampfer MJ, Willett WC, Hennekens CH. A prospective study of exercise and incidence of diabetes among US male physicians. *JAMA* 1992;268(1):63-7.

- Manson JE, Rimm EB, Stampfer MJ, et al. Physical activity and incidence of non-insulin-dependent diabetes mellitus in women. *Lancet* 1991;338:774-8.

- *The Diabetic Reader*, published by Prana Publications and Paraphernalia, 5623 Matilija Avenue, Van Nuys, CA 91401, 1-800-735-7726.

Heart Disease/Hypertension

- Despres, J.-P., Bouchard, C., & Malina, R. (1990). Physical activity and coronary heart disease risk factors during childhood and adolescence. *Exercise and Sport Sciences Reviews*, 18, 243-261.

- Ekelund L-G, Haskell WL, Johnson JL, Whaley FS, Criqui MH, Sheps DS. Physical fitness as a predictor of cardiovascular mortality in asymptomatic North American men. *N Engl J Med* 1988;319(21):1379-84.

- Folsom AR, Prineas RJ, Kaye SA, Munger RG. Incidence of hypertension and stroke in relation to body fat distribution and other risk factors in older women. *Stroke* 1990;21:701-6.

- Gartside PS, Glueck CJ. The important role of modifiable dietary and behavioral characteristics in the causation and prevention of coronary heart disease hospitalization and mortality: the prospective NHANES I follow-up study. *J Am Coll Nutr* 1995;14(1):71-9.

- Hein HO, Suadicani P, Gyntelberg F. Physical fitness or physical activity as a predictor of ischaemic heart disease? A 17-year follow-up in the Copenhagen Male Study. *J Intern Med* 1992;232:471-9.

- Kavanagh T, Yacoub MH, Mertens DJ, Kennedy J, Campbell RB, Sawyer P. Cardiorespiratory responses to exercise training after orthotopic cardiac transplantation. *Circulation* 1988;77:162-71.

- Kostis JB, Rosen RC, Cosgrove NM, Shindler DM, Wilson AC. Nonpharmacologic therapy improves functional and emotional status in congestive heart failure. *Chest* 1994;106:996-1001.

- Lampman RM, Schteingart DE. Effects of exercise training on glucose control, lipid metabolism, and insulin sensitivity in hypertriglyceridemia and non-insulin dependent diabetes mellitus. *Med Sci Sports Exerc* 1991;23:703-12.

- Lapidus L, Bengtsson C. Socioeconomic factors and physical activity in relation to cardiovascular disease and death: a 12 year follow up of participants in a population study of women in Gothenburg, Sweden. *Br Heart J* 1986;55:295-301.

- Lavie CJ, Milani RV. Effects of cardiac rehabilitation programs on exercise capacity, coronary risk factors, behavioral characteristics, and quality of life in a large elderly cohort. *Am J Cardiol* 1995;76:177-9.

- Lavie CJ, Milani RV. Effects of cardiac rehabilitation and exercise training in obese patients with coronary artery disease. *Chest* 1996;109:52-6.

601

- Lavie CJ, Milani RV. Effects of cardiac rehabilitation and exercise training on low-density lipoprotein cholesterol in patients with hypertriglyceridemia and coronary artery disease. *Am J Cardiol* 1994; 74:1192-5.

- Martin JE, Dubbert PM, Cushman WC. Controlled trial of aerobic exercise in hypertension. *Circulation* 1990;81:1560-7.

- Morris JN. Exercise in the prevention of coronary heart disease: today's best buy in public health. *Med Sci Sports Exercise* 1994;26(7):807-14.

- Paffenbarger RS Jr, Wing AL, Hyde RT, Jung DL. Physical activity and incidence of hypertension in college alumni. *Am J Epidemiol* 1983;117(3):245-57.

- Powell, K. E., Thompson, P. D., Caspersen, C. J., & Kendrick, J. S. (1987). Physical activity and the incidence of coronary heart disease. *Annual Reviews of Public Health*, 8, 253-287.

- Raitakari, O. T., Parkka, K. V. K., Taimela, S., Telama, R., Rasanen, L., & Viikari, J. S. A. (1994). Effects of persistent physical activity and inactivity on coronary risk factors. *American Journal of Epidemiology*, 140, 195-205.

- Rodriguez BL, Curb JD, Burchfiel CM, et al. Physical activity and 23-year incidence of coronary heart disease morbidity and mortality among middle-aged men: the Honolulu Heart Program. *Circulation* 1994;89:2540-4.

- Slattery ML, Jacobs DR Jr, Nichaman MZ. Leisure time physical activity and coronary heart disease death: the US Railroad Study. *Circulation* 1989;79:304-11.

- Slattery ML, Jacobs DR Jr. Physical fitness and cardiovascular disease mortality: the US Railroad Study. *Am J Epidemiol* 1988;127(3):571-80.

- Sobolski J, Kornitzer M, De Backer G, et al. Protection against ischemic heart disease in the Belgian Fitness Study: physical fitness rather than physical activity? *Am J Epidemiol* 1987; 125(4):601-10.

- Tipton, C. M: (1991). Exercise, training, and hypertension: An update. *Exercise and Sport Sciences Reviews*, 19, 447-506.

- Yeager KK, Anda RF, Macera CA, Donehoo RS, Eaker ED. Sedentary lifestyle and state variation in coronary heart disease mortality. *Public Health Rep* 1995; 110(1):100-2.

Kidney Disease

- Goldberg, A. P., & Harter, H. R. (1994). Physical activity, fitness, and kidney disease. In C. Bouchard, R. J. Shephard, & T. Stephens (Eds.), *Physical activity, fitness, and health* (pp. 762-773). Champaign, IL: Human Kinetics.

Miscellaneous

- Agre JC. The role of exercise in the patient with post-polio syndrome. *Ann N Y Acad Sci* 1995;753: 321-34.

- Brenner, I., Shek, P. N., & Shephard, R. J. (1994). Infection in athletes. *Sports Medicine*, 17, 86-107.

- Christensen, T. (1994). Physical activity, fitness, and recovery from surgical trauma. In C. Bouchard, R. J. Shephard, & T. Stephens (Eds.), *Physical activity, fitness, and health* (pp. 832-839). Champaign, IL: Human Kinetics.

- Davidoff GN, Lampman RM, Westbury L, Deron J, Finestone HM, Islam S. Exercise testing and training of persons with dysvascular amputation: safety and efficacy of arm ergometry. *Arch Phys Med Rehabil* 1992;73:334-8.

- Evans WJ. Reversing sarcopenia: how weight training can build strength and vitality. *Geriatrics* 1996;51(5):46-7,51-3.

- Lohi EL, Lindberg C, Andersen O. Physical training effects in myasthenia gravis. *Arch Phys Med Rehabil* 1993;74:1178-80.

- Prior JC, Vigna Y, Alojada N. Conditioning exercise decreases premenstrual symptoms. A prospective controlled three month trial. *Eur J Appl Physiol* 1986;55:349-55.

- Regensteiner JG, Steiner JF, Hiatt WR Exercise training improves functional status in patients with peripheral arterial disease. *J Vasc Surg* 1996;23:104-15.

Multiple Sclerosis

- Petajan JH, Gappmaier E, White AT, Spencer MK, Mino L, Hicks RW. Impact of aerobic training on fitness and quality of life in multiple sclerosis. *Ann Neurol* 1996;39:432-41.

Osteoporosis

- Aloia JF, Vaswani AN, Yeh JK, Cohn SH. Premenopausal bone mass is related to physical activity. *Arch Intern Med* 1988;148:121-3.

- Bakker C, Hidding A, van der Linden S, van Doorslaer E. Cost effectiveness of group physical therapy compared to individualized therapy for ankylosing spondylitis. A randomized controlled trial. *J Rheumatol* 1994;21:264-8.

- *Boning Up on Osteoporosis*, a comprehensive 70-page booklet about prevention, diagnosis, and treatment, is available for $4 by writing the National Osteoporosis Foundation, 1150 17th St. NW, Suite 500, Washington, DC 20036-4603.

- Dalsky GP, Stocke KS, Ehsani AA, Slatopolsky E, Lee WC, Birge SJ Jr. Weight-bearing exercise training and lumbar bone mineral content in postmenopausal women. *Ann Intern Med* 1988;108:824-8.

- Dilsen G, Berker C, Oral A, Varan G. The role of physical exercise in prevention and management of osteoporosis. *Clin Rheumatol* 1989;8(Suppl 2):70-5.

- Drinkwater, B. (1994). Physical activity, fitness and osteoporosis. In C. Bouchard, R. J. Shephard, & T. Stephens (Eds.), *Physical activity, fitness, and health* (pp. 724-736). Champaign; IL: Human Kinetics.

- Fisher NM, Pendergast DR. Effects of a muscle exercise program on exercise capacity in subjects with osteoarthritis. *Arch Phys Med Rehabil* 1994; 75:792-7.

- Greendale GA, Barrett-Connor E, Edelstein S, Ingles S, Haile R. Lifetime leisure exercise and osteoporosis: the Rancho Bernardo Study. *Am J Epidemiol* 1995;141(10):951-9.

- Harkcom TM, Lampman RM, Banwell BF, Castor CW. Therapeutic value of graded aerobic exercise training in rheumatoid arthritis. *Arthritis Rheum* 1985;28:32-9.

- Lane NE, Bloch DA, Jones HH, Marshall WH, Wood PD, Fries JF. Long-distance running, bone density, and osteoarthritis. *JAMA* 1986;255(9):1147-51.

- Michel BA, Bloch DA, Fries JF. Weight-bearing exercise, overexercise, and lumbar bone density over age 50 years. *Arch Intern Med* 1989;149:2325-9.

- Nelson, Miriam, with Wernick, Sarah. *Strong Women Stay Young.* Bantam Books, 1997, $23.95.

- Prince RL, Smith M, Dick IM, Price RI, Webb PG, Henderson NK, et al. Prevention of postmenopausal osteoporosis. A comparative study of exercise, calcium supplementation, and hormone-replacement therapy. *N Engl J Med* 1991;325:1189-95.

- Pruitt LA, Jackson RD, Bartels RL, Lehnhard HJ. Weight-training effects on bone mineral density in early postmenopausal women. *J Bone Miner Res* 1992;7(2):179-85.

Parkinson's Disease

- Kuroda K, Tatara K, Takatorige T, Shinsho E Effect of physical exercise on mortality in patients with Parkinson's disease. *Acta Neurol Scand* 1992;86:55-9.

Stroke

- Kohl, H. W., & McKenzie, J. D. (1994). Physical activity, fitness, and stroke. In C. Bouchard, R. J. Shephard, & T. Stephens (Eds.), *Physical activity, fitness, and health* (pp. 609-621). Champaign, IL: Human Kinetics.

Physical Activity and Mental Health

- Biddle, S. (1995). Exercise and psychosocial health. *Research Quarterly for Exercise and Sport*, 66, 292-297.

- Camacho TC, Roberts RE, Lazarus NB, Kaplan GA, Cohen RD. Physical activity and depression: evidence from the Alameda County Study. *Am J Epidemiol* 1991;134(2):220-31.

- Farmer ME, Locke BZ, Mocicki EK, Dannenberg AL, Larson DB, Radloff LS. Physical activity and depressive symptoms: the NHANES I Epidemiologic Follow-up Study. *Am J Epidemiol* 1988;128(6):1340-51.

- North, T.C., McCullagh, P., & Tran, Z. V. (1990). Effect of exercise on depression. *Exercise and Sport Sciences Reviews*, 18, 379-415.

- Ross CE, Hayes D. Exercise and psychologic well-being in the community. *Am J Epidemiol* 1988;127(4):762-71.

- Shephard, R. J., Lavallee, H., Volle, M., LaBarre, R., & Beaucage, C. (1994). Academic skills and required physical education: The Trois Rivieres experience. *CAHPER Research Supplement*, 1(1), 1-12.

- Shields, D. L. L., & Bredemeier, B. J. L. (1995). *Character development and physical activity*. Champaign, IL: Human Kinetics.

- Stephens T. Physical activity and mental health in the United States and Canada: evidence from four population surveys. *Prev Med* 1988;17:35-47.

- Tomporowski, P. D., & Ellis, N. R. (1986). Effects of exercise on cognitive processes: A review. *Psychological Bulletin*, 99, 338-346.

- Weyerer S. Physical inactivity and depression in the community. *Int J Sports Med* 1992:13(6):492-6.

Risks of Physical Activity

- Arraiz GA, Wigle DT, Mao Y. Risk assessment of physical activity and physical fitness in the Canada health survey mortality follow-up study. *J Clin Epidemiol* 1992;45(4):419-28.

- Mueller, F. O., & Cantu, R. C. (1990). Catastrophic injuries in high school and college sports, Fall 1982-Spring 1988. *Medicine and Science in Sports and Exercise*, 22, 737-741.

- Pekkanen, J., Marti, B., Nissinen, A., Tuomilehto, J., Punsar, S., & Karvonen, M. (1987). Reduction of premature mortality by high physical activity: A 20-year follow-up of middle-aged Finnish men. *Lancet*, i, 1473-1477.

- Shephard, R. J. (1994). Physical activity and reduction of health risks. How far are the benefits independent of fat loss? *Journal of Sports Medicine and Physical Fitness*, 34, 91-98.

- Slavin, J. L. (1985). Eating disorders in women athletes. In J. Puhl, C. H. Brown, & R. O. Voy (Eds.), *Sport science perspectives for women* (pp. 189-197). Champaign, IL: Human Kinetics.

- Vuori, I. (1995b). Sudden death and exercise: Effects of age and type of activity. *Sports Science Reviews*, 4, 46-84.

Specific Physical Activities

An Introduction to Running: One Step at a Time, single copy free. President's Council on Physical Fitness and Sports, Room 738-H, 200 Independence Avenue SW, Washington, DC 20201.

AR&FA's Guide to Running and Racing, free with self-addressed, stamped, business-size envelope. American Running and Fitness Association, 4405 East West Highway, Suite 405, Bethesda, MD 20814.

Swimming for a Healthy Heart, (Box S-GL), **Cycling for a Healthy Heart** (Box C-GL), **Walking for a Healthy Heart** (Box W-GL), single copy of each free with self-addressed, stamped business-size envelope for each pamphlet and with box number indicated on request. American Heart Association, National Center, 7272 Greenville Avenue, Dallas, TX 75231-4596.

Aquatics Program, single copy free. American Red Cross, 430 17th Street, NW, Washington, DC 20006.

Index

Index

Health Reference Series
COMPLETE CATALOG

AIDS Sourcebook, 1st Edition

Basic Information about AIDS and HIV Infection, Featuring Historical and Statistical Data, Current Research, Prevention, and Other Special Topics of Interest for Persons Living with AIDS

Along with Source Listings for Further Assistance

Edited by Karen Bellenir and Peter D. Dresser. 831 pages. 1995. 0-7808-0031-1. $78.

"One strength of this book is its practical emphasis. The intended audience is the lay reader . . . useful as an educational tool for health care providers who work with AIDS patients. Recommended for public libraries as well as hospital or academic libraries that collect consumer materials."
— Bulletin of the Medical Library Association, Jan '96

"This is the most comprehensive volume of its kind on an important medical topic. Highly recommended for all libraries." — Reference Book Review, '96

"Very useful reference for all libraries."
— Choice, Association of College and Research Libraries, Oct '95

"There is a wealth of information here that can provide much educational assistance. It is a must book for all libraries and should be on the desk of each and every congressional leader. Highly recommended."
— AIDS Book Review Journal, Aug '95

"Recommended for most collections."
— Library Journal, Jul '95

■

AIDS Sourcebook, 2nd Edition

Basic Consumer Health Information about Acquired Immune Deficiency Syndrome (AIDS) and Human Immunodeficiency Virus (HIV) Infection, Featuring Updated Statistical Data, Reports on Recent Research and Prevention Initiatives, and Other Special Topics of Interest for Persons Living with AIDS, Including New Antiretroviral Treatment Options, Strategies for Combating Opportunistic Infections, Information about Clinical Trials, and More

Along with a Glossary of Important Terms and Resource Listings for Further Help and Information

Edited by Karen Bellenir. 751 pages. 1999. 0-7808-0225-X. $78.

"Highly recommended."
— American Reference Books Annual, 2000

"Excellent sourcebook. This continues to be a highly recommended book. There is no other book that provides as much information as this book provides."
— AIDS Book Review Journal, Dec-Jan 2000

"Recommended reference source."
— Booklist, American Library Association, Dec '99

"A solid text for college-level health libraries."
— The Bookwatch, Aug '99

Cited in Reference Sources for Small and Medium-Sized Libraries, American Library Association, 1999

■

Alcoholism Sourcebook

Basic Consumer Health Information about the Physical and Mental Consequences of Alcohol Abuse, Including Liver Disease, Pancreatitis, Wernicke-Korsakoff Syndrome (Alcoholic Dementia), Fetal Alcohol Syndrome, Heart Disease, Kidney Disorders, Gastrointestinal Problems, and Immune System Compromise and Featuring Facts about Addiction, Detoxification, Alcohol Withdrawal, Recovery, and the Maintenance of Sobriety

Along with a Glossary and Directories of Resources for Further Help and Information

Edited by Karen Bellenir. 613 pages. 2000. 0-7808-0325-6. $78.

"Recommended reference source."
— Booklist, American Library Association, Dec '00

"Presents a wealth of information on alcohol use and abuse and its effects on the body and mind, treatment, and prevention." — SciTech Book News, Dec '00

"Important new health guide which packs in the latest consumer information about the problems of alcoholism." — Reviewer's Bookwatch, Nov '00

SEE ALSO Drug Abuse Sourcebook, Substance Abuse Sourcebook

■

Allergies Sourcebook

Basic Information about Major Forms and Mechanisms of Common Allergic Reactions, Sensitivities, and Intolerances, Including Anaphylaxis, Asthma, Hives and Other Dermatologic Symptoms, Rhinitis, and Sinusitis

Along with Their Usual Triggers Like Animal Fur, Chemicals, Drugs, Dust, Foods, Insects, Latex, Pollen, and Poison Ivy, Oak, and Sumac; Plus Information on Prevention, Identification, and Treatment

Edited by Allan R. Cook. 611 pages. 1997. 0-7808-0036-2. $78.

■

Alternative Medicine Sourcebook

Basic Consumer Health Information about Alternatives to Conventional Medicine, Including Acupressure, Acupuncture, Aromatherapy, Ayurveda, Bioelectromagnetics, Environmental Medicine, Essence

Therapy, Food and Nutrition Therapy, Herbal Therapy, Homeopathy, Imaging, Massage, Naturopathy, Reflexology, Relaxation and Meditation, Sound Therapy, Vitamin and Mineral Therapy, and Yoga, and More

Edited by Allan R. Cook. 737 pages. 1999. 0-7808-0200-4. $78.

"Recommended reference source."
—Booklist, American Library Association, Feb '00

"A great addition to the reference collection of every type of library." —American Reference Books Annual, 2000

■

Alzheimer's, Stroke & 29 Other Neurological Disorders Sourcebook, 1st Edition

Basic Information for the Layperson on 31 Diseases or Disorders Affecting the Brain and Nervous System, First Describing the Illness, Then Listing Symptoms, Diagnostic Methods, and Treatment Options, and Including Statistics on Incidences and Causes

Edited by Frank E. Bair. 579 pages. 1993. 1-55888-748-2. $78.

"Nontechnical reference book that provides reader-friendly information."
—Family Caregiver Alliance Update, Winter '96

"Should be included in any library's patient education section." —American Reference Books Annual, 1994

"Written in an approachable and accessible style. Recommended for patient education and consumer health collections in health science center and public libraries." —Academic Library Book Review, Dec '93

"It is very handy to have information on more than thirty neurological disorders under one cover, and there is no recent source like it." —Reference Quarterly, American Library Association, Fall '93

SEE ALSO Brain Disorders Sourcebook

■

Alzheimer's Disease Sourcebook, 2nd Edition

Basic Consumer Health Information about Alzheimer's Disease, Related Disorders, and Other Dementias, Including Multi-Infarct Dementia, AIDS-Related Dementia, Alcoholic Dementia, Huntington's Disease, Delirium, and Confusional States

Along with Reports Detailing Current Research Efforts in Prevention and Treatment, Long-Term Care Issues, and Listings of Sources for Additional Help and Information

Edited by Karen Bellenir. 524 pages. 1999. 0-7808-0223-3. $78.

"Provides a wealth of useful information not otherwise available in one place. This resource is recommended for all types of libraries."
—American Reference Books Annual, 2000

"Recommended reference source."
—Booklist, American Library Association, Oct '99

Arthritis Sourcebook

Basic Consumer Health Information about Specific Forms of Arthritis and Related Disorders, Including Rheumatoid Arthritis, Osteoarthritis, Gout, Polymyalgia Rheumatica, Psoriatic Arthritis, Spondyloarthropathies, Juvenile Rheumatoid Arthritis, and Juvenile Ankylosing Spondylitis

Along with Information about Medical, Surgical, and Alternative Treatment Options, and Including Strategies for Coping with Pain, Fatigue, and Stress

Edited by Allan R. Cook. 550 pages. 1998. 0-7808-0201-2. $78.

". . . accessible to the layperson."
—Reference and Research Book News, Feb '99

■

Asthma Sourcebook

Basic Consumer Health Information about Asthma, Including Symptoms, Traditional and Nontraditional Remedies, Treatment Advances, Quality-of-Life Aids, Medical Research Updates, and the Role of Allergies, Exercise, Age, the Environment, and Genetics in the Development of Asthma

Along with Statistical Data, a Glossary, and Directories of Support Groups, and Other Resources for Further Information

Edited by Annemarie S. Muth. 628 pages. 2000. 0-7808-0381-7. $78.

"Highly recommended." —The Bookwatch, Jan '01

■

Back & Neck Disorders Sourcebook

Basic Information about Disorders and Injuries of the Spinal Cord and Vertebrae, Including Facts on Chiropractic Treatment, Surgical Interventions, Paralysis, and Rehabilitation

Along with Advice for Preventing Back Trouble

Edited by Karen Bellenir. 548 pages. 1997. 0-7808-0202-0. $78.

"The strength of this work is its basic, easy-to-read format. Recommended."
—Reference and User Services Quarterly, American Library Association, Winter '97

■

Blood & Circulatory Disorders Sourcebook

Basic Information about Blood and Its Components, Anemias, Leukemias, Bleeding Disorders, and Circulatory Disorders, Including Aplastic Anemia, Thalassemia, Sickle-Cell Disease, Hemochromatosis, Hemophilia, Von Willebrand Disease, and Vascular Diseases

Along with a Special Section on Blood Transfusions and Blood Supply Safety, a Glossary, and Source Listings for Further Help and Information

Edited by Karen Bellenir and Linda M. Shin. 554 pages. 1998. 0-7808-0203-9. $78.

"Recommended reference source."
—*Booklist, American Library Association, Feb '99*

"An important reference sourcebook written in simple language for everyday, non-technical users. "
—*Reviewer's Bookwatch, Jan '99*

■

Brain Disorders Sourcebook

Basic Consumer Health Information about Strokes, Epilepsy, Amyotrophic Lateral Sclerosis (ALS/Lou Gehrig's Disease), Parkinson's Disease, Brain Tumors, Cerebral Palsy, Headache, Tourette Syndrome, and More

Along with Statistical Data, Treatment and Rehabilitation Options, Coping Strategies, Reports on Current Research Initiatives, a Glossary, and Resource Listings for Additional Help and Information

Edited by Karen Bellenir. 481 pages. 1999. 0-7808-0229-2. $78.

"Belongs on the shelves of any library with a consumer health collection." —*E-Streams, Mar '00*

"Recommended reference source."
— *Booklist, American Library Association, Oct '99*

SEE ALSO *Alzheimer's, Stroke & 29 Other Neurological Disorders Sourcebook, 1st Edition*

■

Breast Cancer Sourcebook

Basic Consumer Health Information about Breast Cancer, Including Diagnostic Methods, Treatment Options, Alternative Therapies, Self-Help Information, Related Health Concerns, Statistical and Demographic Data, and Facts for Men with Breast Cancer

Along with Reports on Current Research Initiatives, a Glossary of Related Medical Terms, and a Directory of Sources for Further Help and Information

Edited by Edward J. Prucha and Karen Bellenir. 600 pages. 2001. 0-7808-0244-6. $78.

SEE ALSO *Cancer Sourcebook for Women, 1st and 2nd Editions, Women's Health Concerns Sourcebook*

■

Burns Sourcebook

Basic Consumer Health Information about Various Types of Burns and Scalds, Including Flame, Heat, Cold, Electrical, Chemical, and Sun Burns

Along with Information on Short-Term and Long-Term Treatments, Tissue Reconstruction, Plastic Surgery, Prevention Suggestions, and First Aid

Edited by Allan R. Cook. 604 pages. 1999. 0-7808-0204-7. $78.

"This key reference guide is an invaluable addition to all health care and public libraries in confronting this ongoing health issue."
—*American Reference Books Annual, 2000*

"This is an exceptional addition to the series and is highly recommended for all consumer health collections, hospital libraries, and academic medical centers." —*E-Streams, Mar '00*

"Recommended reference source."
—*Booklist, American Library Association, Dec '99*

SEE ALSO *Skin Disorders Sourcebook*

■

Cancer Sourcebook, 1st Edition

Basic Information on Cancer Types, Symptoms, Diagnostic Methods, and Treatments, Including Statistics on Cancer Occurrences Worldwide and the Risks Associated with Known Carcinogens and Activities

Edited by Frank E. Bair. 932 pages. 1990. 1-55888-888-8. $78.

Cited in *Reference Sources for Small and Medium-Sized Libraries, American Library Association, 1999*

"Written in nontechnical language. Useful for patients, their families, medical professionals, and librarians."
—*Guide to Reference Books, 1996*

"Designed with the non-medical professional in mind. Libraries and medical facilities interested in patient education should certainly consider adding the *Cancer Sourcebook* to their holdings. This compact collection of reliable information . . . is an invaluable tool for helping patients and patients' families and friends to take the first steps in coping with the many difficulties of cancer."
—*Medical Reference Services Quarterly, Winter '91*

"Specifically created for the nontechnical reader . . . an important resource for the general reader trying to understand the complexities of cancer."
—*American Reference Books Annual, 1991*

"This publication's nontechnical nature and very comprehensive format make it useful for both the general public and undergraduate students."
—*Choice, Association of College and Research Libraries, Oct '90*

■

New Cancer Sourcebook, 2nd Edition

Basic Information about Major Forms and Stages of Cancer, Featuring Facts about Primary and Secondary Tumors of the Respiratory, Nervous, Lymphatic, Circulatory, Skeletal, and Gastrointestinal Systems, and Specific Organs; Statistical and Demographic Data; Treatment Options; and Strategies for Coping

Edited by Allan R. Cook. 1,313 pages. 1996. 0-7808-0041-9. $78.

"An excellent resource for patients with newly diagnosed cancer and their families. The dialogue is simple, direct, and comprehensive. Highly recommended for patients and families to aid in their understanding of cancer and its treatment."
—*Booklist Health Sciences Supplement, American Library Association, Oct '97*

"The amount of factual and useful information is extensive. The writing is very clear, geared to general readers. Recommended for all levels."

—Choice, Association of College and Research Libraries, Jan '97

■

Cancer Sourcebook, 3rd Edition

Basic Consumer Health Information about Major Forms and Stages of Cancer, Featuring Facts about Primary and Secondary Tumors of the Respiratory, Nervous, Lymphatic, Circulatory, Skeletal, and Gastrointestinal Systems, and Specific Organs

Along with Statistical and Demographic Data, Treatment Options, Strategies for Coping, a Glossary, and a Directory of Sources for Additional Help and Information

Edited by Edward J. Prucha. 1,069 pages. 2000. 0-7808-0227-6. $78.

"**Recommended reference source.**"

—Booklist, American Library Association, Dec '00

■

Cancer Sourcebook for Women, 1st Edition

Basic Information about Specific Forms of Cancer That Affect Women, Featuring Facts about Breast Cancer, Cervical Cancer, Ovarian Cancer, Cancer of the Uterus and Uterine Sarcoma, Cancer of the Vagina, and Cancer of the Vulva; Statistical and Demographic Data; Treatments, Self-Help Management Suggestions, and Current Research Initiatives

Edited by Allan R. Cook and Peter D. Dresser. 524 pages. 1996. 0-7808-0076-1. $78.

"**. . . written in easily understandable, non-technical language. Recommended for public libraries or hospital and academic libraries that collect patient education or consumer health materials.**"

— Medical Reference Services Quarterly, Spring '97

"**Would be of value in a consumer health library. . . . written with the health care consumer in mind. Medical jargon is at a minimum, and medical terms are explained in clear, understandable sentences.**"

— Bulletin of the Medical Library Association, Oct '96

"**The availability under one cover of all these pertinent publications, grouped under cohesive headings, makes this certainly a most useful sourcebook.**"

— Choice, Association of College and Research Libraries, Jun '96

"**Presents a comprehensive knowledge base for general readers. Men and women both benefit from the gold mine of information nestled between the two covers of this book. Recommended.**"

—Academic Library Book Review, Summer '96

"**This timely book is highly recommended for consumer health and patient education collections in all libraries.**" *— Library Journal, Apr '96*

SEE ALSO Breast Cancer Sourcebook, Women's Health Concerns Sourcebook

Cancer Sourcebook for Women, 2nd Edition

Basic Consumer Health Information about Specific Forms of Cancer That Affect Women, Including Cervical Cancer, Ovarian Cancer, Endometrial Cancer, Uterine Sarcoma, Vaginal Cancer, Vulvar Cancer, and Gestational Trophoblastic Tumor; and Featuring Statistical Information, Facts about Tests and Treatments, a Glossary of Cancer Terms, and an Extensive List of Additional Resources

Edited by Karen Bellenir. 600 pages. 2001. 0-7808-0226-8. $78.

SEE ALSO Breast Cancer Sourcebook, Women's Health Concerns Sourcebook

■

Cardiovascular Diseases & Disorders Sourcebook, 1st Edition

Basic Information about Cardiovascular Diseases and Disorders, Featuring Facts about the Cardiovascular System, Demographic and Statistical Data, Descriptions of Pharmacological and Surgical Interventions, Lifestyle Modifications, and a Special Section Focusing on Heart Disorders in Children

Edited by Karen Bellenir and Peter D. Dresser. 683 pages. 1995. 0-7808-0032-X. $78.

"**. . . comprehensive format provides an extensive overview on this subject.**"

—Choice, Association of College and Research Libraries, Jun '96

"**. . . an easily understood, complete, up-to-date resource. This well executed public health tool will make valuable information available to those that need it most, patients and their families. The typeface, sturdy non-reflective paper, and library binding add a feel of quality found wanting in other publications. Highly recommended for academic and general libraries.** "

—Academic Library Book Review, Summer '96

SEE ALSO Healthy Heart Sourcebook for Women, Heart Diseases & Disorders Sourcebook, 2nd Edition

■

Caregiving Sourcebook

Basic Consumer Health Information for Caregivers, Including a Profile of Caregivers, Caregiving Responsibilities and Concerns, Tips for Specific Conditions, Care Environments, and the Effects of Caregiving

Along with Facts about Legal Issues, Financial Information, and Future Planning, a Glossary, and a Listing of Additional Resources

Edited by Joyce Brennfleck Shannon. 550 pages. 2001. 0-7808-0331-0. $78.

Colds, Flu & Other Common Ailments Sourcebook

Basic Consumer Health Information about Common Ailments and Injuries, Including Colds, Coughs, the Flu, Sinus Problems, Headaches, Fever, Nausea and Vomiting, Menstrual Cramps, Diarrhea, Constipation, Hemorrhoids, Back Pain, Dandruff, Dry and Itchy Skin, Cuts, Scrapes, Sprains, Bruises, and More

Along with Information about Prevention, Self-Care, Choosing a Doctor, Over-the-Counter Medications, Folk Remedies, and Alternative Therapies, and Including a Glossary of Important Terms and a Directory of Resources for Further Help and Information

Edited by Chad T. Kimball. 638 pages. 2001. 0-7808-0435-X. $78.

◼

Communication Disorders Sourcebook

Basic Information about Deafness and Hearing Loss, Speech and Language Disorders, Voice Disorders, Balance and Vestibular Disorders, and Disorders of Smell, Taste, and Touch

Edited by Linda M. Ross. 533 pages. 1996. 0-7808-0077-X. $78.

"This is skillfully edited and is a welcome resource for the layperson. It should be found in every public and medical library." *— Booklist Health Sciences Supplement, American Library Association, Oct '97*

◼

Congenital Disorders Sourcebook

Basic Information about Disorders Acquired during Gestation, Including Spina Bifida, Hydrocephalus, Cerebral Palsy, Heart Defects, Craniofacial Abnormalities, Fetal Alcohol Syndrome, and More

Along with Current Treatment Options and Statistical Data

Edited by Karen Bellenir. 607 pages. 1997. 0-7808-0205-5. $78.

"Recommended reference source." *— Booklist, American Library Association, Oct '97*

SEE ALSO *Pregnancy & Birth Sourcebook*

◼

Consumer Issues in Health Care Sourcebook

Basic Information about Health Care Fundamentals and Related Consumer Issues, Including Exams and Screening Tests, Physician Specialties, Choosing a Doctor, Using Prescription and Over-the-Counter Medications Safely, Avoiding Health Scams, Managing Common Health Risks in the Home, Care Options for Chronically or Terminally Ill Patients, and a List of Resources for Obtaining Help and Further Information

Edited by Karen Bellenir. 618 pages. 1998. 0-7808-0221-7. $78.

"Both public and academic libraries will want to have a copy in their collection for readers who are interested in self-education on health issues." *—American Reference Books Annual, 2000*

"The editor has researched the literature from government agencies and others, saving readers the time and effort of having to do the research themselves. Recommended for public libraries." *— Reference and User Services Quarterly, American Library Association, Spring '99*

"Recommended reference source." *— Booklist, American Library Association, Dec '98*

◼

Contagious & Non-Contagious Infectious Diseases Sourcebook

Basic Information about Contagious Diseases like Measles, Polio, Hepatitis B, and Infectious Mononucleosis, and Non-Contagious Infectious Diseases like Tetanus and Toxic Shock Syndrome, and Diseases Occurring as Secondary Infections Such as Shingles and Reye Syndrome

Along with Vaccination, Prevention, and Treatment Information, and a Section Describing Emerging Infectious Disease Threats

Edited by Karen Bellenir and Peter D. Dresser. 566 pages. 1996. 0-7808-0075-3. $78.

◼

Death & Dying Sourcebook

Basic Consumer Health Information for the Layperson about End-of-Life Care and Related Ethical and Legal Issues, Including Chief Causes of Death, Autopsies, Pain Management for the Terminally Ill, Life Support Systems, Insurance, Euthanasia, Assisted Suicide, Hospice Programs, Living Wills, Funeral Planning, Counseling, Mourning, Organ Donation, and Physician Training

Along with Statistical Data, a Glossary, and Listings of Sources for Further Help and Information

Edited by Annemarie S. Muth. 641 pages. 1999. 0-7808-0230-6. $78.

"Recommended reference source." *—Booklist, American Library Association, Aug '00*

"This book is a definite must for all those involved in end-of-life care." *— Doody's Review Service, 2000*

◼

Diabetes Sourcebook, 1st Edition

Basic Information about Insulin-Dependent and Non-insulin-Dependent Diabetes Mellitus, Gestational Diabetes, and Diabetic Complications, Symptoms, Treatment, and Research Results, Including Statistics on Prevalence, Morbidity, and Mortality

Along with Source Listings for Further Help and Information

Edited by Karen Bellenir and Peter D. Dresser. 827 pages. 1994. 1-55888-751-2. $78.

"... very informative and understandable for the layperson without being simplistic. It provides a comprehensive overview for laypersons who want a general understanding of the disease or who want to focus on various aspects of the disease."
— *Bulletin of the Medical Library Association, Jan '96*

■

Diabetes Sourcebook, 2nd Edition

Basic Consumer Health Information about Type 1 Diabetes (Insulin-Dependent or Juvenile-Onset Diabetes), Type 2 (Noninsulin-Dependent or Adult-Onset Diabetes), Gestational Diabetes, and Related Disorders, Including Diabetes Prevalence Data, Management Issues, the Role of Diet and Exercise in Controlling Diabetes, Insulin and Other Diabetes Medicines, and Complications of Diabetes Such as Eye Diseases, Periodontal Disease, Amputation, and End-Stage Renal Disease

Along with Reports on Current Research Initiatives, a Glossary, and Resource Listings for Further Help and Information

Edited by Karen Bellenir. 688 pages. 1998. 0-7808-0224-1. $78.

"This comprehensive book is an excellent addition for high school, academic, medical, and public libraries. This volume is highly recommended."
— *American Reference Books Annual, 2000*

"An invaluable reference." — *Library Journal, May '00*

Selected as one of the 250 "Best Health Sciences Books of 1999." — *Doody's Rating Service, Mar-Apr 2000*

"Recommended reference source."
— *Booklist, American Library Association, Feb '99*

"... provides reliable mainstream medical information ... belongs on the shelves of any library with a consumer health collection." — *E-Streams, Sep '99*

"Provides useful information for the general public."
— *Healthlines, University of Michigan Health Management Research Center, Sep/Oct '99*

■

Diet & Nutrition Sourcebook, 1st Edition

Basic Information about Nutrition, Including the Dietary Guidelines for Americans, the Food Guide Pyramid, and Their Applications in Daily Diet, Nutritional Advice for Specific Age Groups, Current Nutritional Issues and Controversies, the New Food Label and How to Use It to Promote Healthy Eating, and Recent Developments in Nutritional Research

Edited by Dan R. Harris. 662 pages. 1996. 0-7808-0084-2. $78.

"Useful reference as a food and nutrition sourcebook for the general consumer." — *Booklist Health Sciences Supplement, American Library Association, Oct '97*

"Recommended for public libraries and medical libraries that receive general information requests on nutrition. It is readable and will appeal to those interested in learning more about healthy dietary practices."
— *Medical Reference Services Quarterly, Fall '97*

"An abundance of medical and social statistics is translated into readable information geared toward the general reader." — *Bookwatch, Mar '97*

"With dozens of questionable diet books on the market, it is so refreshing to find a reliable and factual reference book. Recommended to aspiring professionals, librarians, and others seeking and giving reliable dietary advice. An excellent compilation." — *Choice, Association of College and Research Libraries, Feb '97*

SEE ALSO *Digestive Diseases & Disorders Sourcebook, Gastrointestinal Diseases & Disorders Sourcebook*

■

Diet & Nutrition Sourcebook, 2nd Edition

Basic Consumer Health Information about Dietary Guidelines, Recommended Daily Intake Values, Vitamins, Minerals, Fiber, Fat, Weight Control, Dietary Supplements, and Food Additives

Along with Special Sections on Nutrition Needs throughout Life and Nutrition for People with Such Specific Medical Concerns as Allergies, High Blood Cholesterol, Hypertension, Diabetes, Celiac Disease, Seizure Disorders, Phenylketonuria (PKU), Cancer, and Eating Disorders, and Including Reports on Current Nutrition Research and Source Listings for Additional Help and Information

Edited by Karen Bellenir. 650 pages. 1999. 0-7808-0228-4. $78.

"This book is an excellent source of basic diet and nutrition information." — *Booklist Health Sciences Supplement, American Library Association, Dec '00*

"This reference document should be in any public library, but it would be a very good guide for beginning students in the health sciences. If the other books in this publisher's series are as good as this, they should all be in the health sciences collections."
— *American Reference Books Annual, 2000*

"This book is an excellent general nutrition reference for consumers who desire to take an active role in their health care for prevention. Consumers of all ages who select this book can feel confident they are receiving current and accurate information."
— *Journal of Nutrition for the Elderly, Vol. 19, No. 4, '00*

"Recommended reference source."
— *Booklist, American Library Association, Dec '99*

SEE ALSO *Digestive Diseases & Disorders Sourcebook, Gastrointestinal Diseases & Disorders Sourcebook*

Digestive Diseases & Disorders Sourcebook

Basic Consumer Health Information about Diseases and Disorders that Impact the Upper and Lower Digestive System, Including Celiac Disease, Constipation, Crohn's Disease, Cyclic Vomiting Syndrome, Diarrhea, Diverticulosis and Diverticulitis, Gallstones, Heartburn, Hemorrhoids, Hernias, Indigestion (Dyspepsia), Irritable Bowel Syndrome, Lactose Intolerance, Ulcers, and More

Along with Information about Medications and Other Treatments, Tips for Maintaining a Healthy Digestive Tract, a Glossary, and Directory of Digestive Diseases Organizations

Edited by Karen Bellenir. 335 pages. 1999. 0-7808-0327-2. $48.

"This title is recommended for public, hospital, and health sciences libraries with consumer health collections." — *E-Streams, Jul-Aug '00*

"Recommended reference source."
— *Booklist, American Library Association, May '00*

SEE ALSO *Diet & Nutrition Sourcebook, 1st and 2nd Editions, Gastrointestinal Diseases & Disorders Sourcebook*

■

Disabilities Sourcebook

Basic Consumer Health Information about Physical and Psychiatric Disabilities, Including Descriptions of Major Causes of Disability, Assistive and Adaptive Aids, Workplace Issues, and Accessibility Concerns

Along with Information about the Americans with Disabilities Act, a Glossary, and Resources for Additional Help and Information

Edited by Dawn D. Matthews. 616 pages. 2000. 0-7808-0389-2. $78.

"An excellent source book in easy-to-read format covering many current topics; highly recommended for all libraries."
— *Choice, Association of College and Research Libraries, Jan '01*

"Recommended reference source."
— *Booklist, American Library Association, Jul '00*

"An involving, invaluable handbook."
— *The Bookwatch, May '00*

■

Domestic Violence & Child Abuse Sourcebook

Basic Consumer Health Information about Spousal/Partner, Child, Sibling, Parent, and Elder Abuse, Covering Physical, Emotional, and Sexual Abuse, Teen Dating Violence, and Stalking; Includes Information about Hotlines, Safe Houses, Safety Plans, and Other Resources for Support and Assistance, Community Initiatives, and Reports on Current Directions in Research and Treatment

Along with a Glossary, Sources for Further Reading, and Governmental and Non-Governmental Organizations Contact Information

Edited by Helene Henderson. 1,064 pages. 2000. 0-7808-0235-7. $78.

■

Drug Abuse Sourcebook

Basic Consumer Health Information about Illicit Substances of Abuse and the Diversion of Prescription Medications, Including Depressants, Hallucinogens, Inhalants, Marijuana, Narcotics, Stimulants, and Anabolic Steroids

Along with Facts about Related Health Risks, Treatment Issues, and Substance Abuse Prevention Programs, a Glossary of Terms, Statistical Data, and Directories of Hotline Services, Self-Help Groups, and Organizations Able to Provide Further Information

Edited by Karen Bellenir. 629 pages. 2000. 0-7808-0242-X. $78.

"Highly recommended." — *The Bookwatch, Jan '01*

SEE ALSO *Alcoholism Sourcebook, Substance Abuse Sourcebook*

■

Ear, Nose & Throat Disorders Sourcebook

Basic Information about Disorders of the Ears, Nose, Sinus Cavities, Pharynx, and Larynx, Including Ear Infections, Tinnitus, Vestibular Disorders, Allergic and Non-Allergic Rhinitis, Sore Throats, Tonsillitis, and Cancers That Affect the Ears, Nose, Sinuses, and Throat

Along with Reports on Current Research Initiatives, a Glossary of Related Medical Terms, and a Directory of Sources for Further Help and Information

Edited by Karen Bellenir and Linda M. Shin. 576 pages. 1998. 0-7808-0206-3. $78.

"Overall, this sourcebook is helpful for the consumer seeking information on ENT issues. It is recommended for public libraries."
— *American Reference Books Annual, 1999*

"Recommended reference source."
— *Booklist, American Library Association, Dec '98*

■

Eating Disorders Sourcebook

Basic Consumer Health Information about Eating Disorders, Including Information about Anorexia Nervosa, Bulimia Nervosa, Binge Eating, Body Dysmorphic Disorder, Pica, Laxative Abuse, and Night Eating Syndrome

Along with Information about Causes, Adverse Affects, and Treatment and Prevention Issues, and Featuring a Section on Concerns Specific to Children and Adolescents, a Glossary, and Resources for Further Help and Information

Edited by Dawn D. Matthews. 350 pages. 2001. 0-7808-0335-3. $48.

Endocrine & Metabolic Disorders Sourcebook

Basic Information for the Layperson about Pancreatic and Insulin-Related Disorders Such as Pancreatitis, Diabetes, and Hypoglycemia; Adrenal Gland Disorders Such as Cushing's Syndrome, Addison's Disease, and Congenital Adrenal Hyperplasia; Pituitary Gland Disorders Such as Growth Hormone Deficiency, Acromegaly, and Pituitary Tumors; Thyroid Disorders Such as Hypothyroidism, Graves' Disease, Hashimoto's Disease, and Goiter; Hyperparathyroidism; and Other Diseases and Syndromes of Hormone Imbalance or Metabolic Dysfunction

Along with Reports on Current Research Initiatives

Edited by Linda M. Shin. 574 pages. 1998. 0-7808-0207-1. $78.

"Omnigraphics has produced another needed resource for health information consumers."
— *American Reference Books Annual, 2000*

"Recommended reference source."
— *Booklist, American Library Association, Dec '98*

■

Environmentally Induced Disorders Sourcebook

Basic Information about Diseases and Syndromes Linked to Exposure to Pollutants and Other Substances in Outdoor and Indoor Environments Such as Lead, Asbestos, Formaldehyde, Mercury, Emissions, Noise, and More

Edited by Allan R. Cook. 620 pages. 1997. 0-7808-0083-4. $78.

"Recommended reference source."
— *Booklist, American Library Association, Sep '98*

"This book will be a useful addition to anyone's library." — *Choice Health Sciences Supplement, Association of College and Research Libraries, May '98*

". . . a good survey of numerous environmentally induced physical disorders . . . a useful addition to anyone's library."
— *Doody's Health Sciences Book Reviews, Jan '98*

". . . provide[s] introductory information from the best authorities around. Since this volume covers topics that potentially affect everyone, it will surely be one of the most frequently consulted volumes in the *Health Reference Series*." — *Rettig on Reference, Nov '97*

■

Ethnic Diseases Sourcebook

Basic Consumer Health Information for Ethnic and Racial Minority Groups in the United States, Including General Health Indicators and Behaviors, Ethnic Diseases, Genetic Testing, the Impact of Chronic Diseases, Women's Health, Mental Health Issues, and Preventive Health Care Services

Along with a Glossary and a Listing of Additional Resources

Edited by Joyce Brennfleck Shannon. 664 pages. 2001. 0-7808-0336-1. $78.

Family Planning Sourcebook

Basic Consumer Health Information about Planning for Pregnancy and Contraception, Including Traditional Methods, Barrier Methods, Hormonal Methods, Permanent Methods, Future Methods, Emergency Contraception, and Birth Control Choices for Women at Each Stage of Life

Along with Statistics, a Glossary, and Sources of Additional Information

Edited by Amy Marcaccio Keyzer. 520 pages. 2001. 0-7808-0379-5. $78.

SEE ALSO *Pregnancy & Birth Sourcebook*

■

Fitness & Exercise Sourcebook, 1st Edition

Basic Information on Fitness and Exercise, Including Fitness Activities for Specific Age Groups, Exercise for People with Specific Medical Conditions, How to Begin a Fitness Program in Running, Walking, Swimming, Cycling, and Other Athletic Activities, and Recent Research in Fitness and Exercise

Edited by Dan R. Harris. 663 pages. 1996. 0-7808-0186-5. $78.

"A good resource for general readers."
— *Choice, Association of College and Research Libraries, Nov '97*

"The perennial popularity of the topic . . . make this an appealing selection for public libraries."
— *Rettig on Reference, Jun/Jul '97*

■

Fitness & Exercise Sourcebook, 2nd Edition

Basic Consumer Health Information about the Fundamentals of Fitness and Exercise, Including How to Begin and Maintain a Fitness Program, Fitness as a Lifestyle, the Link between Fitness and Diet, Advice for Specific Groups of People, Exercise as It Relates to Specific Medical Conditions, and Recent Research in Fitness and Exercise

Along with a Glossary of Important Terms and Resources for Additional Help and Information

Edited by Kristen M. Gledhill. 646 pages. 2001. 0-7808-0334-5. $78.

■

Food & Animal Borne Diseases Sourcebook

Basic Information about Diseases That Can Be Spread to Humans through the Ingestion of Contaminated Food or Water or by Contact with Infected Animals and Insects, Such as Botulism, E. Coli, Hepatitis A, Trichinosis, Lyme Disease, and Rabies

Along with Information Regarding Prevention and Treatment Methods, and Including a Special Section for

International Travelers Describing Diseases Such as Cholera, Malaria, Travelers' Diarrhea, and Yellow Fever, and Offering Recommendations for Avoiding Illness

Edited by Karen Bellenir and Peter D. Dresser. 535 pages. 1995. 0-7808-0033-8. $78.

"Targeting general readers and providing them with a single, comprehensive source of information on selected topics, this book continues, with the excellent caliber of its predecessors, to catalog topical information on health matters of general interest. Readable and thorough, this valuable resource is highly recommended for all libraries."
— Academic Library Book Review, Summer '96

"A comprehensive collection of authoritative information."
— Emergency Medical Services, Oct '95

■

Food Safety Sourcebook

Basic Consumer Health Information about the Safe Handling of Meat, Poultry, Seafood, Eggs, Fruit Juices, and Other Food Items, and Facts about Pesticides, Drinking Water, Food Safety Overseas, and the Onset, Duration, and Symptoms of Foodborne Illnesses, Including Types of Pathogenic Bacteria, Parasitic Protozoa, Worms, Viruses, and Natural Toxins

Along with the Role of the Consumer, the Food Handler, and the Government in Food Safety; a Glossary, and Resources for Additional Help and Information

Edited by Dawn D. Matthews. 339 pages. 1999. 0-7808-0326-4. $48.

"This book is recommended for public libraries and universities with home economic and food science programs."
— E-Streams, Nov '00

"This book takes the complex issues of food safety and foodborne pathogens and presents them in an easily understood manner. [It does] an excellent job of covering a large and often confusing topic."
— American Reference Books Annual, 2000

"Recommended reference source."
— Booklist, American Library Association, May '00

■

Forensic Medicine Sourcebook

Basic Consumer Information for the Layperson about Forensic Medicine, Including Crime Scene Investigation, Evidence Collection and Analysis, Expert Testimony, Computer-Aided Criminal Identification, Digital Imaging in the Courtroom, DNA Profiling, Accident Reconstruction, Autopsies, Ballistics, Drugs and Explosives Detection, Latent Fingerprints, Product Tampering, and Questioned Document Examination

Along with Statistical Data, a Glossary of Forensics Terminology, and Listings of Sources for Further Help and Information

Edited by Annemarie S. Muth. 574 pages. 1999. 0-7808-0232-2. $78.

"There are several items that make this book attractive to consumers who are seeking certain forensic data. . . .

This is a useful current source for those seeking general forensic medical answers."
— American Reference Books Annual, 2000

"Recommended for public libraries."
— Reference & User Services Quarterly, American Library Association, Spring 2000

"Recommended reference source."
— Booklist, American Library Association, Feb '00

"A wealth of information, useful statistics, references are up-to-date and extremely complete. This wonderful collection of data will help students who are interested in a career in any type of forensic field. It is a great resource for attorneys who need information about types of expert witnesses needed in a particular case. It also offers useful information for fiction and nonfiction writers whose work involves a crime. A fascinating compilation. All levels."
— Choice, Association of College and Research Libraries, Jan 2000

■

Gastrointestinal Diseases & Disorders Sourcebook

Basic Information about Gastroesophageal Reflux Disease (Heartburn), Ulcers, Diverticulosis, Irritable Bowel Syndrome, Crohn's Disease, Ulcerative Colitis, Diarrhea, Constipation, Lactose Intolerance, Hemorrhoids, Hepatitis, Cirrhosis, and Other Digestive Problems, Featuring Statistics, Descriptions of Symptoms, and Current Treatment Methods of Interest for Persons Living with Upper and Lower Gastrointestinal Maladies

Edited by Linda M. Ross. 413 pages. 1996. 0-7808-0078-8. $78.

". . . very readable form. The successful editorial work that brought this material together into a useful and understandable reference makes accessible to all readers information that can help them more effectively understand and obtain help for digestive tract problems."
— Choice, Association of College and Research Libraries, Feb '97

SEE ALSO Diet & Nutrition Sourcebook, 1st and 2nd Editions, Digestive Diseases & Disorders Sourcebook

■

Genetic Disorders Sourcebook, 1st Edition

Basic Information about Heritable Diseases and Disorders Such as Down Syndrome, PKU, Hemophilia, Von Willebrand Disease, Gaucher Disease, Tay-Sachs Disease, and Sickle-Cell Disease, Along with Information about Genetic Screening, Gene Therapy, Home Care, and Including Source Listings for Further Help and Information on More Than 300 Disorders

Edited by Karen Bellenir. 642 pages. 1996. 0-7808-0034-6. $78.

"Recommended for undergraduate libraries or libraries that serve the public."
— Science & Technology Libraries, Vol. 18, No. 1, '99

"Provides essential medical information to both the general public and those diagnosed with a serious or fatal genetic disease or disorder."
—Choice, Association of College and Research Libraries, Jan '97

"Geared toward the lay public. It would be well placed in all public libraries and in those hospital and medical libraries in which access to genetic references is limited." — Doody's Health Sciences Book Review, Oct '96

■

Genetic Disorders Sourcebook, 2nd Edition

Basic Consumer Health Information about Hereditary Diseases and Disorders, Including Cystic Fibrosis, Down Syndrome, Hemophilia, Huntington's Disease, Sickle Cell Anemia, and More; Facts about Genes, Gene Research and Therapy, Genetic Screening, Ethics of Gene Testing, Genetic Counseling, and Advice on Coping and Caring

Along with a Glossary of Genetic Terminology and a Resource List for Help, Support, and Further Information

Edited by Kathy Massimini. 768 pages. 2001. 0-7808-0241-1. $78.

■

Head Trauma Sourcebook

Basic Information for the Layperson about Open-Head and Closed-Head Injuries, Treatment Advances, Recovery, and Rehabilitation

Along with Reports on Current Research Initiatives

Edited by Karen Bellenir. 414 pages. 1997. 0-7808-0208-X. $78.

■

Health Insurance Sourcebook

Basic Information about Managed Care Organizations, Traditional Fee-for-Service Insurance, Insurance Portability and Pre-Existing Conditions Clauses, Medicare, Medicaid, Social Security, and Military Health Care

Along with Information about Insurance Fraud

Edited by Wendy Wilcox. 530 pages. 1997. 0-7808-0222-5. $78.

"Particularly useful because it brings much of this information together in one volume. This book will be a handy reference source in the health sciences library, hospital library, college and university library, and medium to large public library."
— Medical Reference Services Quarterly, Fall '98

Awarded "Books of the Year Award"
— American Journal of Nursing, 1997

"The layout of the book is particularly helpful as it provides easy access to reference material. A most useful addition to the vast amount of information about health insurance. The use of data from U.S. government agencies is most commendable. Useful in a library or learning center for healthcare professional students."
— Doody's Health Sciences Book Reviews, Nov '97

Healthy Aging Sourcebook

Basic Consumer Health Information about Maintaining Health through the Aging Process, Including Advice on Nutrition, Exercise, and Sleep, Help in Making Decisions about Midlife Issues and Retirement, and Guidance Concerning Practical and Informed Choices in Health Consumerism

Along with Data Concerning the Theories of Aging, Different Experiences in Aging by Minority Groups, and Facts about Aging Now and Aging in the Future; and Featuring a Glossary, a Guide to Consumer Help, Additional Suggested Reading, and Practical Resource Directory

Edited by Jenifer Swanson. 536 pages. 1999. 0-7808-0390-6. $78.

"Recommended reference source."
—Booklist, American Library Association, Feb '00

SEE ALSO Physical & Mental Issues in Aging Sourcebook

■

Healthy Heart Sourcebook for Women

Basic Consumer Health Information about Cardiac Issues Specific to Women, Including Facts about Major Risk Factors and Prevention, Treatment and Control Strategies, and Important Dietary Issues

Along with a Special Section Regarding the Pros and Cons of Hormone Replacement Therapy and Its Impact on Heart Health, and Additional Help, Including Recipes, a Glossary, and a Directory of Resources

Edited by Dawn D. Matthews. 336 pages. 2000. 0-7808-0329-9. $48.

"Contains very important information about coronary artery disease that all women should know. The information is current and presented in an easy-to-read format. The book will make a good addition to any library."
— American Medical Writers Association Journal, Summer '00

"Important, basic reference."
— Reviewer's Bookwatch, Jul '00

SEE ALSO Cardiovascular Diseases & Disorders Sourcebook, 1st Edition, Heart Diseases & Disorders Sourcebook, 2nd Edition, Women's Health Concerns Sourcebook

■

Heart Diseases & Disorders Sourcebook, 2nd Edition

Basic Consumer Health Information about Heart Attacks, Angina, Rhythm Disorders, Heart Failure, Valve Disease, Congenital Heart Disorders, and More, Including Descriptions of Surgical Procedures and Other Interventions, Medications, Cardiac Rehabilitation, Risk Identification, and Prevention Tips

Along with Statistical Data, Reports on Current Research Initiatives, a Glossary of Cardiovascular Terms, and Resource Directory

Edited by Karen Bellenir. 612 pages. 2000. 0-7808-0238-1. $78.

"Recommended reference source."
—*Booklist, American Library Association, Dec '00*

"Provides comprehensive coverage of matters related to the heart. This title is recommended for health sciences and public libraries with consumer health collections."
—*E-Streams, Oct '00*

SEE ALSO *Cardiovascular Diseases & Disorders Sourcebook, 1st Edition, Healthy Heart Sourcebook for Women*

■

Immune System Disorders Sourcebook

Basic Information about Lupus, Multiple Sclerosis, Guillain-Barré Syndrome, Chronic Granulomatous Disease, and More

Along with Statistical and Demographic Data and Reports on Current Research Initiatives

Edited by Allan R. Cook. 608 pages. 1997. 0-7808-0209-8. $78.

■

Infant & Toddler Health Sourcebook

Basic Consumer Health Information about the Physical and Mental Development of Newborns, Infants, and Toddlers, Including Neonatal Concerns, Nutrition Recommendations, Immunization Schedules, Common Pediatric Disorders, Assessments and Milestones, Safety Tips, and Advice for Parents and Other Caregivers

Along with a Glossary of Terms and Resource Listings for Additional Help

Edited by Jenifer Swanson. 585 pages. 2000. 0-7808-0246-2. $78.

■

Kidney & Urinary Tract Diseases & Disorders Sourcebook

Basic Information about Kidney Stones, Urinary Incontinence, Bladder Disease, End Stage Renal Disease, Dialysis, and More

Along with Statistical and Demographic Data and Reports on Current Research Initiatives

Edited by Linda M. Ross. 602 pages. 1997. 0-7808-0079-6. $78.

■

Learning Disabilities Sourcebook

Basic Information about Disorders Such as Dyslexia, Visual and Auditory Processing Deficits, Attention Deficit/Hyperactivity Disorder, and Autism

Along with Statistical and Demographic Data, Reports on Current Research Initiatives, an Explanation of the Assessment Process, and a Special Section for Adults with Learning Disabilities

Edited by Linda M. Shin. 579 pages. 1998. 0-7808-0210-1. $78.

Named "Outstanding Reference Book of 1999."
—*New York Public Library, Feb 2000*

"An excellent candidate for inclusion in a public library reference section. It's a great source of information. Teachers will also find the book useful. Definitely worth reading."
—*Journal of Adolescent & Adult Literacy, Feb 2000*

"Readable . . . provides a solid base of information regarding successful techniques used with individuals who have learning disabilities, as well as practical suggestions for educators and family members. Clear language, concise descriptions, and pertinent information for contacting multiple resources add to the strength of this book as a useful tool."
—*Choice, Association of College and Research Libraries, Feb '99*

"Recommended reference source."
—*Booklist, American Library Association, Sep '98*

"This is a useful resource for libraries and for those who don't have the time to identify and locate the individual publications."
—*Disability Resources Monthly, Sep '98*

■

Liver Disorders Sourcebook

Basic Consumer Health Information about the Liver and How It Works; Liver Diseases, Including Cancer, Cirrhosis, Hepatitis, and Toxic and Drug Related Diseases; Tips for Maintaining a Healthy Liver; Laboratory Tests, Radiology Tests, and Facts about Liver Transplantation

Along with a Section on Support Groups, a Glossary, and Resource Listings

Edited by Joyce Brennfleck Shannon. 591 pages. 2000. 0-7808-0383-3. $78.

"This title is recommended for health sciences and public libraries with consumer health collections."
—*E-Streams, Oct '00*

"Recommended reference source."
—*Booklist, American Library Association, Jun '00*

■

Medical Tests Sourcebook

Basic Consumer Health Information about Medical Tests, Including Periodic Health Exams, General Screening Tests, Tests You Can Do at Home, Findings of the U.S. Preventive Services Task Force, X-ray and Radiology Tests, Electrical Tests, Tests of Blood and Other Body Fluids and Tissues, Scope Tests, Lung Tests, Genetic Tests, Pregnancy Tests, Newborn Screening Tests, Sexually Transmitted Disease Tests, and Computer Aided Diagnoses

Along with a Section on Paying for Medical Tests, a Glossary, and Resource Listings

Edited by Joyce Brennfleck Shannon. 691 pages. 1999. 0-7808-0243-8. $78.

"A valuable reference guide."
—*American Reference Books Annual, 2000*

"Recommended for hospital and health sciences libraries with consumer health collections."
—*E-Streams, Mar '00*

"This is an overall excellent reference with a wealth of general knowledge that may aid those who are reluctant to get vital tests performed."
—*Today's Librarian, Jan 2000*

■

Men's Health Concerns Sourcebook

Basic Information about Health Issues That Affect Men, Featuring Facts about the Top Causes of Death in Men, Including Heart Disease, Stroke, Cancers, Prostate Disorders, Chronic Obstructive Pulmonary Disease, Pneumonia and Influenza, Human Immuno-deficiency Virus and Acquired Immune Deficiency Syndrome, Diabetes Mellitus, Stress, Suicide, Accidents and Homicides; and Facts about Common Concerns for Men, Including Impotence, Contraception, Circumcision, Sleep Disorders, Snoring, Hair Loss, Diet, Nutrition, Exercise, Kidney and Urological Disorders, and Backaches

Edited by Allan R. Cook. 738 pages. 1998. 0-7808-0212-8. $78.

"This comprehensive resource and the series are highly recommended."
—*American Reference Books Annual, 2000*

"Recommended reference source."
—*Booklist, American Library Association, Dec '98*

■

Mental Health Disorders Sourcebook, 1st Edition

Basic Information about Schizophrenia, Depression, Bipolar Disorder, Panic Disorder, Obsessive-Compulsive Disorder, Phobias and Other Anxiety Disorders, Paranoia and Other Personality Disorders, Eating Disorders, and Sleep Disorders

Along with Information about Treatment and Therapies

Edited by Karen Bellenir. 548 pages. 1995. 0-7808-0040-0. $78.

"This is an excellent new book . . . written in easy-to-understand language." —*Booklist Health Sciences Supplement, American Library Association, Oct '97*

". . . useful for public and academic libraries and consumer health collections."
—*Medical Reference Services Quarterly, Spring '97*

"The great strengths of the book are its readability and its inclusion of places to find more information. Especially recommended." —*Reference Quarterly, American Library Association, Winter '96*

". . . a good resource for a consumer health library."
—*Bulletin of the Medical Library Association, Oct '96*

"The information is data-based and couched in brief, concise language that avoids jargon. . . . a useful reference source." —*Readings, Sep '96*

"The text is well organized and adequately written for its target audience." —*Choice, Association of College and Research Libraries, Jun '96*

". . . provides information on a wide range of mental disorders, presented in nontechnical language."
—*Exceptional Child Education Resources, Spring '96*

"Recommended for public and academic libraries."
—*Reference Book Review, 1996*

■

Mental Health Disorders Sourcebook, 2nd Edition

Basic Consumer Health Information about Anxiety Disorders, Depression and Other Mood Disorders, Eating Disorders, Personality Disorders, Schizophrenia, and More, Including Disease Descriptions, Treatment Options, and Reports on Current Research Initiatives

Along with Statistical Data, Tips for Maintaining Mental Health, a Glossary, and Directory of Sources for Additional Help and Information

Edited by Karen Bellenir. 605 pages. 2000. 0-7808-0240-3. $78.

"Recommended reference source."
—*Booklist, American Library Association, Jun '00*

■

Mental Retardation Sourcebook

Basic Consumer Health Information about Mental Retardation and Its Causes, Including Down Syndrome, Fetal Alcohol Syndrome, Fragile X Syndrome, Genetic Conditions, Injury, and Environmental Sources

Along with Preventive Strategies, Parenting Issues, Educational Implications, Health Care Needs, Employment and Economic Matters, Legal Issues, a Glossary, and a Resource Listing for Additional Help and Information

Edited by Joyce Brennfleck Shannon. 642 pages. 2000. 0-7808-0377-9. $78.

"The strength of this work is that it compiles many basic fact sheets and addresses for further information in one volume. It is intended and suitable for the general public. The sourcebook is relevant to any collection providing health information to the general public."
—*E-Streams, Nov '00*

"From preventing retardation to parenting and family challenges, this covers health, social and legal issues and will prove an invaluable overview."
—*Reviewer's Bookwatch, Jul '00*

Obesity Sourcebook

Basic Consumer Health Information about Diseases and Other Problems Associated with Obesity, and Including Facts about Risk Factors, Prevention Issues, and Management Approaches

Along with Statistical and Demographic Data, Information about Special Populations, Research Updates, a Glossary, and Source Listings for Further Help and Information

Edited by Wilma Caldwell and Chad T. Kimball. 376 pages. 2001. 0-7808-0333-7. $48.

Ophthalmic Disorders Sourcebook

Basic Information about Glaucoma, Cataracts, Macular Degeneration, Strabismus, Refractive Disorders, and More

Along with Statistical and Demographic Data and Reports on Current Research Initiatives

Edited by Linda M. Ross. 631 pages. 1996. 0-7808-0081-8. $78.

Oral Health Sourcebook

Basic Information about Diseases and Conditions Affecting Oral Health, Including Cavities, Gum Disease, Dry Mouth, Oral Cancers, Fever Blisters, Canker Sores, Oral Thrush, Bad Breath, Temporomandibular Disorders, and other Craniofacial Syndromes

Along with Statistical Data on the Oral Health of Americans, Oral Hygiene, Emergency First Aid, Information on Treatment Procedures and Methods of Replacing Lost Teeth

Edited by Allan R. Cook. 558 pages. 1997. 0-7808-0082-6. $78.

"Unique source which will fill a gap in dental sources for patients and the lay public. A valuable reference tool even in a library with thousands of books on dentistry. Comprehensive, clear, inexpensive, and easy to read and use. It fills an enormous gap in the health care literature." —Reference and User Services Quarterly, American Library Association, Summer '98

"Recommended reference source."
—Booklist, American Library Association, Dec '97

Osteoporosis Sourcebook

Basic Consumer Health Information about Primary and Secondary Osteoporosis and Juvenile Osteoporosis and Related Conditions, Including Fibrous Dysplasia, Gaucher Disease, Hyperthyroidism, Hypophosphatasia, Myeloma, Osteopetrosis, Osteogenesis Imperfecta, and Paget's Disease

Along with Information about Risk Factors, Treatments, Traditional and Non-Traditional Pain Management, a Glossary of Related Terms, and a Directory of Resources

Edited by Allan R. Cook. 584 pages. 2001. 0-7808-0239-X. $78.

SEE ALSO Women's Health Concerns Sourcebook

Pain Sourcebook

Basic Information about Specific Forms of Acute and Chronic Pain, Including Headaches, Back Pain, Muscular Pain, Neuralgia, Surgical Pain, and Cancer Pain

Along with Pain Relief Options Such as Analgesics, Narcotics, Nerve Blocks, Transcutaneous Nerve Stimulation, and Alternative Forms of Pain Control, Including Biofeedback, Imaging, Behavior Modification, and Relaxation Techniques

Edited by Allan R. Cook. 667 pages. 1997. 0-7808-0213-6. $78.

"The text is readable, easily understood, and well indexed. This excellent volume belongs in all patient education libraries, consumer health sections of public libraries, and many personal collections."
—American Reference Books Annual, 1999

"A beneficial reference." —Booklist Health Sciences Supplement, American Library Association, Oct '98

"The information is basic in terms of scholarship and is appropriate for general readers. Written in journalistic style ... intended for non-professionals. Quite thorough in its coverage of different pain conditions and summarizes the latest clinical information regarding pain treatment." —Choice, Association of College and Research Libraries, Jun '98

"Recommended reference source."
—Booklist, American Library Association, Mar '98

Pediatric Cancer Sourcebook

Basic Consumer Health Information about Leukemias, Brain Tumors, Sarcomas, Lymphomas, and Other Cancers in Infants, Children, and Adolescents, Including Descriptions of Cancers, Treatments, and Coping Strategies

Along with Suggestions for Parents, Caregivers, and Concerned Relatives, a Glossary of Cancer Terms, and Resource Listings

Edited by Edward J. Prucha. 587 pages. 1999. 0-7808-0245-4. $78.

"A valuable addition to all libraries specializing in health services and many public libraries."
—American Reference Books Annual, 2000

"Recommended reference source."
—Booklist, American Library Association, Feb '00

"An excellent source of information. Recommended for public, hospital, and health science libraries with consumer health collections." —E-Streams, Jun '00

Physical & Mental Issues in Aging Sourcebook

Basic Consumer Health Information on Physical and Mental Disorders Associated with the Aging Process, Including Concerns about Cardiovascular Disease, Pulmonary Disease, Oral Health, Digestive Disorders, Musculoskeletal and Skin Disorders, Metabolic Changes, Sexual and Reproductive Issues, and Changes in Vision, Hearing, and Other Senses

643

Along with Data about Longevity and Causes of Death, Information on Acute and Chronic Pain, Descriptions of Mental Concerns, a Glossary of Terms, and Resource Listings for Additional Help

Edited by Jenifer Swanson. 660 pages. 1999. 0-7808-0233-0. $78.

"Recommended for public libraries."
— American Reference Books Annual, 2000

"This is a treasure of health information for the layperson."
— Choice Health Sciences Supplement, Association of College & Research Libraries, May 2000

"Recommended reference source."
— Booklist, American Library Association, Oct '99

SEE ALSO Healthy Aging Sourcebook

■

Podiatry Sourcebook

Basic Consumer Health Information about Foot Conditions, Diseases, and Injuries, Including Bunions, Corns, Calluses, Athlete's Foot, Plantar Warts, Hammertoes and Clawtoes, Club Foot, Heel Pain, Gout, and More

Along with Facts about Foot Care, Disease Prevention, Foot Safety, Choosing a Foot Care Specialist, a Glossary of Terms, and Resource Listings for Additional Information

Edited by M. Lisa Weatherford. 600 pages. 2001. 0-7808-0215-2. $78.

■

Pregnancy & Birth Sourcebook

Basic Information about Planning for Pregnancy, Maternal Health, Fetal Growth and Development, Labor and Delivery, Postpartum and Perinatal Care, Pregnancy in Mothers with Special Concerns, and Disorders of Pregnancy, Including Genetic Counseling, Nutrition and Exercise, Obstetrical Tests, Pregnancy Discomfort, Multiple Births, Cesarean Sections, Medical Testing of Newborns, Breastfeeding, Gestational Diabetes, and Ectopic Pregnancy

Edited by Heather E. Aldred. 737 pages. 1997. 0-7808-0216-0. $78.

"A well-organized handbook. Recommended."
— Choice, Association of College and Research Libraries, Apr '98

"Recommended reference source."
— Booklist, American Library Association, Mar '98

"Recommended for public libraries."
— American Reference Books Annual, 1998

SEE ALSO Congenital Disorders Sourcebook, Family Planning Sourcebook

■

Prostate Cancer Sourcebook

Basic Consumer Health Information about Prostate Cancer, Including Information about the Associated Risk Factors, Detection, Diagnosis, and Treatment of Prostate Cancer

Along with Information on Non-Malignant Prostate Conditions, and Featuring a Section Listing Support and Treatment Centers and a Glossary of Related Terms

Edited by Dawn D. Matthews. 300 pages. 2001. 0-7808-0324-8. $78.

■

Public Health Sourcebook

Basic Information about Government Health Agencies, Including National Health Statistics and Trends, Healthy People 2000 Program Goals and Objectives, the Centers for Disease Control and Prevention, the Food and Drug Administration, and the National Institutes of Health

Along with Full Contact Information for Each Agency

Edited by Wendy Wilcox. 698 pages. 1998. 0-7808-0220-9. $78.

"Recommended reference source."
— Booklist, American Library Association, Sep '98

"This consumer guide provides welcome assistance in navigating the maze of federal health agencies and their data on public health concerns."
— SciTech Book News, Sep '98

■

Reconstructive & Cosmetic Surgery Sourcebook

Basic Consumer Health Information on Cosmetic and Reconstructive Plastic Surgery, Including Statistical Information about Different Surgical Procedures, Things to Consider Prior to Surgery, Plastic Surgery Techniques and Tools, Emotional and Psychological Considerations, and Procedure-Specific Information

Along with a Glossary of Terms and a Listing of Resources for Additional Help and Information

Edited by M. Lisa Weatherford. 374 pages. 2001. 0-7808-0214-4. $48.

■

Rehabilitation Sourcebook

Basic Consumer Health Information about Rehabilitation for People Recovering from Heart Surgery, Spinal Cord Injury, Stroke, Orthopedic Impairments, Amputation, Pulmonary Impairments, Traumatic Injury, and More, Including Physical Therapy, Occupational Therapy, Speech/ Language Therapy, Massage Therapy, Dance Therapy, Art Therapy, and Recreational Therapy

Along with Information on Assistive and Adaptive Devices, a Glossary, and Resources for Additional Help and Information

Edited by Dawn D. Matthews. 531 pages. 1999. 0-7808-0236-5. $78.

"Recommended reference source."
— Booklist, American Library Association, May '00

Respiratory Diseases & Disorders Sourcebook

Basic Information about Respiratory Diseases and Disorders, Including Asthma, Cystic Fibrosis, Pneumonia, the Common Cold, Influenza, and Others, Featuring Facts about the Respiratory System, Statistical and Demographic Data, Treatments, Self-Help Management Suggestions, and Current Research Initiatives

Edited by Allan R. Cook and Peter D. Dresser. 771 pages. 1995. 0-7808-0037-0. $78.

"Designed for the layperson and for patients and their families coping with respiratory illness. . . . an extensive array of information on diagnosis, treatment, management, and prevention of respiratory illnesses for the general reader." —*Choice, Association of College and Research Libraries, Jun '96*

"A highly recommended text for all collections. It is a comforting reminder of the power of knowledge that good books carry between their covers." —*Academic Library Book Review, Spring '96*

"A comprehensive collection of authoritative information presented in a nontechnical, humanitarian style for patients, families, and caregivers." —*Association of Operating Room Nurses, Sep/Oct '95*

■

Sexually Transmitted Diseases Sourcebook, 1st Edition

Basic Information about Herpes, Chlamydia, Gonorrhea, Hepatitis, Nongonoccocal Urethritis, Pelvic Inflammatory Disease, Syphilis, AIDS, and More

Along with Current Data on Treatments and Preventions

Edited by Linda M. Ross. 550 pages. 1997. 0-7808-0217-9. $78.

■

Sexually Transmitted Diseases Sourcebook, 2nd Edition

Basic Consumer Health Information about Sexually Transmitted Diseases, Including Information on the Diagnosis and Treatment of Chlamydia, Gonorrhea, Hepatitis, Herpes, HIV, Mononucleosis, Syphilis, and Others

Along with Information on Prevention, Such as Condom Use, Vaccines, and STD Education; And Featuring a Section on Issues Related to Youth and Adolescents, a Glossary, and Resources for Additional Help and Information

Edited by Dawn D. Matthews. 538 pages. 2001. 0-7808-0249-7. $78.

Skin Disorders Sourcebook

Basic Information about Common Skin and Scalp Conditions Caused by Aging, Allergies, Immune Reactions, Sun Exposure, Infectious Organisms, Parasites, Cosmetics, and Skin Traumas, Including Abrasions, Cuts, and Pressure Sores

Along with Information on Prevention and Treatment

Edited by Allan R. Cook. 647 pages. 1997. 0-7808-0080-X. $78.

". . . comprehensive, easily read reference book." —*Doody's Health Sciences Book Reviews, Oct '97*

SEE ALSO Burns Sourcebook

■

Sleep Disorders Sourcebook

Basic Consumer Health Information about Sleep and Its Disorders, Including Insomnia, Sleepwalking, Sleep Apnea, Restless Leg Syndrome, and Narcolepsy

Along with Data about Shiftwork and Its Effects, Information on the Societal Costs of Sleep Deprivation, Descriptions of Treatment Options, a Glossary of Terms, and Resource Listings for Additional Help

Edited by Jenifer Swanson. 439 pages. 1998. 0-7808-0234-9. $78.

"This text will complement any home or medical library. It is user-friendly and ideal for the adult reader." —*American Reference Books Annual, 2000*

"Recommended reference source." —*Booklist, American Library Association, Feb '99*

"A useful resource that provides accurate, relevant, and accessible information on sleep to the general public. Health care providers who deal with sleep disorders patients may also find it helpful in being prepared to answer some of the questions patients ask." —*Respiratory Care, Jul '99*

■

Sports Injuries Sourcebook

Basic Consumer Health Information about Common Sports Injuries, Prevention of Injury in Specific Sports, Tips for Training, and Rehabilitation from Injury

Along with Information about Special Concerns for Children, Young Girls in Athletic Training Programs, Senior Athletes, and Women Athletes, and a Directory of Resources for Further Help and Information

Edited by Heather E. Aldred. 624 pages. 1999. 0-7808-0218-7. $78.

"Public libraries and undergraduate academic libraries will find this book useful for its nontechnical language." —*American Reference Books Annual, 2000*

"While this easy-to-read book is recommended for all libraries, it should prove to be especially useful for public, high school, and academic libraries; certainly it should be on the bookshelf of every school gymnasium." —*E-Streams, Mar '00*

Substance Abuse Sourcebook

Basic Health-Related Information about the Abuse of Legal and Illegal Substances Such as Alcohol, Tobacco, Prescription Drugs, Marijuana, Cocaine, and Heroin; and Including Facts about Substance Abuse Prevention Strategies, Intervention Methods, Treatment and Recovery Programs, and a Section Addressing the Special Problems Related to Substance Abuse during Pregnancy

Edited by Karen Bellenir. 573 pages. 1996. 0-7808-0038-9. $78.

"A valuable addition to any health reference section. Highly recommended."
— *The Book Report, Mar/Apr '97*

". . . a comprehensive collection of substance abuse information that's both highly readable and compact. Families and caregivers of substance abusers will find the information enlightening and helpful, while teachers, social workers and journalists should benefit from the concise format. Recommended."
— *Drug Abuse Update, Winter '96/'97*

SEE ALSO Alcoholism Sourcebook, Drug Abuse Sourcebook

■

Traveler's Health Sourcebook

Basic Consumer Health Information for Travelers, Including Physical and Medical Preparations, Transportation Health and Safety, Essential Information about Food and Water, Sun Exposure, Insect and Snake Bites, Camping and Wilderness Medicine, and Travel with Physical or Medical Disabilities

Along with International Travel Tips, Vaccination Recommendations, Geographical Health Issues, Disease Risks, a Glossary, and a Listing of Additional Resources

Edited by Joyce Brennfleck Shannon. 613 pages. 2000. 0-7808-0384-1. $78.

■

Women's Health Concerns Sourcebook

Basic Information about Health Issues That Affect Women, Featuring Facts about Menstruation and Other Gynecological Concerns, Including Endometriosis, Fibroids, Menopause, and Vaginitis; Reproductive Concerns, Including Birth Control, Infertility, and Abortion; and Facts about Additional Physical, Emotional, and Mental Health Concerns Prevalent among Women Such as Osteoporosis, Urinary Tract Disorders, Eating Disorders, and Depression

Along with Tips for Maintaining a Healthy Lifestyle

Edited by Heather E. Aldred. 567 pages. 1997. 0-7808-0219-5. $78.

"Handy compilation. There is an impressive range of diseases, devices, disorders, procedures, and other physical and emotional issues covered . . . well organized, illustrated, and indexed." — *Choice, Association of College and Research Libraries, Jan '98*

SEE ALSO Breast Cancer Sourcebook, Cancer Sourcebook for Women, 1st and 2nd Editions, Healthy Heart Sourcebook for Women, Osteoporosis Sourcebook

■

Workplace Health & Safety Sourcebook

Basic Consumer Health Information about Workplace Health and Safety, Including the Effect of Workplace Hazards on the Lungs, Skin, Heart, Ears, Eyes, Brain, Reproductive Organs, Musculoskeletal System, and Other Organs and Body Parts

Along with Information about Occupational Cancer, Personal Protective Equipment, Toxic and Hazardous Chemicals, Child Labor, Stress, and Workplace Violence

Edited by Chad T. Kimball. 626 pages. 2000. 0-7808-0231-4. $78.

"Highly recommended." — *The Bookwatch, Jan '01*

■

Worldwide Health Sourcebook

Basic Information about Global Health Issues, Including Malnutrition, Reproductive Health, Disease Dispersion and Prevention, Emerging Diseases, Risky Health Behaviors, and the Leading Causes of Death

Along with Global Health Concerns for Children, Women, and the Elderly, Mental Health Issues, Research and Technology Advancements, and Economic, Environmental, and Political Health Implications, a Glossary, and a Resource Listing for Additional Help and Information

Edited by Joyce Brennfleck Shannon. 614 pages. 2001. 0-7808-0330-2. $78.

■

Health Reference Series Cumulative Index 1999

A Comprehensive Index to the Individual Volumes of the Health Reference Series, Including a Subject Index, Name Index, Organization Index, and Publication Index

Along with a Master List of Acronyms and Abbreviations

Edited by Edward J. Prucha, Anne Holmes, and Robert Rudnick. 990 pages. 2000. 0-7808-0382-5. $78.

"Essential for collections that hold any of the numerous *Health Reference Series* titles."
— *Choice, Association of College and Research Libraries, Nov '00*

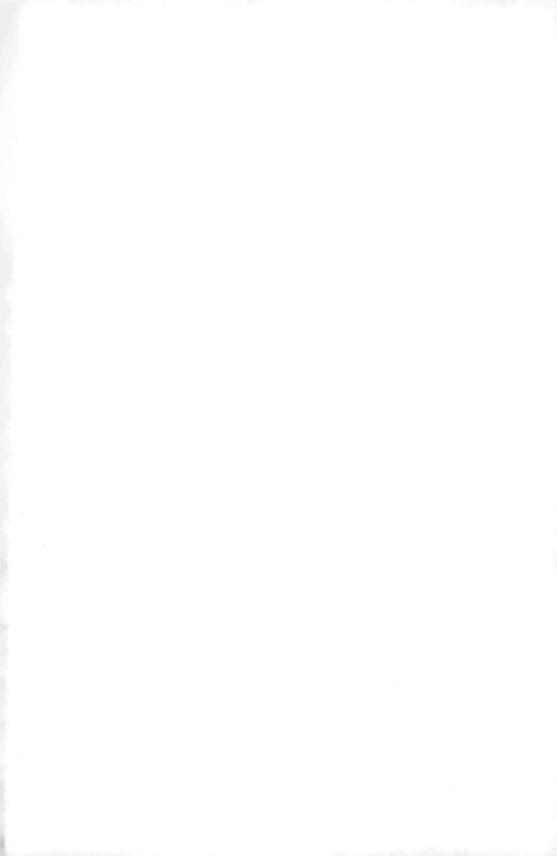

		DATE DUE	